Third Edition

Appleton & Lange's Review for the
PHYSICIAN ASSISTANT

Anthony A. Miller, MEd, PA-C
Director
Physician Assistant Program
School of Allied Health
Medical College of Ohio
Toledo, Ohio

Albert F. Simon, MEd, PA-C
Chairman
Physician Assistant Studies
Saint Francis College
Loretto, Pennsylvania

Patrick J. Cafferty, PA-C
Neurosurgical Associates of Western Kentucky
Paducah, Kentucky

Appleton & Lange
Stamford, Connecticut

Copyright © 1998 by Appleton & Lange
A Simon & Schuster Company

98 99 00 01 / 10 9 8 7 6 5 4 3 2 1

Prentice Hall International (UK) Limited, *London*
Prentice Hall of Australia Pty. Limited, *Sydney*
Prentice Hall Canada, Inc., *Toronto*
Prentice Hall Hispanoamericana, S.A., *Mexico*
Prentice Hall of India Private Limited, *New Delhi*
Prentice Hall of Japan, Inc., *Tokyo*
Simon & Schuster Asia Pte. Ltd., *Singapore*
Editora Prentice Hall do Brasil Ltda., *Rio de Janeiro*
Prentice Hall, *Upper Saddle River, New Jersey*

ISBN 0-8385-0279-2
90000
9 780838 502792

Acquisitions Editor: Marinita Timban
Production Editor: Eileen L. Pendagast
Designer: Libby Schmitz

PRINTED IN THE UNITED STATES OF AMERICA

Contributors

William H. Fenn, MM, PA-C
Chairman and Associate Professor
Physician Assistant Department
Western Michigan University
Kalamazoo, Michigan

Steve B. Fisher, BHS, PA-C
Clinical Physician Assistant
Division of Neurosurgery
University of Kentucky Medical Center
President-elect, Kentucky Academy of Physician
    Assistants
Lexington, Kentucky

Ronald P. Grimm, BHS, PA-C
Geisinger Medical Center
Danville, Pennsylvania

Scott B. Harp, EMT-P, PA-C
Jackson Purchase Emergency Medicine Physicians
Paducah, Kentucky

Nancy Ivansek, MA, PA-C
Director, Occupational Health
University Health Center at LanderBrook
Mayfield Heights, Ohio

Deborah Jalbert, MBA, PA-C
Assistant Professor and Associate Director
Physician Assistant Program
University of Texas Southwestern Medical Center
Dallas, Texas

Robert W. Jarski, PhD, PA-C
Associate Professor
School of Health Sciences
Oakland University
Rochester, Michigan

Brenda L. Jasper, PA-C
Renal-Endocrine Associates, PC
Monroeville, Pennsylvania

Catherine Judd, PA-C
Faculty Associate
Department of Psychiatry
Assistant Professor of Health Care Sciences
Physician Assistant Program
University of Texas Southwestern Medical Center
Dallas, Texas

Peter Juergensen, BS, PA-C
Adjunct Clinical Assistant Professor
Quinnipiac College
Lecturer in Internal Medicine
Yale University School of Medicine
New Haven, Connecticut

Timothy J. Kappes, BHS, PA-C
Central Regional Chairperson
Kentucky Academy of Physician Assistants
Lexington, Kentucky

Ricky E. Kortyna, MHS, PA-C
Division of Pediatric Neurosurgery
Department of Neurosurgery
Allegheny University of the Health Sciences
Pittsburgh, Pennsylvania
Adjunct Clinical Instructor
Department of Physician Assistant
Duquesne University
Pittsburgh, Pennsylvania

Denyse M. Mahoney, PA-C
New York Hospital, Queens
Department of Obstetrics & Gynecology
Flushing, New York

Marsha R. Mayo-Adams, PA-C
Primary Care Medical Center
Murray, Kentucky

Richard E. Murphy, PA-C
Senior Physician Assistant
Departments of Surgery and Cardiothoracic Surgery
New England Medical Center
Boston, Massachusetts

Doris Rapp, PharmD, PA-C
Associate Professor
University of Kentucky Physician Assistant
    Program and College of Pharmacology
Lexington, Kentucky

Janean R. Schepp, BS, PA-C
Medical Associates
Menomonee Falls, Wisconsin

Rebecca Lovell Scott, PhD, PA-C
Academic Coordinator
Physician Assistant Program
College of Health Sciences
Roanoke, Virginia

Henry W. Stoll, PA-C
Senior Lecturer
MEDEX School of Medicine
Physician Assistant Program
University of Washington
Seattle, Washington

Joseph H. Thornton, MPH, PA-C
Assistant Professor
Department of Primary Care
School of Health Related Professions
Program Director
Physician Assistant Program
Seton Hall University
University of Medicine and Dentistry of
    New Jersey
Newark, New Jersey

Tim Thurston, BHS, PA-C
Grogan & Howard, PSC
Paducah, Kentucky

Contents

Preface

The physician assistant profession has witnessed significant changes in the health care industry over the past few years. Our profession has not been immune to the experiences of dramatic shifts in health care delivery, financing, and in some cases, rationing. Rapid changes in technology have also had a significant impact on health care.

We have attempted to respond to the changing aspects of health care by including new treatments and diagnostic testing in updated questions and references while maintaining the basic format and quality PA students and graduates have grown to expect since Patrick Cafferty's first edition. In addition, revisions have been made to respond to recently announced changes in the format of the NCCPA certification examination.

We believe that you will find this review book a helpful and useful resource as you prepare for your initial or recertification examination. Your comments and constructive criticisms are welcome and will be considered in future editions.

We would like to thank our families, friends, and coworkers for their support, encouragement, and patience during the long hours spent working on this project. We also wish to thank Marinita Timban from Appleton & Lange for her editorial assistance, and our contributors for their hard work and dedication. Finally, we thank you, the readers, for choosing this book as one of your resources. We wish you success on the examination.

Anthony A. Miller, MEd, PA-C
Albert F. Simon, MEd, PA-C

To PJS, you are always there for me, AFS.
To KHM, thank you for your love and support, AAM.

Introduction

This book has been designed as a study aid to review for the Physician Assistant National Certification and Recertification Examination. Here, in one package, is a comprehensive review resource with more than 1000 questions presented in the same format as those seen in the national examinations. Each question is answered with a referenced, paragraph-length answer. In addition, the final section of the book contains a 200-question Practice Test for self-assessment purposes. The entire book has been organized by specialty area to help evaluate your areas of relative strength and weakness and to further direct your study effort with the available references.

ORGANIZATION

This book is divided into 9 chapters. Chapter 1 provides helpful hints on how to prepare for and take certification examinations. Chapters 2 through 8 review the major areas of medicine using the question-and-answer format. Chapter 5, Internal Medicine, is subdivided into 11 sections covering its subspecialties. The final chapter is a 200-question Practice Test.

This introduction provides information on question types, methods for using this book, and specific information on the national certifying and recertifying examinations.

QUESTIONS

The National Certifying Examination contains two different types of questions. In the past, about 40% of these have been "one best answer–single item"

questions and "one best answer–matching set." In some cases, a group of two or three questions may be related to a situational theme. In addition, some questions have illustrative material (graphs, x-rays, tables) that require understanding and interpretation on your part. Finally, some of the items are stated in the negative. In such instances, we have printed the negative word in capital letters (eg, "All of the following are correct EXCEPT"; "Which of the following choices is NOT correct"; and "Which of the following is LEAST correct").

One Best Answer–Single Item Question

This type of question presents a problem or asks a question and is followed by five choices, only one of which is entirely correct. The directions preceding this type of question will generally appear as below:

DIRECTIONS (Questions 1 through 7): Each of the numbered items or incomplete statements in this section is followed by answers or by completions of the statement. Select the ONE lettered answer or completion that is BEST in each case.

An example for this item type follows:

1. An obese 21-year-old woman complains of increased growth of coarse hair on her lip, chin, chest, and abdomen. She also notes menstrual irregularity with periods of amenorrhea. The most likely cause is

   (A) polycystic ovary disease
   (B) an ovarian tumor
   (C) an adrenal tumor
   (D) Cushing's disease
   (E) familial hirsutism

In this type of question, choices other than the correct answer may be partially correct, but there can only be one best answer. In the question above, the key word is "most." Although ovarian tumors, adrenal tumors, and Cushing's disease are causes of hirsutism (described in the stem of the question), polycystic ovary disease is a much more common cause. Familial hirsutism is not associated with the menstrual irregularities mentioned. Thus, the most likely cause of the manifestations described can only be "(A) polycystic ovary disease."

One Best Answer–Matching Sets

These questions are essentially matching questions that are usually accompanied by the following general directions:

DIRECTIONS (Questions 2 through 6): Each group of items in this section consists of lettered headings followed by a set of numbered words or phrases. For each numbered word or phrase, select the ONE lettered heading that is most closely associated with it. Each lettered heading may be selected once, more than once, or not at all.

Any number of questions (usually two to six) may follow the five headings.

Questions 2 through 4

For each adverse drug reaction listed below, select the antibiotic with which it is most closely associated.

    (A) tetracycline
    (B) chloramphenicol
    (C) Clindamycin
    (D) cefotaxime
    (E) gentamicin

  2. Bone marrow suppression

  3. Pseudomembranous enterocolitis

  4. Acute fatty necrosis of liver

Note that, unlike the single-item questions, the choices in the matching sets questions precede the actual questions. As with the single-item questions, however, only one choice can be correct for a given question.

Any number of questions (usually two to six) may follow the four headings.

Questions 5 and 6

    (A) polymyositis
    (B) polymyalgia rheumatica
    (C) both
    (D) neither

  5. Pain is a prominent syndrome

  6. Associated with internal malignancy in adults

Note that, as with the other matching-set questions, the choices precede the actual questions. Once again, only one choice can be correct for a given question.

Answers, Explanations, and References

In each of the sections of this book, the question sections are followed by a section containing the answers, explanations, and references for the questions. This section (1) tells you the answer to each question; (2) gives you an explanation and reviews the reason the answer is correct, background information on the subject matter, and the reason the other answers are incorrect; and (3) tells you where you can find more in-depth information on the subject matter in other books and journals. We encourage you to use this section as a basis for further study and understanding.

If you choose the correct answer to a question, you can the read the explanation (1) for reinforcement and (2) to add to your knowledge of the subject matter (remember that the explanations usually tell not only why the answer is correct, but often also why the other choices are incorrect). If you choose the wrong answer to a question, you can read the explanation for an instructional review of the material in the question. Furthermore, you can note the reference cited, look up the complete source in the references at the end of the chapter (eg, Cunningham FG: Williams Obstetrics, 20th ed. Stamford, CT., Appleton & Lange, 1997), and refer to the pages cited for a more in-depth discussion.

Practice Test

The 200-question Practice Test at the end of the book covers and reviews all the topics covered in

Chapters 2 through 8. The questions are grouped according to question type, with the subject areas integrated. Specific instructions for how to take the Practice Test are given later.

HOW TO USE THIS BOOK

There are two logical ways to get the most value from this book. We will call them Plan A and Plan B.

In Plan A, you go straight to the Practice Test and complete it according to the instructions given. This will be a good indicator of your initial knowledge of the subject and will help to identify specific areas for preparation and review. You can now use the earlier chapters of the book to help you improve your relative weak points.

In Plan B, you go through Chapters 2 through 8 checking off your answers, and then comparing your choices with the answers and discussions in the book. Once you have completed this process, you can take the Practice Test and see how well prepared you are. If you still have a major weakness, it should be apparent in time for you to take remedial action.

In Plan A, by taking the Practice Test first, you get quick feedback regarding your initial areas of strength and weakness. You may find that you have a good command of the material, indicating that perhaps only a cursory review of the first eight chapters is necessary. This, of course, would be good to know early in your exam preparation. On the other hand, you may find that you have many areas of weakness. In this case, you could then focus on these areas in your review—not just with this book, but also with appropriate textbooks. (It is, however, unlikely that you will not study prior to taking the National Boards, especially since you have this book.) Therefore, it may be more realistic to take the Practice Test after you have reviewed the first eight chapters (as in Plan B). This is likely to provide you with a more realistic type of testing situation, as very few of us merely sit down to a test without studying. In this case, you will have done some reviewing (from superficial to in-depth), and your Practice Test will reflect this study time. If, after reviewing the first eight chapters and taking the Practice Test, you still have

some weaknesses, you can then go back to the first of these chapters and supplement your review with the reference texts.

We hope that through careful use of this book, whether through Plan A or Plan B, you find this text a useful and beneficial study guide.

SPECIFIC INFORMATION ON THE EXAMINATIONS

The official source for all information on the Certification or Recertification process is the National Commission on Certification of Physician Assistants, Inc. (NCCPA), 6849-B2 Peachtree Dunwoody Rd., Atlanta, Georgia 30328. This organization is comprised of representatives from the major organizations of medicine, including the American Academy of Physician Assistants and the Association of Physician Assistant Programs. Their function is to formulate and administer the annual certification examination and to provide the means for recertification.

Eligibility requires completion or near completion of a Physician Assistant or Surgeon's Assistant program that is accredited by the Commission on Accreditation of Allied Health Educational Programs (CAAHEP). Details regarding registration are available from the NCCPA.

The entry-level examination (PANCE) consists of a 360-question examination addressing all aspects of Physician Assistant education, including anatomy, physiology, history taking, physical examination, laboratory and radiographic interpretation, as well as treatment modalities. For an additional fee, candidates may elect to take an extended examination in the area of surgery. This optional examination consists of 180 questions. Successful candidates will be provided a special recognition noting their proficiency in the area of surgery. Tips for improving your score on the exam are provided in Chapter 1. The future of the recertification examination (PANRE) is not clear as of this revision. However, as of this printing, the recertification examination consists of 300 questions constructed in a similar format as the entry-level examination. Plans for an alternative pathway for recertification are in the trial phase and may provide practicing PAs with a choice for recertification.

CHAPTER 1

Test-Taking Skills: Tips and Techniques

Robert W. Jarski, PhD, PA-C

Machine-scorable written exams measure not only medical knowledge but also test-taking skills. Through examples, practice, and explanations, this section is designed to help the physician assistant student or graduate use appropriate methods for answering the types of written questions found on standardized Board exams. Information on preparing for Board exams is also included.

To pass written Board exams, three conditions are generally necessary: (1) knowing about or recognizing the medical information contained in the questions; (2) using appropriate test-taking skills; and (3) avoiding situations that are likely to cause mistakes or impede performance. Test anxiety is an example.

Standardized exams can be intimidating and result in test anxiety. However, remembering that most test questions were created by well-intentioned clinicians can help keep the exam's purpose in perspective. In addition, multiple choice questions are limited in what they can evaluate; they generally assess only fundamental cognitive knowledge. Test-wise individuals use strategies that enable them to perform their best in responding to questions on fundamental knowledge.

The fact is, written tests—even at their "state-of-the-art" best—are crude evaluation devices (Snelbecker, 1985; Maatsch, 1983). Multiple-choice questions cannot reflect a clinician's total fund of medical skills. For example, patient rapport and the mechanics of examining patients are not accurately measured through multiple-choice questions. Multiple-choice questions can, however, successfully measure certain cognitive or knowledge skills. Ma-

chine-scored exams have limited assessment capabilities. Test taking is a discrete skill that is different from clinical skills, and expert clinicians are not necessarily expert test takers.

Test takers should master the skill of test taking the same way they have mastered the skill of physical examination. This may be accomplished by practicing the methods suggested in this section, answering the questions that follow in the text, and completing the Practice Test at the end of the book.

This section primarily presents information based on objective studies and sound psychological theories of test taking, perception, and recall (Snelbecker, 1985; U.S. Department of Education, 1986; DeCecco and Crawford, 1974; Carman, 1984; Phipps, 1983). The chapter is organized in four sections: (1) what to do when preparing for the exam; (2) what to do during the exam; (3) illustrative questions; and (4) do's and don'ts that bring together the strategies explained in the previous three sections.

Objectives

In this chapter the student or graduate physician assistant will

1. Identify proven techniques from the psychology of learning and educational measurement that will enhance test performance
2. Identify information from testing theory that will help avoid "careless" errors
3. Practice using clues to help identify correct and incorrect responses to exam questions

WHAT TO DO WHEN PREPARING FOR THE EXAM

Getting into Practice

To develop test-taking skills, you must *actively* practice what you will be doing on the test, that is, answering multiple-choice and matching questions. Reading and reviewing texts are rarely enough. To become proficient in suturing wounds, you not only read about suturing, but also practice suturing. Some physician assistants have not taken a written exam in weeks, months, or years. Do not attempt to sit for Board exams without practicing answering multiple-choice questions any sooner than you would suture a facial laceration without having sutured skin in weeks, months, or years. Responding to questions similar to those encountered on the Boards is invaluable for exam preparation. The book is designed for this purpose.

Areas to Emphasize

Direct your studying to the primary care areas with which you are least familiar. Although you may enjoy studying the areas relating directly to your practice, the task at hand is to pass the Boards. This is best accomplished by achieving a fundamental knowledge of each medical discipline appearing on the exam.

Write several of your own test questions. Those who do so frequently comment that their questions were surprisingly similar to those on the boards. This is probably so because only a limited amount of knowledge is amenable to the written exam format. In addition to identifying clinical information that is likely to be tested, you will gain valuable insight into the logic of test item construction, which in turn helps you to select correct answers.

Scheduling Preparation Time

Using a calendar, schedule specific periods for test preparation, setting aside specific times for reviewing and answering multiple-choice questions. Regular preparation over several months is preferred to cramming; studying just before the exam is usually nonproductive.

For the recertification exam, the amount of preparation needed depends largely on your practice setting. If your knowledge in primary care family medicine is current, you probably need less preparation than a physician assistant in a subspe-

cialty practice. Although an attempt is made to compare a physician assistant's practice profile to board scores by discipline, primary care knowledge will enhance test performance. It is assumed that all physician assistants should have fundamental knowledge in primary care. In addition to primary care knowledge, preparation in specialty disciplines is encouraged for graduates sitting for specialty Board exams.

The usual learning aids, such as the use of mnemonics, are highly recommended. The reader is referred to appropriate references (Carman, 1984; Phipps, 1983) for general information about study skills. The remainder of this chapter addresses specific information about the Board exams.

WHAT TO DO DURING THE EXAM

Physical Needs

Find a seat with few or no distractions, avoiding places near doorways and thoroughfares. Repeated interference can hinder your test performance. Take your watch in case a clock is not easily visible. If the exam is held in a facility that permits smoking, nonsmokers should ascertain through the proctor that they will have a smoke-free environment.

Speak with the proctor about any reasonable specific needs you may have. Consider the proctor your advocate. He or she is there to provide a favorable testing environment. It is the proctor's responsibility to provide it.

Consider nutritional and other personal needs. It is recommended that a heavy meal not be eaten within 2 hours prior to the exam, but a complex carbohydrate snack approximately 30 minutes before test time may be beneficial. You may also wish to bring with you packaged drinks and other supplies, such as tissues and cough drops. Keep food and drinks handy for breaks if consuming them during the exam is restricted. Get adequate sleep and rest before the exam.

Time Allowance

Before beginning each section of the exam, calculate the amount of time you can spend on each question. Never go over the calculated time limit on your first attempt at each question. If you do not know an answer, come back to it at the end. When calculating your time allotment, allow for a few extra minutes at the end so you can return to skipped items. Your subconscious will process those items while you work on the other questions. Also, hints often appear in other test items. (See Test Mechanics later.) Time is usually not an obstacle in the Board exam; you probably will have more time than needed.

Attitude

During the test, maintain a positive, confident attitude. Remind yourself that you prepared as best you could, and use some other effective techniques such as those we describe.

Do not become discouraged by questions you cannot answer. Many test items are, by design, those that have been answered incorrectly by a large number of test takers. Test questions with a predetermined discrimination level are retained for use in future exams. If too many test takers answer a particular test item correctly, it is not used again. Therefore, many of the items you will be answering are those that test takers have failed. So keep in mind that there will be a number of questions you are not expected to answer correctly.

Also be aware that numerous experimental questions are found on most standardized exams. Experimental questions are those being field-tested, and they are not counted in your score. Because you do not know which items these are, assume that any absurd question is experimental. Try not to become irate or unnecessarily concerned about any question.

Self-coaching and imaging or visualization techniques may be helpful for all test takers (Davis et al, 1995; Rossman, 1987). Stress management methods may be especially useful for anxious test takers (Davis et al, 1995; Benson and Stuart, 1992; Hiebert et al, 1983; Benson, 1975). Most professional athletes and stage performers master and routinely use these techniques to avoid situations likely to interfere with optimal performance.

These techniques will not bring to mind medical knowledge never encountered, but they may help you retrieve learned information and avoid exam errors due to extreme stress. Managing stress generally results in improved concentration and the ability to reason logically. The suggested techniques may be learned through special courses and by consulting appropriate references (Davis et al,

1995; Benson and Stuart, 1992; Rossman, 1987; Hiebert et al, 1983; Benson, 1975). Techniques should be learned and practiced several weeks before the exam and used the day of the exam; certain brief imaging procedures may be used for relaxing and improving concentration during the exam.

Concentration

During the exam, think of nothing except the questions in front of you. When working in the operating room, you concentrate on the operative field. Similarly, give the exam your full, serious, and undivided attention. Problems at work or home should be left at the exam room doorstep; your one and only task during the exam period is to answer questions to the best of your ability.

Test Mechanics

Before beginning each section of the exam, always read the instructions. Formats could change. Never find yourself having answered an entire section incorrectly because you failed to read the instructions.

You are allowed to mark on the test booklet unless instructed otherwise. It has been found that errors can be minimized by marking your answers in the test booklet, and then marking the machine-scorable answer sheet after every 20 to 30 questions. This process varies the task, allows some psychological rest, and forces you to periodically check for accuracy in marking the correct item number on the answer sheet.

If you do not know the answer to a question, skip it and continue answering the questions you know. Frequently, you will find clues in other questions that will help you answer those you left blank. In addition, your subconscious will have processed the questions you skipped. It has been found that a great deal of information is stored in memory, but information retrieval is often faulty. Methods such as rest and varying mental tasks enhance retrieval. Come back later to the questions you left blank.

Changing Your Answer

Contrary to some popular misconceptions, if you doubt an answer selection and want to change it, it is suggested that you do so. In numerous studies across disciplines examining thousands of changed responses, answers were changed approximately twice as often from incorrect responses to correct ones (Welch and Leichner, 1988; Fabrey and Case, 1985; Shababudin, 1983). If you really have no idea which response is correct and you find yourself purely guessing, perhaps your first instinct is accurate. However, if you have a reason to change your answer, you will probably change from an incorrect to a correct response.

Answering by Elimination
Selecting your answer by the process of elimination increases the probability of choosing the correct response. Using the stem of the question, form a sentence with each choice provided. Be cautioned against selecting the first answer you think is correct; consider *all* possibilities before making a final selection.

Most test questions have in common the following anatomic features: (1) one choice is easily recognized as an outlier and incorrect; (2) two choices appear plausible as either slightly off the topic or the opposite of the correct answer (e.g., artery versus arteriole, left versus right hemithorax); and (3) two choices are correct, but one is better than the other.

The test taker's job is to (1) eliminate the outlier; (2) identify the two plausible choices and reject them after weighing them against the two that are more likely to be correct; and then (3) select the better answer of the remaining two. As with a differential diagnosis, this job is accomplished effectively through the process of elimination.

By using the process of elimination, almost anyone can eliminate the outlier. In doing so, the probability of selecting the wrong answer by guessing alone is decreased by 20%. If the two plausible but incorrect choices are identified, the test taker then has two remaining items and a 50–50 chance of guessing the correct answer.

Always Triage First
On some exams, points for selecting unnecessarily dangerous, invasive, expensive, or potentially harmful choices are tallied separately. On the exam, as in real life, you are allowed very few such errors. Screen each and every question for potentially harmful or invasive choices. Just as patients are triaged, you should similarly triage each test item encountered. There are three question categories that should be identified.

The first is the "friendly" question—the one that assesses your medical knowledge simply by asking for information. The second category includes those questions designed to trap. Unlike the "friendly" question, the item designed to trap has a preconceived attractor or distractor that may catch the test taker off guard. The third type of question is the one containing a potentially harmful choice. It may refer to a treatment, procedure, finding, or diagnosis.

The third category might not be necessarily tricky, but the test item writer had in mind a possible pitfall that must not be selected. This pitfall should be identified in your triaging. As you read each test item, place it into one of the three categories before selecting your answer.

Detailed examples of each question type are presented in the Illustrative Questions section.

About Matching Questions
In general, matching questions should be treated as multiple-choice questions. Although most of the same tips and techniques can be applied, the main difference is that matching questions use a common set of item choices for each "stem." Identify (match) the choice or choices of which you are most certain. As always, read the instructions to ascertain the purpose of each set of matching questions.

Some General Hints
Certain "hints" of test taking apply to most multiple-choice and matching questions. These hints are not, however, as likely to work on standardized exams as on other tests, but they may be useful as a last resort for answering some test items.

The choices "all of the above" or "none of the above" have an increased probability of being correct. If a single-answer multiple-choice question contains two alternatives that mean exactly the same thing, they probably are both incorrect.

Finally, if you must make a pure guess, (C) is most likely the correct choice. The next most likely choice is (B). Board exam test writers try to guard against these probabilities, but the odds might prove useful to you if all else fails.

ILLUSTRATIVE QUESTIONS

You will encounter the following types of questions on Board exams. Each example presented illustrates a strategy to help identify correct choices.

As always, first triage each question and identify its category.

The Oversimplification

Some questions appear tricky because you think "no question could be this simple!" If you really know the answer to a question, answer it without belaboring or looking for booby traps that are not there. The following is an example.

A 22-year-old woman presents with abdominal pain and fever of 2 days duration. During the digital pelvic exam, she experiences exquisite pain when the cervix is moved. This suggests a diagnosis of

- (A) uterine fibroids
- (B) vaginitis
- (C) peritonitis
- (D) cystitis
- (E) cervical carcinoma

The item least likely to cause pain, (E), is eliminated. Any of the remaining four are possibilities, but peritonitis of any etiology is usually a safe diagnostic consideration. Do not get bogged down considering the unlikely diagnostic possibilities when an obvious choice is present. The oversimplification in this case is the correct answer, (C).

The Oversimplification That Is Dangerous by Omission

As always, triage questions for traps. In the following question, the correct choice is an oversimplification that is dangerous by omission.

A painless testicular mass is found in an otherwise normal 29-year-old. Which of the following diagnoses should be pursued?

- (A) varicocele
- (B) carcinoma
- (C) furuncle
- (D) torsion
- (E) strangulation

Choices (C), (D), and (E) are ruled out because they usually are painful. (A) and (B), however, usually

are painless. Because of its prognosis if left untreated, a testicular mass should be considered cancer until proven otherwise. Not to do so would be considered a life-threatening omission. The correct choice is (B).

Always screen questions for dangerous or critical choices whether harmful by omission or commission. A potentially harmful choice may present itself as an oversimplification.

Clues from Logic

Sometimes a logical (and correct) answer is contained in the stem, as shown in the following example.

The diagnosis of congenital hip dislocation is made

- (A) in utero
- (B) at birth
- (C) at 6 weeks of age
- (D) at 6 months of age
- (E) fluoroscopically

The term *congenital* means "present at birth." This is when the diagnosis of congenital hip dislocation is made. The correct choice is (B).

Clues from Related Areas

Similar to clues from logic, knowledge about related disciplines can provide additional hints.

An obese 45-year-old woman presents with acute genital pain. Upon examination you find a 2- to 3-cm soft mass in the right labia majora. This is most likely

- (A) marked lymphadenopathy
- (B) an inguinal hernia
- (C) a femoral hernia
- (D) a femoral aneurysm
- (E) neurofibroma

If the mass were located in the scrotum of an obese man, you would probably not miss the common diagnosis of inguinal hernia. Remembering from developmental anatomy that the labia majora and scrotum are corresponding tissues, (B) would be selected as the correct response, even if the test taker had minimal knowledge about surgical emergencies.

The "Odd" Choice

This test-taking clue is demonstrated by way of two examples. The first example comes from psychiatry.

Which of the following is not a sign of transsexualism?

- (A) rejecting one's anatomic sex
- (B) sex identity problems during childhood
- (C) dressing in clothing of the opposite sex
- (D) aversion toward one's own genitalia
- (E) sex identity problems during adolescence

Transsexualism is considered pathological because the patient considers a mutilating procedure preferable to living as his/her designated sex. Each choice except (C) implies pathology—rejecting one's own anatomy, sex identity problems, and aversion. The odd choice, (C), has, however, no associated pathology and is the correct response.

The second example follows.

A 65-year-old man complains of burning pain in the distal extremities especially upon exposure to heat. Upon examination, the hands and feet are warm and erythematous. The findings are most consistent with

- (A) diabetes mellitus
- (B) arteriosclerosis
- (C) Raynaud's phenomenon
- (D) thromboembolism
- (E) erythromelalgia

With the limited amount of information provided in the stem, it is unlikely that you can differentiate precisely among the choices provided. Your only clue is the odd choice. Even if you are unfamiliar with the infrequently seen problem of erythromelalgia, notice that choices A through D are associated with problems causing impaired circulation and cold extremities. "Erythro" or "red" implies *increased* circulation and warmth. (E), the odd choice among the options provided, is the correct answer.

Qualifying Words

Test-item stems containing qualifying words such as most, more, usually, often, less seldom, few will sometimes lead you to the correct answer.

You see in the outpatient clinic a 32-year-old man whom you suspect is suffering from alcohol withdrawal. The most likely finding would be

- (A) visual hallucinations
- (B) auditory hallucinations
- (C) fine motor tremors
- (D) major motor seizures
- (E) autonomic hyperactivity

Any of the above may be seen with alcohol withdrawal. However, fine motor tremors are the most common by far. The stem contains a qualifying word suggesting (C) as the correct choice.

If a qualifying word appears among the choices presented, it deserves special attention. Words such as *best, entirely, completely, always,* and *all* imply that something is always true; words such as *worst, never, no,* and *none* imply that something is never true. In clinical practice, *always* and *never* are rarely correct.

The Overqualified Choice

To make an answer acceptable, test-item writers sometimes must qualify a choice to the point at which the test taker recognizes the ploy. The following example illustrates an overqualified choice.

In a 66-year-old emphysematous man with a 100-pack-per-year smoking history, clubbing is most appropriately described as

- (A) discoloration
- (B) a flattened angle between the dorsal surface of the distal phalanx and the proximal nail
- (C) an abnormal inwardly curved nail
- (D) a pack/year history
- (E) a measurably increased eponychium

The overqualified (lengthy) choice, (B), is likely to be correct, as in this example.

However, remember the "odd choice" described above! Sometimes the very short "odd choice" is correct. You will recognize this variation because it will be attractively precise and succinct.

Having at least some knowledge of the item, you will identify it as accurate.

Strange Terms

Choices containing completely unfamiliar words are likely to be distractors. Do not assume that you somehow missed an important chapter of Harrison's or that there is a gap in your education. If the choice appears completely bizarre, the test-item writer was probably scraping the barrel for a distractor.

On a routine peripheral blood smear from a 13-year-old boy, you see a nucleated cell that is filled with bright red granules and is approximately three times the diameter of a typical red blood cell. This should be recognized as a (an)

(A) Franz–Kulig cell
(B) myelocyte
(C) eosinophil
(D) Olson cell
(E) Kupffer cell

Choices A, D, and E are completely fictitious. The test-item writer obviously did not lack imagination. B is familiar—remember basic anatomy or hematology? However, identifying a myelocyte on the peripheral smear is not basic primary care, which the Board exam covers. Physician assistants should recognize the morphology and significance of an eosinophil, thus, the correct response is (C).

"Apple Pie" Choices

There are some responses to which no one would object. Consider the following test question.

When evaluating a 23-year-old woman with vaginal bleeding, the most important clinical information is gained from the

(A) prothrombin time
(B) partial thromboplastin time
(C) CBC and iron studies
(D) physical exam
(E) detailed history

A patient's history provides a clinician's best information and is almost never incorrect. (E) is an "apple pie" choice.

The "apple pie" choice, however, can also be used by test-item writers to set traps.

The most important physical exam component(s) in the emergency evaluation of an unconscious patient is (are)

(A) body symmetry
(B) a carefully performed and prompt neurological exam
(C) the cardiopulmonary exam
(D) vital signs
(E) blood gases

The initial triage of this question would identify it as a "trap" question because of the critical nature of the scenario combined with an incorrect "apple pie" choice. Blood gases are promptly dismissed because they are not physical exam components, for which the stem asks. (B) appears attractive because of its "apple pie" component. Nevertheless, remember your ABCs of emergency care! The correct response is (D).

Hints from Inconsistencies in Terminology

Grammar inconsistencies between the stem and a choice (e.g., tense, number, gender) are usually recognized by expert educational evaluators who screen Board exam test questions. You will, therefore, seldom encounter this type of "hint" on Board exams, although it will be found more frequently in classroom situations. Hints due to inconsistencies in terminology are more frequent than other types of hints because expert test-item reviewers frequently lack a medical background. Therefore, you may benefit from recognizing inconsistencies in terminology.

A 19-year-old unconscious motorcycle accident victim with suspected multiple trauma is brought to the emergency room. The most significant physical findings usually will result from

(A) undressing the patient
(B) a prompt neurological exam
(C) interviewing the family
(D) interviewing a witness to the accident
(E) all the above

Choices (C) and (D) can be excluded because they refer to historical, not physical findings. This also excludes foil (E). Although indicated, at this point of presentation, the neurological exam is too focused. A more general, overall assessment provides the best clinical information. Therefore, critical, life-saving information across organ systems may be gained from observing the patient. Choice (A) is correct. Similarly, choice (E), blood gases, in the previous example was eliminated because it was inconsistent with the information asked for in the stem.

Rank Orders

When given a list of numbers or other rank orders, the correct response most often occurs somewhere between the extremes, as shown in these examples.

A 17-year-old woman presents with a history of pelvic discomfort during menses. Through questioning, you determine that the amount of blood lost during each cycle is normal. The amount of her blood loss would be approximately

(A) 25 mL
(B) 35 mL
(C) 70 mL
(D) 100 mL
(E) 125 mL

Here is the second example.

In reviewing the chart of a 45-year-old man, you notice a past diagnosis of chronic schizophrenia. To be termed *chronic*, this disorder was present for at least

(A) 3 months
(B) 1 year
(C) 2 years
(D) 3 years
(E) 4 years

Most test-item writers try to bury the correct answer somewhere in the middle. (C) is the correct answer in each example.

As with hints from inconsistencies in terminology, this clue does not work as often on board exams as it does on classroom tests. Educational

evaluators try to randomize the position of correct responses as much as possible. However, when in doubt, it is better to avoid the extremes when presented with rank-ordered options.

DO'S AND DON'TS

The following do's and don'ts summarize some of the important points made earlier in this section.

DO practice what you will be doing during the exam, that is, answering multiple-choice and matching questions. Answering these questions is a skill different from knowing clinical information. Get into practice for answering exam questions by actually answering them. This is imperative for the clinician who has not taken a written, machine-scorable exam recently.

DO direct your studying to the primary care areas with which you are *least* familiar. Passing the Boards is best accomplished by achieving a fundamental knowledge level in each medical discipline assessed on the exam.

DO write your own multiple-choice and matching questions. Not only will you gain insights into the mechanics of test-item writing and correctly answering questions, but also it is likely that many of your items will resemble actual Board exam questions.

DO get adequate sleep and rest before the exam.

DO relate test questions to your own practice and experience. Test-item writers are people who have derived many test questions from their own clinical experience. What would *you* expect a primary care physician assistant to know? Use this mind-set to understand the goal of a question and to keep a positive attitude throughout the exam.

DO change your answer if you have a good reason to do so. You are twice as likely to change from an incorrect response to a correct one. However, if you are only playing a hunch with no information about the topic at all, your first "gut" reaction might be correct.

DO triage each and every question before selecting your answer. Evaluate it as a question designed to (1) test knowledge in a "friendly" way; (2) trap by including common pitfalls; or (3) trap by including potentially dangerous choices. In the first case, the apparent oversimplification is probably the correct choice. In questions designed to trap, beware of the "apple pie" choice—by omission or commission. On the test, as in real clinical life, you cannot afford to make many dangerous errors.

DO use the process of elimination. Your job is to find the single best answer. As with a patient's differential diagnosis, this usually is done by *elimination*. Avoid choosing an answer until after you have considered all choices.

DO read the question stem and combine it with each foil to form a sentence. After doing this, use the process of elimination to arrive at the final answer.

DO mark your answers in the test booklet and transfer them to the machine-scorable answer sheet after every 20 to 30 questions. This procedure tends to minimize errors and provide psychological rest.

DO consider the proctor your colleague. He or she is there to support you and to facilitate your best performance on the exam. Expect and demand this kind of treatment.

DO leave items blank if you are not sure of the answer. Return to these items when you finish the rest of the exam or at a time when you gain information from other questions.

DO pace yourself, allowing a calculated amount of time per question. In your time allocation, allow for some extra minutes at the end for returning to items left blank.

DO make *educated* guesses, if you must guess. Use the information provided in this section to help in your decision. By also using your medical knowledge and judgment, your chances will be much improved.

DO be alert for qualifying words such as most, more, usually, often, less, seldom, few, which will sometimes lead you to the correct answer.

DO eliminate choices containing completely unfamiliar words as distractors. If the choice appears completely unfamiliar, it is probably incorrect.

DO consider "apple pie" choices as probably correct. However, beware that they may also be used to trap.

DO consider choices that are different from the others—the "odd choice." This may involve the choice having the "odd" meaning or the "odd"

length—long or short. The overqualified choice often is correct.

DO select item (C) when purely guessing. It is most frequently the correct response on many one-choice-only multiple-choice questions. If you eliminate (C) as a possibility, (B) is the next most likely choice. This is a "last-ditch" strategy that works more often on classroom tests than on Board exams.

DO select "all the above" or "none of the above" as a last-ditch strategy. When appearing as choices, they are likely to be correct.

DO read all instructions for each section of the exam. Be aware of any change in format.

DO use the hints in this chapter pertaining to single-answer multiple-choice questions for answering matching questions. As with other formats on the Board exam, triage each item and beware of dangerous or potentially harmful responses.

DO avoid situations that might put you in an unfavorable mind-set before the exam. For example, if you anticipate heavy highway traffic, arrive at the exam site a day early. If disturbances bother you during an exam, come early and select a seat in a far corner of the testing room. Let nothing interfere with your best possible performance on the day of the exam.

DO consider taking the exam a positive experience. Keep your motivation high through self-coaching and imaging techniques. Use recommended stress management techniques, especially if you are anxious when taking tests.

DO plan to reward yourself for a good performance after the exam. This facilitates a positive attitude.

DO dress comfortably in layers. Bring a sweater or loose jacket to use if the room temperature is uncomfortably cold.

DO remember to bring needed supplies (pencils and erasers) and admissions materials (such as identification cards). If allowed, hard candy may help if you begin to feel hungry or develop a "tickle" in your throat.

DO reread instructions provided by the testing agency the night before to ensure you arrive on time, at the right place, and with the right supplies. Recheck directions to the test center.

DON'T cram at the last minute. This kind of preparation will not be adequate for an exam that covers mostly primary care breadth rather than depth.

DON'T eat a large meal within 2 hours of the beginning of the exam. Be well nourished, but not full.

DON'T think of anything except the exam in front of you. Think of it as your "operative field." Concentrate on giving your best possible performance.

DON'T become irate over seemingly absurd questions. Answer them to the best of your ability, realizing that they probably are experimental questions that will not affect your score. Other test takers probably will also consider them absurd.

DON'T guess randomly. Even if you are completely unsure of the answer to a question, use the hints suggested to increase the probability of guessing the correct response. Make educated, not random guesses.

DON'T leave any item blank at the end of the exam. Unanswered items will be counted wrong.

DON'T discuss the examination during the administration or during breaks, which adds to anxiety and may result in disqualification.

REFERENCES

Benson H. *The Relaxation Response.* New York: Avon Books; 1975.

Benson H, Stuart EM. *The Wellness Book.* New York: Birch Lane Press; 1992.

Carman RA. *Study Skills: A Student's Guide for Survival,* 2nd ed. New York: Wiley; 1984.

Davis M, Eshelman ER, McKay M. *The Relaxation and Stress Reduction Workbook.* Oakland, CA: New Harbinger Publications; 1995.

DeCecco JP, Crawford WR. *The Psychology of Learning and Instruction,* 2nd ed. Englewood Cliffs, NJ: Prentice-Hall; 1974.

Fabrey L, Case SM. Further support for changing multiple-choice answers. *J Med Educ.* June 1985: 488–490.

Hiebert B, Cardinal J, Dumka L, Marx RW. Self-instructed relaxation: A therapeutic alternative. *Biofeedback Self-Regul.* December 1983: 601–617.

Maatsch JL. *The Predictive Value of Medical Specialty Examinations: Final Report.* Washington, DC: National Center for Health Services Research, Contract No. HS-02-038-04; 1983.

Phipps R. *The Successful Student's Handbook: A Step-by-Step Guide to Study, Reading and Thinking Skills.* Seattle, WA: University of Washington Press; 1983.

Rossman ML. *Healing Yourself.* New York: Simon and Schuster; 1987.

Shababudin SH. Pattern of answer changes to multiple-choice questions in physiology. *Med Educ.* March 1983: 316–318.

Snelbecker GE. *Learning Theory, Instructional Theory and Psychoeducational Design.* Lanham, MD: University Printers of America; 1985.

U.S. Department of Education. *What Works: Research about Teaching and Learning.* Washington, DC: U.S. Department of Education; 1986.

Welch J, Leichner P. Analysis of changing answers on multiple-choice examination for nationwide sample of Canadian psychiatry residents. *J Med Educ.* February 1988: 133–135.

CHAPTER 2

Surgery
Questions

Steve B. Fisher, BHS, PA-C, Timothy J. Kappes, BHS, PA-C, and Tim Thurston, BHS, PA-C

DIRECTIONS (Question 1): Each of the numbered items or incomplete statements in this section is followed by answers or by completions of the statement. Select the ONE lettered answer or completion that is BEST in each case.

Question 1

1. Which of the following disorders of hemostasis is most commonly seen in the bleeding surgical patient?

   (A) thrombocytopenia
   (B) disseminated intravascular coagulopathy (DIC)
   (C) Von Willebrand's disease (Factor VIII)
   (D) Christmas disease (Factor IX)
   (E) classical hemophilia (Factor VIII)

DIRECTIONS (Questions 2 through 5): Each group of items in this section consists of lettered headings followed by a set of numbered words or phrases. For each numbered word or phrase, select the ONE lettered heading that is most closely associated with it. Each lettered heading may be selected once, more than once, or not at all.

Questions 2 through 5

Match the following symptoms or signs with the most likely diagnosis.

   (A) neurogenic shock
   (B) septic shock
   (C) insulin shock
   (D) hypovolemic shock
   (E) cardiogenic shock

2. Lower-extremity paresthesias

3. Muffled heart sounds

4. Fracture of the femur

5. Tachycardia and warm skin

DIRECTIONS (Questions 6 through 21): Each of the numbered items or incomplete statements in this section is followed by answers or by completions of the statement. Select the ONE lettered answer or completion that is BEST in each case.

Questions 6 through 21

6. Which of the following symptoms are LEAST likely to be associated with carcinoma of the breast?

   (A) nipple retraction
   (B) erythema or skin discoloration
   (C) skin dimpling
   (D) breast pain
   (E) axillary lymphadenopathy

7. Mammography is indicated

   (A) annually in all women of child-bearing age
   (B) annually in women more than 35 years of age
   (C) at 40 years of age and then annually after the age of 50
   (D) annually, beginning at 30 years of age for women on oral contraceptives
   (E) none of the above

8. All of the following are of historical importance in the evaluation of a patient with a breast mass EXCEPT

   (A) use of oral contraceptives
   (B) age of the first childbirth
   (C) family history of breast cancer
   (D) history of benign breast mass
   (E) history of endometriosis

9. Diffuse abdominal pain that is "wave-like" and associated with vomiting is most likely

   (A) pancreatitis
   (B) peptic ulcer disease
   (C) appendicitis
   (D) bowel obstruction
   (E) cholelithiasis

10. Abdominal pain that is sudden in onset and severe is NOT associated with

    (A) perforated peptic ulcer
    (B) ureteral colic
    (C) biliary colic
    (D) ruptured abdominal aneurysm
    (E) pancreatitis

11. If intestinal obstruction is suspected, which radiological procedure is indicated initially?

    (A) barium enema
    (B) abdominal ultrasound
    (C) abdominal CAT scan
    (D) flat and upright abdomen
    (E) upper gastrointestinal series with small bowel follow-through

12. Pain out of proportion with physical findings is associated with which diagnosis?

    (A) perforated peptic ulcer
    (B) peritonitis
    (C) mesenteric occlusion
    (D) Crohn's disease
    (E) cecal volvulus

13. Which nervous structure is at greater risk during anterior cervical microdiscectomy?

    (A) superior laryngeal nerve
    (B) recurrent laryngeal nerve
    (C) cervical sympathetic chain
    (D) vagus nerve
    (E) inferior laryngeal nerve

14. The most useful diagnostic test in the preoperative evaluation of a solid thyroid mass is

    (A) ultrasound
    (B) thyroid function test
    (C) needle aspiration
    (D) radioactive scan
    (E) needle biopsy

15. Which thyroid malignancy has the best prognosis following surgical excision?

    (A) follicular carcinoma
    (B) papillary carcinoma
    (C) medullary carcinoma
    (D) anaplastic carcinoma
    (E) lymphoma

16. Which of the following might be associated with thyroid carcinoma?

    (A) hoarseness
    (B) dysphagia
    (C) palpable mass
    (D) Delphian node
    (E) all of the above

17. Which factor is most significant as a precursor to thyroid carcinoma?

    (A) appearance of thyroid nodule
    (B) history of hyperthyroidism

(C) irradiation of the neck

(D) history of goiter

(E) abnormal thyroid function tests

18. Primary hyperparathyroidism is NOT caused by

(A) parathyroid adenoma

(B) hyperplasia of the parathyroid

(C) carcinoma of the parathyroid

(D) vitamin D deficiency

(E) MEN (multiple endocrine neoplasia) type I and II

19. The most common cause of hypoparathyroidism is

(A) idiopathic

(B) metastatic carcinoma

(C) I^{131} therapy for Graves' disease

(D) surgery

(E) renal failure

20. Which of the following are branches of the superior mesenteric artery?

(A) right colic, middle colic, and ileocolic

(B) left colic, sigmoid, and hemorrhoid

(C) right and left gastric

(D) common hepatic, splenic, and left gastric

(E) none of the above

21. The following are characteristic features of the colon EXCEPT

(A) taenia coli

(B) appendices epiploicae

(C) haustra

(D) ligament of Treitz

(E) marginal artery of Drummond

DIRECTIONS (Questions 22 through 26): Each group of items in this section consists of lettered headings followed by a set of numbered words or phrases. For each numbered word or phrase, select the ONE lettered heading that is most closely associated with it. Each lettered heading may be selected once, more than once, or not at all.

Questions 22 through 26

Match the following sign/symptom with the most commonly associated form of colitis:

(A) Crohn's colitis

(B) ulcerative colitis

22. Discontinuous involvement

23. Transmural involvement

24. Bleeding

25. Anal fissures

26. Abdominal mass

DIRECTIONS (Questions 27 through 56): Each of the numbered items or incomplete statements in this section is followed by answers or by completions of the statement. Select the ONE lettered answer or completion that is BEST in each case.

Questions 27 through 56

27. Antibiotic-induced colitis results from overgrowth of

(A) *Bacteroides fragilis*

(B) *Escherichia coli*

(C) *Clostridium tetani*

(D) *Clostridium difficile*

(E) *Bacteroides vulgatus*

28. Treatment of pseudomembranous colitis consists of

(A) steroids

(B) sulfasalazine

(C) ampicillin

(D) metronidazole

(E) colectomy

29. Radiographic findings in Crohn's colitis include only

(A) cobblestoning

(B) concentric involvement

(C) findings only in the colon

(D) lead pipe appearance

(E) calcium deposits

30. Complications of ulcerative colitis include

    (A) juvenile polyposis coli
    (B) mesenteric ischemia
    (C) Peutz–Jeghers syndrome
    (D) carcinoma
    (E) superimposed Crohn's colitis

31. Initial treatment of colitis includes

    (A) nasogastric suction
    (B) parenteral nutrition
    (C) corticosteroids
    (D) surgical resection
    (E) oral ampicillin

32. Surgical management of ulcerative colitis includes

    (A) abdominoperineal resection
    (B) regional resection
    (C) low anterior resection
    (D) total colectomy with ileostomy
    (E) arteriographic embolization

33. Bleeding from diverticulosis is

    (A) rare
    (B) commonly diagnosed with a barium enema
    (C) often the only symptom
    (D) associated with abdominal pain
    (E) never life-threatening

34. The traditional diagnostic procedure of choice for massive lower gastrointestinal bleeding is

    (A) CT scan
    (B) colonoscopy
    (C) barium enema
    (D) mesenteric angiography
    (E) radionucleotide imaging

35. Which is NOT a complication of diverticulitis?

    (A) obstruction
    (B) perforation
    (C) fistula
    (D) carcinoma
    (E) bleeding

36. Which procedure should NOT be performed with diverticulitis?

    (A) placement of a nasogastric tube
    (B) barium enema
    (C) insertion of a Foley catheter
    (D) CT of the abdomen and pelvis
    (E) ultrasound of the pelvis

37. Anal fissure is NOT associated with

    (A) Crohn's disease
    (B) tuberculosis
    (C) trauma
    (D) diabetes
    (E) syphilis

38. A 45-year-old male presents to the ER after an explosive gasoline accident. When examined, he is noted to have third-degree burns to the posterior chest wall, posterior lower extremities bilaterally, and the palm of the right hand. What percentage of total body surface is affected?

    (A) 36%
    (B) 54%
    (C) 55%
    (D) 37%
    (E) 45%

39. Diverticular abscess is best treated by

    (A) antibiotic and observation
    (B) percutaneous drainage
    (C) resection and primary anastomosis
    (D) transanal drainage
    (E) resection, drainage, and colostomy

40. Screening for carcinoma of the colon should NOT include

    (A) complete blood count and liver function tests
    (B) hemoccult

(C) endoscopy

(D) digital rectal exam

(E) carcinoembryonic antigen titers

41. The following are characteristic of esophageal achalasia EXCEPT

(A) incomplete relaxation of lower esophageal sphincter

(B) absence of esophageal peristalsis

(C) gastroesophageal reflux

(D) elevated lower esophageal sphincter pressure

(E) relative increase of the intraesophageal baseline pressures

42. Surgical treatment for failed medical management of gastroesophageal reflux disease consists of

(A) antrectomy and vagotomy

(B) esophageal dilation

(C) esophagomyotomy

(D) Nissen fundoplication

(E) highly selective vagotomy

43. In the diagnosis of esophageal motility disorders, the best initial confirming test is

(A) pH monitoring

(B) endoscopy

(C) barium swallow

(D) CT scanning

(E) physical examination

44. Diaphragmatic hernias are NOT associated with

(A) volvulus with acute gastric obstruction

(B) hematemesis

(C) gastric ischemia

(D) carcinoma

(E) recurrent pneumonia

45. The diagnosis of acute pancreatitis is based on

(A) elevated serum amylase

(B) 2 hour urine amylase

(C) subnormal lipase

(D) elevated calcium

(E) leukocytosis

46. Initial treatment of pancreatitis consists of

(A) IV fluids and NPO

(B) clear liquid diet

(C) IV antibiotics

(D) exploratory laparotomy

(E) cholecystectomy

47. The complications of gastroesophageal reflux include all the following EXCEPT

(A) bleeding

(B) Barrett's esophagus

(C) esophageal contractures

(D) esophageal ulceration

(E) Mallory–Weiss syndrome

48. The earliest feature of esophageal carcinoma is

(A) dyspnea

(B) hematemesis

(C) pain

(D) dysphagia

(E) weight loss

49. The main duct emptying the pancreas is the

(A) ampulla of Vater

(B) duct of Sylvius

(C) duct of Wirsung

(D) duct of Santorini

(E) ampulla of Laffaye

50. The most common complication of acute pancreatitis is

(A) pseudocyst

(B) abscess

(C) diabetes

(D) steatorrhea

(E) chronic pancreatitis

51. Diagnosis of chronic pancreatitis has been easier with the advent of

    (A) CT scan
    (B) ultrasound
    (C) MRI (magnetic resonance imaging)
    (D) ERCP (endoscopic retrograde chole-cystopancreatography)
    (E) radionucleotide imaging

52. Initial treatment of a mature pancreatic pseudocyst consists of

    (A) observation
    (B) total pancreatectomy
    (C) endoscopic cannulation and drainage
    (D) Whipple procedure
    (E) percutaneous drainage under CT scan

53. Classic findings in a patient with chronic pancreatitis include

    (A) diabetes
    (B) hypocalcemia
    (C) weight gain
    (D) fever
    (E) intractable abdominal pain

54. Symptoms of carcinoma of the pancreas may include

    (A) pruritis
    (B) periumbilical pain
    (C) weight gain
    (D) fever with chills
    (E) melanic stool

55. Which of the following is not removed in the Whipple procedure?

    (A) head of the pancreas
    (B) gallbladder
    (C) duodenum
    (D) spleen
    (E) distal stomach

56. A "free-floating" prostate noted after a motor vehicle accident is indicative of what injury?

    (A) bladder injury
    (B) urethral injury
    (C) renal injury
    (D) ureteral injury
    (E) acetabular injury

DIRECTIONS (Questions 57 through 61): Each group of items in this section consists of lettered headings followed by a set of numbered words or phrases. For each numbered word or phrase, select the ONE lettered heading that is most closely associated with it. Each lettered heading may be selected once, more than once, or not at all.

Questions 57 through 61

Match the following hernias to their definitions.

    (A) organ involved in the hernia
    (B) incarcerated
    (C) ischemia
    (D) patent tunica vaginalis
    (E) Hesselbach's triangle

57. Strangulated hernia

58. Incarcerated hernia

59. Direct hernia

60. Indirect hernia

61. Sliding hernia

DIRECTIONS (Questions 62 through 83): Each of the numbered items or incomplete statements in this section is followed by answers or by completions of the statement. Select the ONE lettered answer or completion that is BEST in each case.

Questions 62 through 83

62. The most common type of hernia in females is

    (A) indirect hernia
    (B) direct hernia
    (C) femoral hernia
    (D) ventral hernia
    (E) spigelian hernia

63. Which of the following is the most common primary tumor of the brain?

    (A) glioblastoma
    (B) meningioma
    (C) astrocytoma
    (D) medulloblastoma
    (E) acoustic neuroma

64. A 29-year-old male presents with complaints of severe low-back and leg pain following a sneeze. His pain extends from the buttocks posteriorly to the sole of the foot. On examination you note an absent ankle jerk and weakness of plantar flexion. The most likely diagnosis is

    (A) spinal cord tumor
    (B) S1 radiculopathy
    (C) L5 radiculopathy
    (D) pulled hamstring
    (E) spondylolysis

65. Uncommon complications of groin hernioplasty include

    (A) ischemic orchiditis
    (B) recurrence
    (C) hemorrhage
    (D) ileoinguinal nerve injury
    (E) infection

66. What procedure should NOT be performed if a basilar skull fracture is noted?

    (A) insertion of a nasogastric tube
    (B) CT scan of the head
    (C) skull roentgenograms
    (D) cerebral arteriogram
    (E) lumbar puncture

67. Which of the following statements about melena is true?

    (A) Melena usually indicates lower gastrointestinal tract bleeding.
    (B) It may indicate only hemorrhoidal disease.
    (C) As little as 50 mL of blood may produce melena.

    (D) Only blood produces black stools.
    (E) Medications can never produce positive melenic stool.

68. Which of the following is true regarding proximal gastric ulcers?

    (A) Stress is often a precipitating factor.
    (B) Incidence decreases with age.
    (C) Acid hypersecretion is an associated factor.
    (D) In the United States, gastric ulcers are much less common than duodenal ulcers.
    (E) Gastric ulcers are not affected by nonsteroidal anti-inflammatory drugs.

69. Which of the following procedures would decrease gastric acid production?

    (A) parietal cell vagotomy
    (B) antrectomy and selective vagotomy
    (C) proximal gastrectomy
    (D) pyloroplasty
    (E) truncal vagotomy

70. The most common abnormal physiological mechanism of duodenal ulcer formation is

    (A) increased secretion of gastric acid
    (B) rapid gastric emptying
    (C) fasting hypergastrinemia
    (D) hyperpepsinogenemia
    (E) deficient duodenal buffers

71. A 70-year-old female presents with massive melena and associated hypotension corrected with IV fluid and blood. Which of the following should be done first to determine the source of gastrointestinal bleeding?

    (A) a lower gastrointestinal barium enema
    (B) sigmoidoscopy
    (C) colonoscopy
    (D) radionucleotide imaging
    (E) selective arteriography

72. A 60-year-old diabetic male presents with a bleeding duodenal ulcer. He is treated with nasogastric suctioning, saline lavage, and blood transfusions as needed. However, he continues to bleed actively and requires more than 12 units of blood in the first 24 hours. Prior to this he was otherwise healthy. The treatment of choice is

    (A) systemic infusion of vasopressin (pitressin)
    (B) angiographic catheterization of the gastroduodenal artery and gelfoam embolization
    (C) proximal gastric vagotomy
    (D) oversewing the ulcer, bilateral truncal vagotomy, and pyloroplasty
    (E) bilateral truncal vagotomy, antrectomy, and Billroth II gastrojejunostomy

73. The treatment of choice for a 50-year-old male with biopsy-documented gastric lymphoma would be

    (A) wide local excision
    (B) chemotherapy
    (C) subtotal gastrectomy and radiotherapy
    (D) subtotal gastrectomy
    (E) radiotherapy

74. Which of the following statements regarding gallstones is NOT correct?

    (A) There are two basic types of gallstones.
    (B) In the United States, cholesterol gallstones account for 70% of all cases.
    (C) The three major components of bile are bile salts, lecithin, and cholesterol.
    (D) Worldwide, pigmented stones are the most common type.
    (E) Gallstones greater than 2.5 cm are not determinant of cancer risk.

75. Pigmented gallstone formation has been associated with

    (A) hemolytic disease
    (B) coronary artery bypass with graft
    (C) colon carcinomas

(D) subtotal colectomy
(E) atherosclerotic cardiovascular disease

76. Which statement regarding the use of HIDA isotope scans to define gallbladder function is correct?

    (A) They can be used to define obstruction of the pancreatic ducts.
    (B) They are seldom effective when the patient's serum bilirubin level is higher than 3.5 mg/100 mL.
    (C) They are the diagnostic tools of choice for defining acute cholecystitis secondary to cystic duct obstruction.
    (D) Their toxicity is approximately the same as that of IV cholangiography.
    (E) It is contraindicated for acalculus cholecystitis.

77. Which statement regarding sclerosing cholangitis is true?

    (A) Individuals with sclerosing cholangitis have stones in their common bile duct.
    (B) It occurs more frequently in females than males.
    (C) It has been seen in association with ulcerative colitis.
    (D) It is thought to result from trauma during the passage of gallstones.
    (E) The gallbladder is always involved.

78. Lithogenic bile is characterized by a low ratio of concentration of

    (A) cholesterol to bile salts
    (B) cholesterol to lecithin and bile salts
    (C) cholesterol to lecithin
    (D) bilirubinate to cholesterol
    (E) lecithin and bile salts to cholesterol

79. The major stimulus for gallbladder emptying is mediated by

    (A) stimulation of the sympathetic system
    (B) release of cholecystokinin
    (C) stimulation of the parasympathetic (vagal) system

(D) release of secretin

(E) secretion of hydrochloric acid

80. The treatment of radiolucent gallstones with chenodeoxycholic acid for 2 years results in a complete dissolution in what percentage of patients?

(A) less than 5

(B) 15

(C) 25

(D) 35

(E) greater than 40

81. In patients with asymptomatic gallstones who were treated without surgery, symptoms developed in what percentage of patients?

(A) less than 10

(B) 20

(C) 30

(D) 40

(E) 50

82. A 40-year-old female complains of recurrent postprandial attacks of colicky right upper quadrant pain. Ultrasonography does not demonstrate gallstones. She presently is pain free. The next diagnostic test should be

(A) flat plate of the abdomen

(B) oral cholecystography

(C) HIDA scan

(D) CT scan of the gallbladder

(E) percutaneous transhepatic cholangiography (PTC)

83. A 65-year-old male who has previously undergone cholecystectomy presents in the ER with jaundice, fever, and right upper-quadrant abdominal pain. Initial treatment should be

(A) antibiotics

(B) endoscopic sphincterotomy

(C) percutaneous transhepatic drainage

(D) T-tube decompression of the common bile duct

(E) emergency exploratory laparotomy

DIRECTIONS (Questions 84 through 87): Each group of items in this section consists of lettered headings followed by a set of numbered words or phrases. For each numbered word or phrase, select the ONE lettered heading that is most closely associated with it. Each lettered heading may be selected once, more than once, or not at all.

Questions 84 through 87

(A) acute cholecystitis

(B) chronic cholecystitis

(C) both

(D) neither

84. Cystic duct obstruction

85. Empyema

86. May require immediate operation

87. HIDA scan is the specific diagnostic test

Questions 88 through 90

Match the following physical exam findings with the diagnosis.

(A) basal skull fracture

(B) subarachnoid hemorrhage

(C) neither

(D) both

88. Ecchymosis in the postauricular region

89. "Raccoon eyes" and hemotympanum

90. Nuchal rigidity and cranial nerve palsies with motor abnormalities

DIRECTIONS (Questions 91 through 96): Each of the numbered items or incomplete statements in this section is followed by answers or by completions of the statement. Select the ONE lettered answer or completion that is BEST in each case.

Questions 91 through 96

91. The most common primary tumor site associated with hepatic metastases is

    (A) pancreas
    (B) stomach
    (C) colon
    (D) breast
    (E) lung

92. Which of the following is true regarding the treatment of primary hepatocellular carcinoma?

    (A) Most lesions are amenable to resection with a resulting 5-year survival rate of approximately 30%.
    (B) Most lesions are NOT amenable to partial resection and are best treated with radiation.
    (C) Orthotopic liver transplantation has become the treatment of choice.
    (D) Mean survival of untreated patients is 3 to 4 months from the time of onset of the symptoms.
    (E) Both systemic chemotherapy and hepatic arterial chemotherapy produce a response rate of approximately 60%.

93. An elevated level of alpha-fetoprotein in the serum of an adult suggests the diagnosis of

    (A) metastatic cancer of the liver
    (B) primary cancer of the liver
    (C) focal nodular hyperplasia of the liver
    (D) pyogenic liver abscess
    (E) biliary cirrhosis

94. The most common cause of portal hypertension is related to

    (A) extrahepatic venous outflow obstruction
    (B) intrahepatic portal venous obstruction (presinusoidal)

    (C) increased hepatopedal blood flow
    (D) extrahepatic portal venous obstruction
    (E) intrahepatic-hepatic venous obstruction (postsinusoidal)

95. Which of the following best determines long-term survival following a shunting procedure of an alcoholic patient with cirrhosis of the liver?

    (A) control of ascites
    (B) a low-protein diet
    (C) a low-salt intake
    (D) use of lactulose
    (E) abstinence from alcohol

96. Which of the following criteria in a patient with alcoholic cirrhosis provides the most acceptable indication for portal systemic shunting with the best chance of survival?

    (A) documented varices that have never bled but are large
    (B) documented varices that have bled several times in the recent past and have not responded to endoscopic variceal sclerosis
    (C) documented acutely bleeding varices that have not stopped after 10 units of transfused blood
    (D) large esophageal varices and mild encephalopathy
    (E) very high portal pressure discovered during abdominal surgery

DIRECTIONS (Questions 97 through 101): Each group of items in this section consists of lettered headings followed by a set of numbered words or phrases. For each numbered word or phrase, select the ONE lettered heading that is most closely associated with it. Each lettered heading may be selected once, more than once, or not at all.

Questions 97 through 101

Select the type of hepatic abscess described best by the following statements.

- (A) amebic liver abscess
- (B) pyogenic liver abscess
- (C) both
- (D) neither

97. Usually single

98. Predominantly involves the right lobe of the liver

99. The cultures are usually sterile

100. Treatment is primarily medical

101. Treatment is primarily surgical

DIRECTIONS (Questions 102 through 105): Each of the numbered items or incomplete statements in this section is followed by answers or by completions of the statement. Select the ONE lettered answer or completion that is BEST in each case.

Questions 102 through 105

102. What suture would best serve a ruptured distal joint extensor tendon of one of the fingers?

- (A) 6-0 nylon
- (B) 6-0 vicryl
- (C) 2-0 prolene
- (D) 5-0 dexon
- (E) 5-0 monocryl

103. True statements regarding malignant small bowel tumors include

- (A) Carcinoid is the most common malignancy of the small intestine.
- (B) They account for a small percentage of all gastrointestinal malignancies.
- (C) Five-year survival is highest with adenocarcinoma followed by lymphoma, and still lower with leiomyosarcoma.
- (D) Lymphomas are not treated with radiation treatment.
- (E) Pancreaticoduodenectomy is never indicated for duodenal lesions.

104. True statements regarding carcinoid tumors of the gastrointestinal tract include

- (A) They are rarely encountered in an appendix.
- (B) The cell of origin is the Kupffer cell.
- (C) Prognosis is related to tumor size, location, and histological pattern.
- (D) The rectum is the most common site of origin.
- (E) Prognosis is always poor.

105. True statements regarding Meckel's diverticula include

- (A) They occur in 50% of the population in one form or another.
- (B) They are true diverticula.
- (C) Diverticulitis is the most common complication.
- (D) It is never visualized with technetium pertechnetate scans.
- (E) It is usually located 5 feet from the ileocecal valve.

DIRECTIONS (Questions 106 through 109): Each group of items in this section consists of lettered headings followed by a set of numbered phrases. For each numbered phrase, select the ONE lettered heading that is most closely associated with it. Each lettered heading may be selected once, more than once, or not at all.

Questions 106 through 109

- (A) thrombophlebitis
- (B) deep-vein thrombosis
- (C) urinary tract infection
- (D) pulmonary atelectasis
- (E) wound infection

106. Fever within 24 to 48 hours of surgery

107. Fever after the fifth postoperative day

108. Fever occurring 3–5 days after operation with poor postoperative ambulation

109. Fever occurring 3–5 days with an indwelling catheter

DIRECTIONS (Questions 110 through 118): Each of the numbered items or incomplete statements in this section is followed by answers or by completions of the statement. Select the ONE lettered answer or completion that is BEST in each case.

Questions 110 through 118

110. In the evaluation of a female patient with right lower-quadrant pain, which of the following should be included in the differential diagnosis?

    (A) twisted ovarian cyst or tumor
    (B) diverticulitis of the sigmoid colon
    (C) ruptured ectopic pregnancy
    (D) epiploic appendicitis
    (E) all of the above

111. Which of the following radiological findings is/are associated with acute appendicitis?

    (A) distended loop of small bowel in the right lower quadrant
    (B) partial filling of the appendix on barium enema
    (C) a gas-filled appendix
    (D) a mass effect in the cecum on barium enema
    (E) all of the above

112. For which of the following patients would initial nonoperative treatment of appendicitis be appropriate?

    (A) pregnant woman during her first trimester
    (B) 35-year-old patient with subsiding symptoms and a right lower-quadrant mass
    (C) elderly patient with coexisting cardiac disease
    (D) 20-year-old woman with Crohn's disease
    (E) 9-year-old male

113. The most useful screening test for prostate cancer is

    (A) acid phosphatase
    (B) digital rectal examination
    (C) prostate-specific antigen (PSA)
    (D) both rectal exam and PSA
    (E) alkaline phosphatase

114. A male patient in good health presents with an asymptomatic prostate nodule. Biopsy reveals adenocarcinoma. The metastatic workup is negative. Which of the following therapies would be appropriate?

    (A) transurethral prostate resection (TURP)
    (B) radical prostatectomy
    (C) orchiectomy
    (D) estrogen therapy
    (E) prostatectomy with pelvic node dissection

115. A 30-year-old male presents with a nontender hard testicular lump. Appropriate treatment includes which one of the following?

    (A) observation for 3 months
    (B) incisional biopsy via a scrotal incision
    (C) radical orchiectomy
    (D) incisional biopsy via an inguinal incision
    (E) radiation therapy

116. An adolescent male presents with a 3-hour history of severe scrotal pain. The examination reveals scrotal swelling and tenderness that does not permit discrete palpation of the epididymis. The best treatment at this point is

    (A) heat, scrotal elevation, and antibiotics
    (B) manual attempt at detorsion
    (C) analgesics and reexamination
    (D) surgical exploration
    (E) observation for at least 12 hours

117. The preferred method of treatment for urinary tract calculi is

    (A) ureterorenoscopy
    (B) extracorporeal shock wave lithotripsy
    (C) percutaneous nephrolithotomy
    (D) open surgical procedure
    (E) chemical lysis

118. Urinary tract calculi are most commonly composed of

    (A) uric acid
    (B) cystine
    (C) calcium oxalate
    (D) ammonium magnesium phosphate
    (E) pure calcium phosphate

DIRECTIONS (Questions 119 through 125): Each group of items in this section consists of lettered headings followed by a set of numbered words or phrases. For each numbered word or phrase, select the ONE lettered heading that is most closely associated with it. Each lettered heading may be selected once, more than once, or not at all.

Questions 119 through 121

Match the type of joint with its appropriate example.

    (A) elbow
    (B) skull sutures
    (C) pubic symphysis

119. Fibrous joint

120. Fibrocartilaginous joint

121. Diarthroidal joint

Questions 122 through 125

Match the following primary shoulder disorders with their appropriate clinical characteristic.

    (A) pain extending along the proximal humeral groove
    (B) unrelenting pain not relieved by change in position
    (C) limitation of internal rotation and full abduction
    (D) surgical repair may be required

122. Subacromial bursitis

123. Bicipital tendonitis

124. Supraspinatus tendonitis

125. Rotator cuff tear

DIRECTIONS (Questions 126 through 129): Each of the numbered items or incomplete statements in this section is followed by answers or by completions of the statement. Select the ONE lettered answer or completion that is BEST in each case.

Questions 126 through 129

126. Physiological interruption of nerve conduction caused by a transient incomplete or complete paralysis of a peripheral nerve is

    (A) axonopraxia
    (B) neuroapraxia
    (C) axonotmesis
    (D) Wallerian degeneration
    (E) neurotmesis

127. A tear of the lateral meniscus is best diagnosed by means of

    (A) accurate history
    (B) physical examination
    (C) arthroscopy
    (D) MRI
    (E) arthrography

128. Regarding chondromalacia of the patella, which of the following statements is true?

    (A) Radiographs show characteristic changes early in the course of the disease.
    (B) The pain is aggravated by knee flexion, kneeling, and ascending stairs.
    (C) The progressive nature of the disease warrants early surgical intervention.
    (D) The initial changes usually occur on the lateral aspect of the patella.
    (E) Patellectomy is the only proven form of successful surgical therapy.

129. Which of the following is most sensitive to anoxia?

    (A) peripheral nerves
    (B) striated muscle
    (C) skin
    (D) tendon
    (E) bone

DIRECTIONS (Questions 130 through 133): Each group of items in this section consists of a list of lettered headings followed by a set of numbered words or phrases. For each numbered word or phrase, select the ONE lettered heading that is most closely associated with it. Each lettered heading may be selected once, more than once, or not at all.

Questions 130 and 131

    (A) pain in the calf
    (B) pain in the buttock
    (C) both
    (D) neither

130. Aortic occlusion

131. Superficial femoral artery occlusion

Questions 132 and 133

    (A) gangrenous digits
    (B) trophic ulcers
    (C) both
    (D) neither

132. Diabetes mellitus

133. Buerger's disease

DIRECTIONS (Questions 134 through 141): Each of the numbered items or incomplete statements in this section is followed by answers or by completions of the statement. Select the ONE lettered answer or completion that is BEST in each case.

Questions 134 through 141

134. A patient presenting with bilateral leg pain, rubor on dependency, atrophic skin, and decreased skin temperature has

    (A) acute arterial occlusion
    (B) chronic venous insufficiency
    (C) thromboangiitis obliterans
    (D) peripheral artery insufficiency
    (E) popliteal artery entrapment syndrome

135. Which of the following abnormal findings produced by arterial injury is most important?

    (A) pain
    (B) paralysis and paresthesia
    (C) poikilothermia
    (D) pulselessness
    (E) pallor

136. The following statements about congenital arteriovenous fistula are correct EXCEPT

    (A) A simple port-wine stain constitutes one manifestation.
    (B) It is frequently discovered by a parent noticing that one of their child's extremities is larger than the other.
    (C) It may be associated with a thrill or bruit.
    (D) It should be treated aggressively.
    (E) Ulceration and bleeding may occur.

137. Following arterial repair from trauma of the femoral artery, postoperative pulses are now absent. What is the recommended course of action?

    (A) conservative therapy—wait and see if pulses return
    (B) anticoagulant therapy
    (C) vasodilators
    (D) re-exploration and thrombectomy
    (E) amputation

138. Which of the following is the best method to control bleeding in an emergency setting?

    (A) tourniquet
    (B) tourniquet and direct digital pressure
    (C) direct digital pressure
    (D) tourniquet and packing the wound with gauze and applying a pressure dressing
    (E) placing a hemostat on the vessel

139. The following statements about compartment syndromes are true EXCEPT

    (A) Elevated pressure within the compartment compromises arterial inflow.

(B) Sustained pressures above 30 mm Hg indicate impending compartment syndrome.

(C) Following disappearance of pulses, it is best treated by decompression fasciotomy.

(D) Common causes are supracondylar fractures of the humerus and tibial fractures.

(E) Early treatment may result in complete return of function.

140. Which of the following statements concerning diagnosis of arterial occlusive disease of the lower extremities by means of noninvasive testing is false?

(A) Patients without arterial disease will have an ankle/brachial index of 1 or higher.

(B) Patients with advanced ischemia generally will have an ankle/brachial index lower than 0.5.

(C) Diabetic patients may have low ankle/brachial indices because of calcification of arterial walls.

(D) The use of stress testing can increase the sensitivity of testing.

(E) Determination of pressures and waveforms at different levels can define the location of the disease.

141. The most important laboratory examination in arterial occlusive disease is

(A) arteriography

(B) B-mode ultrasonography

(C) Doppler ultrasound

(D) plethysmography

(E) magnetic resonance imaging

DIRECTIONS (Questions 142 through 143): Each group of items in this section consists of lettered headings followed by a set of numbered words or phrases. For each numbered word or phrase, select the ONE lettered heading that is most closely associated with it. Each lettered heading may be selected once, more than once, or not at all.

Questions 142 and 143

(A) are the first sign of unrecognized heart disease

(B) are hypercoagulable state

(C) both

(D) neither

142. Thrombi

143. Emboli

DIRECTIONS (Questions 144 through 146): Each of the numbered items or incomplete statements in this section is followed by answers or by completions of the statement. Select the ONE lettered answer or completion that is BEST in each case.

Questions 144 through 146

144. A patient presents with complaints of swollen legs that have become increasingly brown in color. The patient is likely to have

(A) chronic venous insufficiency

(B) venous thrombosis

(C) varicose veins

(D) lymphedema

(E) atherosclerotic occlusive disease

145. Which atherosclerotic aneurysm is most common?

(A) abdominal aortic aneurysm

(B) carotid artery aneurysm

(C) popliteal aneurysm

(D) femoral aneurysm

(E) subclavian artery aneurysm

146. What treatment course(s) should be taken for patients with an embolic event to their lower extremity?

(A) prompt administration of IV heparin

(B) under local anesthesia, removal of emboli with Fogarty balloon catheter through a short incision

(C) fasciotomy

(D) operative angiography

(E) all of the above

DIRECTIONS (Questions 147 through 158): Each group of items in this section consists of lettered headings followed by a set of numbered words or phrases. For each numbered word or phrase, select the ONE lettered heading that is most closely associated with it. Each lettered heading may be selected once, more than once, or not at all.

Questions 147 and 148

(A) proliferative reaction in the media causing narrowing of the arterial lumen
(B) degenerative changes in the media
(C) both
(D) neither

147. Abdominal aortic aneurysm

148. Atherosclerotic occlusive disease

Questions 149 and 150

(A) impotence
(B) claudication
(C) both
(D) neither

149. Abdominal aortic aneurysm

150. Aortoiliac occlusive disease

Questions 151 through 153

For each set of symptoms, select the associated disorder.

(A) painless, cold cyanosis of the hands and feet
(B) red, warm, painful extremities
(C) persistent mottled reddish-blue discoloration of the skin of the extremities

151. Livedo reticularis

152. Erythromelalgia

153. Acrocyanosis

Questions 154 through 156

(A) recurrent episodes of vasoconstriction in the upper extremities initiated by exposure to cold or emotional stress
(B) secondary manifestation of a more serious disorder of the vascular system
(C) both
(D) neither

154. Raynaud's phenomenon

155. Raynaud's disease

156. Buerger's disease

Questions 157 and 158

(A) edema and redness of the affected part without necrosis of the skin
(B) formation of blisters
(C) both
(D) neither

157. First-degree frostbite injury

158. Second-degree frostbite injury

DIRECTIONS (Questions 159 through 165): Each of the numbered items or incomplete statements in this section is followed by answers or by completions of the statement. Select the ONE lettered answer or completion that is BEST in each case.

Questions 159 through 165

159. The best temperature range for rewarming cold exposed tissue should be

(A) 25–30°C
(B) 32–36°C
(C) 40–44°C
(D) 48–52°C
(E) 55–60°C

160. The following statements about Buerger's disease are correct EXCEPT

(A) The distribution of arterial involvement is the same as that of atherosclerosis.

(B) The distribution of the disease in the lower extremity is similar to the typical arterial involvement in the diabetic.

(C) Early in the course of the disease, the superficial veins undergo recurrent superficial thrombophlebitis.

(D) It is most often seen in men who are between the ages of 20 and 40.

(E) A history of at least a 20-cigarettes-per-day habit is present.

161. Diminution or absence of femoral pulses combined with absence of popliteal and pedal pulses is most likely to occur in patients with

(A) abdominal aortic aneurysm
(B) diabetes mellitus
(C) Buerger's disease
(D) aortoiliac occlusive disease
(E) acute arterial thrombosis

162. The rationale behind education of diabetics to the importance of proper foot care includes which of the following?

(A) It is likely that diabetics will develop atherosclerosis in their lower extremities.

(B) Diabetics may not notice minor trauma.

(C) Diabetics have a propensity for developing infections.

(D) Diabetics are predisposed to ulceration and gangrene of the foot, with relatively rapid progression to limb loss.

(E) All of the above.

163. The following are risk factors for peripheral atherosclerosis EXCEPT

(A) hypertension
(B) female
(C) tobacco use
(D) diabetes mellitus
(E) hyperlipidemia

164. Which of the following is usually implicated in the development of venous stasis ulcers at the ankle?

(A) greater saphenous vein
(B) lesser saphenous vein
(C) perforating or communicating vein
(D) spider veins
(E) none of the above

165. The following statements about ischemic stroke are true EXCEPT

(A) refers to cerebral infarction occurring as a result of impairment to regional blood flow

(B) may be secondary to cerebral embolization of thrombi that originate in the heart

(C) may be due to fibromuscular hyperplasia

(D) may be associated with obliterative arteritis of the great vessels

(E) have not been associated with dissecting thoracic aortic aneurysms

DIRECTIONS (Questions 166 through 168): Each group of items in this section consists of lettered headings followed by a set of numbered words or phrases. For each numbered word or phrase, select the ONE lettered heading that is most closely associated with it. Each lettered heading may be selected once, more than once, or not at all.

Questions 166 through 168

Select the study that will be helpful in establishing the diagnosis of the following diseases.

(A) Adson's maneuver
(B) Allen's test
(C) submersion test
(D) exercise stress test
(E) Valsalva's maneuver

166. Raynaud's disease

167. Thoracic outlet syndrome

168. Femoropopliteal disease

DIRECTIONS (Questions 169 through 174): Each of the numbered items or incomplete statements in this section is followed by answers or by completions of the statement. Select the ONE lettered answer or completion that is BEST in each case.

Questions 169 through 174

169. The statements below are true EXCEPT

(A) Venous valves ensure proximal flow and prevent distal reflux.
(B) The number of venous valves increase the greater the distance from the heart.
(C) Venous valves have little, if any, role in venous disease.
(D) Venous valves may be weakened in patients with varicose veins.
(E) Venous valves are absent from the vena cava and the common iliac veins.

170. The most common cause of secondary lymphedema in the United States is

(A) radiation
(B) malignancy
(C) trauma or surgical excision
(D) inflammation or parasitic invasion
(E) paralysis

171. Which maternal disease is known to cause congenital heart disease?

(A) varicella
(B) rubella
(C) diphtheria
(D) rubeola
(E) tuberculosis

172. The tetrology of Fallot is a classic example of a(n)

(A) left-to-right shunt
(B) right-to-left shunt
(C) left-sided obstruction
(D) noncyanotic malformation
(E) atrial septal defect combination

173. Important principles in a pediatric intensive care unit include all of the following EXCEPT

(A) intravenous fluid intake
(B) monitoring of the electrocardiogram
(C) continuous measurement of central venous, left atrial, and arterial pressure
(D) routine measurement of blood-gas tensions and urine output
(E) constant observation

174. All the following physical findings can point to a severe congenital cardiac malformation EXCEPT

(A) hepatic enlargement
(B) clubbing of the fingers and toes
(C) cyanosis
(D) normal growth and development
(E) fatigue

DIRECTIONS (Questions 175 through 178): Each group of matching questions in this section consists of lettered headings followed by a set of numbered words or phrases. For each numbered word or phrase, select the ONE lettered heading that is most closely associated with it. Each lettered heading may be selected once, more than once, or not at all.

Questions 175 through 178

(A) acyanotic
(B) cyanotic
(C) both
(D) neither

175. Tetralogy of Fallot

176. Ventricular septal defect

177. Atrial septal defect

178. Transposition of the great vessels

DIRECTIONS (Questions 179 through 197): Each of the numbered items or incomplete statements in this section is followed by answers or by completions of the statement. Select the ONE lettered answer or completion that is BEST in each case.

Questions 179 through 197

179. Which noninvasive procedure has become the most valuable test in congenital heart disease?

    (A) electrocardiogram
    (B) chest radiograph
    (C) echocardiogram
    (D) MRI

180. Which item is NOT an essential finding in diagnosis of coarctation of the aorta?

    (A) harsh systolic murmur heard in the back
    (B) systolic pressure higher in upper extremities than in lower extremities
    (C) absent or weak femoral pulses
    (D) soft diastolic murmur at apex
    (E) infants may have severe heart failure; children are usually asymptomatic

181. All of the following are late signs of advanced cardiac disease EXCEPT

    (A) angina
    (B) dyspnea
    (C) edema
    (D) syncope
    (E) hepatomegaly

182. Which symptom is the most common manifestation of coronary artery disease?

    (A) dyspnea
    (B) syncope
    (C) arrhythmia
    (D) angina
    (E) palpitation

183. The most common coexisting disease in patients with descending thoracic aortic surgery is

    (A) coronary artery disease
    (B) chronic obstructive pulmonary disease
    (C) previous surgery for another aneurysm
    (D) previous CABG
    (E) preexisting hypertension

184. Tolerance for periods of perfusion are surprisingly good up to a maximum of

    (A) less than 1 hour
    (B) 2 to 3 hours
    (C) 4 to 5 hours
    (D) 6 to 7 hours
    (E) 8 hours or more

185. The major concern in using percutaneous transluminal coronary angioplasty (PTCA) is

    (A) significant restenosis within first year
    (B) high complication rate
    (C) frequent procedure-related MI and death
    (D) low successful dilation rates per stenosis
    (E) intraprocedure cerebrovascular symptoms

186. A complication that most likely would NOT occur early in the postoperative cardiac surgery course is

    (A) postoperative bleeding
    (B) cardiac arrhythmias
    (C) stroke
    (D) postpericardiotomy syndrome
    (E) graft occlusion

187. The cerebral anoxia following circulatory arrest produces brain damage within

    (A) 30 to 60 seconds
    (B) 1 to 2 minutes
    (C) 3 to 4 minutes
    (D) 5 to 7 minutes
    (E) 6 to 8 minutes

188. Firm indications for operative intervention in mitral stenosis include all EXCEPT

    (A) onset of atrial fibrillation
    (B) NYHA class III or IV symptoms
    (C) minimal reduction of valve area at catheterization
    (D) infective endocarditis
    (E) worsening pulmonary hypertension

189. A late and especially ominous sign in aortic stenosis is

   (A) angina
   (B) congestive heart failure
   (C) exertional syncope
   (D) narrowed pulse pressure
   (E) mid-systolic murmur

190. The myocardial ischemia produced by coronary artery disease can cause one or more of the following events

   (A) angina pectoris
   (B) sudden death
   (C) myocardial infarction
   (D) congestive heart failure
   (E) all of the above

191. Therapy for acute myocardial infarction includes

   (A) angioplasty
   (B) IV administration of a thrombolytic agent
   (C) intracoronary administration of a thrombolytic agent
   (D) immediate bypass preceded by intra-aortic balloon support
   (E) all of the above

192. The following are potential causes of vein graft occlusion within the first 5 years following coronary bypass grafting EXCEPT

   (A) anastomotic technique
   (B) trauma to the vein graft at the time of operation
   (C) intimal hyperplasia
   (D) the use of dipyridamole and aspirin
   (E) poor runoff of recipient coronary artery

193. Which is the best coronary artery bypass grafting material?

   (A) brachial vein
   (B) greater saphenous vein
   (C) lesser saphenous vein
   (D) internal mammary artery
   (E) polytetrafluorethylene (PTFE)

194. In the majority of patients, the cause of chronic constrictive pericarditis is

   (A) viral pericarditis
   (B) *Haemophilus influenzae*
   (C) intensive radiation
   (D) *Staphylococcus*
   (E) unknown

195. Which procedure most commonly causes surgical trauma producing complete heart block?

   (A) repair of ventricular septal defect
   (B) prosthetic valve replacement
   (C) annular abscess excision from endocarditis
   (D) coronary artery bypass graft
   (E) none of the above

196. Surgical treatment of cardiac arrhythmias is done for all the following clinical entities EXCEPT

   (A) Wolff-Parkinson-White (WPW) syndrome
   (B) paroxysmal supraventricular tachycardia (PSVT)
   (C) sustained ventricular tachycardia
   (D) acute atrial fibrillation
   (E) chronic atrial fibrillation

197. The statements about left ventricular aneurysms are true EXCEPT

   (A) Chest x-ray shows a localized ventricular bulge.
   (B) They are due to a severe transmural myocardial infarction.
   (C) The aneurysm undergoes progressive enlargement and rupture.
   (D) More than 80% of aneurysms are in the anteroseptal left ventricle.
   (E) Posterior aneurysms are uncommon.

DIRECTIONS (Questions 198 through 200): Each group of items in this section consists of a list of lettered headings followed by several numbered words or phrases. For each numbered word or phrase, select the ONE lettered heading that is most closely associated with it. Each lettered heading may be selected once, more than once, or not at all.

Questions 198 through 200

    (A) penetrating cardiac trauma

    (B) blunt cardiac trauma

    (C) both

    (D) neither

198. Steering wheel injury

199. Tamponade and hemorrhage

200. Pericardial effusion and chest pain

Answers and Explanations

1. **(A)** Thrombocytopenia is by far the most common bleeding disorder seen in the postoperative patient. This results from platelet consumption in the control of bleeding or from drug interaction or massive blood transfusion. The most common cause of bleeding in a surgical patient is poor local control. This should be suspected in patients who are bleeding from a single site, not multiple sites. *(Schwartz, 1994, pp. 95–118)*

2. **(A)** Lower-extremity paresthesia is most commonly associated with neurogenic shock, as the symptom of paresthesias is associated with a neurologic injury. This causes interruption of the sympathetic innervation responsible for vasoconstriction and results in hypotension. *(Shires et al, 1989, pp. 139–140)*

3. **(E)** Cardiogenic shock. Muffled heart sounds, especially in the hypotensive patient with distended neck veins, should suggest the presence of cardiac tamponade. *(Shires et al, 1989, pp. 138–139)*

4. **(D)** Hypovolemic shock. The fracture of a femur is associated with a large loss of blood into the surrounding tissue and depletes the intravascular space. This in turn causes the reduction in the volume the heart can pump and decreases the systemic blood pressure. *(Shires et al, 1989, pp. 137–180)*

5. **(B)** Septic shock. The individual with an overwhelming infection becomes hyperdynamic, meaning that his or her heart is working very hard; however, the toxins produced by the bacteria, notably gram-negative, will cause a vasodilation. This vasodilation is responsible for the decrease in blood pressure and also the warmth of skin, because there is more blood flowing there. *(Shires et al, 1989, pp. 140–142)*

6. **(D)** Pain is not a symptom associated with carcinoma of the breast. This is more commonly seen in mastitis, pregnancy, or in fat necrosis following trauma. The remainder of the symptoms are all suspicious of carcinoma and should be thoroughly evaluated. *(Bland and Copeland, pp. 552–592)*

7. **(C)** Mammography is indicated initially at the age of 40. All women should be encouraged to have annual or biannual examinations up to the age of 50, at which point the indication is an annual examination. This examination should consist of a physician or physician assistant breast examination as well as mammography. Studies have documented that the early findings on mammogram have led to earlier detection of malignant lesions. *(Bland and Copeland, pp. 540–544)*

8. **(E)** History of endometriosis has not been identified as an established risk factor for

breast cancer. Other choices are important historical points ascertained in the evaluation of the patient with a breast mass. There are associated risks of breast carcinoma in females who have had no children or their first child after the age of 30. In addition, there is an increased risk of breast cancer in those patients with a family history of carcinoma and in those people with benign breast lesions. *(Bland and Copeland, p. 555)*

9. **(D)** Diffuse abdominal pain that is "wave-like" and associated with vomiting is most likely the result of a luminal-type obstruction. Generally, this is a bowel obstruction, either small or large. Pancreatitis, which also is associated with diffuse abdominal pain, generally is a constant pain that often radiates into the back. The remaining choices are occasionally colicky or "wave-like," although they are generally not diffuse in nature. *(McFadden and Zinner, p. 1017)*

10. **(C)** Biliary colic is often an insidious pain that is postprandial in its onset. Perforation of viscus, ureteral colic, the rupturing of an abdominal aneurysm, or severe pancreatitis can be severe in onset and, in fact, can cause a patient to collapse. *(McFadden and Zinner, p. 1017)*

11. **(D)** When evaluating a patient with abdominal pain that you suspect to be an intestinal obstruction, a flat and upright radiograph of the abdomen will provide sufficient information to differentiate a simple obstruction or a dynamic ileus from a perforation of a viscus by the demonstration of free air. Further radiographic investigation would involve the use of a barium enema that would outline the inferior margins of an obstructing lesion. *(McFadden and Zinner, pp. 1028–1031)*

12. **(C)** Pain out of proportion to physical findings is a clue to an underlying vascular etiology. The ischemic pain resulting from either a venous or arterial occlusive process is significant with minimal signs, such as peritonitis or localized tenderness. This unfortunately often is a diagnosis of exclusion that is made only via arteriography. *(Adams, pp. 1495–1499)*

13. **(B)** The recurrent laryngeal nerve lies in the tracheoesophageal groove bilaterally and is responsible for innervation of the vocal cord on the ipsilateral side. It must be identified during anterior cervical microdiscectomy to avoid iatrogenic injury. The cervical sympathetic chain and vagus nerve lie along the path of the carotid artery and jugular vein and are not usually encountered during disc surgery. The laryngeal nerves lie adjacent to the superior and inferior thyroid arteries and are not in the field of surgery for this procedure. *(Weinstein and Hoff, pp. 852–854)*

14. **(E)** The most useful diagnostic test in the preoperative evaluation of a solid thyroid mass is a needle biopsy. Ultrasound and needle aspiration are useful in determining cystic lesions. The radioactive scan is important in differentiating a cold or nonfunctioning nodule; however, the majority of benign lesions also are cold, and this is not in any way diagnostic of carcinoma. In addition, thyroid function tests have no role, because the majority of patients with thyroid carcinoma are found to be euthyroid. *(Kaplan, pp. 1629–1633)*

15. **(B)** Papillary carcinoma of the thyroid has an excellent prognosis following surgical excision. In recent studies, 10-year survival rates were approximately 89%. Follicular carcinoma has a propensity for a multicentric focus of carcinoma. Studies have shown a 10-year survival rate of between 44% and 86% based on the apparent invasiveness of the original tumor. *(Kaplan, pp. 1633–1640)*

16. **(E)** Findings associated with thyroid carcinoma include those of pressure within the neck, such as dysphagia, which may be the result of pressure on the esophagus. In addition, tumor invasion may result in injury to the recurrent laryngeal nerve with resultant vocal cord paralysis and hoarseness. A palpable mass is associated with both benign and malignant processes within the thyroid but should certainly be suspect for a malignant process. A Delphian node is usually palpable on the trachea just above the thyroid isthmus and usually is associated with malig-

nant disease or thyroiditis. *(Kaplan, pp. 1629–1630)*

17. **(C)** The most important factor is a history of external radiation to the head or neck, for in the presence of either a single nodule or multiple thyroid nodules with radiation exposure, 35% to 40% of patients are found to have carcinoma within the thyroid gland. Often the cancer is not present in the palpable nodule. Thyroid function tests are not very useful as diagnostic tests as most patients with thyroid cancer are euthyroid. *(Kaplan, pp. 1629–1630)*

18. **(D)** Vitamin D deficiency is not a cause of primary hyperparathyroidism. Parathyroid adenomas, hyperplasia of the parathyroid gland, as well as carcinoma of the parathyroid gland are all cited in the etiology of primary hyperparathyroidism. In addition, nonparathyroid tumors can secrete a parathyroid hormone-like substance that can mimic primary hyperparathyroidism. *(Clark, pp. 283–290)*

19. **(D)** The most common causes of hypoparathyroidism are related to surgery. This is the result of either surgical removal, trauma, or devascularization during thyroid surgery. Metastatic carcinoma and renal failure generally are associated with elevation of the serum calcium level. Idiopathic hypoparathyroidism is an exceedingly rare condition and would present prior to the age of 16. Idiopathic hypoparathyroidism and hypoparathyroidism after I^{131} therapy for Graves' disease is exceedingly rare. *(Clark, p. 290)*

20. **(A)** The superior mesenteric artery gives rise to the right colic, middle colic, and ileocolic vessels. The inferior mesenteric artery gives rise to the left colic, sigmoid, and hemorrhoidal vessels. Collateral circulation is provided by the marginal artery of Drummond, which traverses the mesenteric border of the colon. *(Schrock, p. 644)*

21. **(D)** The taenia coli, which are longitudinal muscles of the colon, and the haustra, which are outpouchings between the taenia, give the colon its classic appearance. Valvulae conniventes are semicircular valves seen in the small intestine. The ligament of Treitz is a landmark denoting the end of the duodenum and the start of the jejunum. *(Schrock, p. 644)*

22. **(A), 23. (A), 24. (B), 25. (A), 26. (A).** Crohn's colitis is associated with a number of anorectal complications, including anal fistulae and fissures. It is a disease of the entire alimentary tract that can be seen in different sections with normal tissue between the involved areas. Crohn's is almost always a full-thickness disease in contrast to ulcerative colitis, which generally involves the mucosa and submucosa only. Because of Crohn's transmural involvement, it can cause localized perforation and inflammatory masses in the abdomen.

The indications for surgery in the treatment of ulcerative colitis include *active disease unresponsive to medical therapy, risk of cancer,* and *severe bleeding.* Because only the large intestine is involved, a proctocolectomy should cure the patient of intestinal disease. Patients requiring operation because of active disease usually have extensive edema and ulceration of the intestine, fluid, electrolyte, and blood loss, and sometimes dilatation of the colon with possible perforation. These patients with *toxic colitis* or *toxic megacolon* must be treated aggressively with bowel rest, antibiotics, and corticosteroids. Should their clinical situation deteriorate, they should have emergency abdominal colectomy or, if walled-off perforation is encountered, a diverting loop ileostomy combined with a decompressing colostomy, as described for fulminant Crohn's colitis. Barium enema, antidiarrheal agents, and morphine should be avoided because they might intensify the colonic dilation. Careful observation of the patient is more important than serial radiographs of the abdomen looking for an arbitrary limit to cecal dilatation as an indication for surgery. *(Kodner et al, pp. 1238–1253)*

27. **(D)** Antibiotics alter the normal colonic bacterial population and allow an overgrowth of a pathogen called *Clostridium difficile.* The pathogen releases two types of exotoxin, cytopathic toxin and enteropathic toxin. The

screening consists of sending stool for *C. difficile* toxin. The cytopathic toxin is screened for in this specific test. Antidiarrheal medications should be avoided because of increasing the chances for toxic megacolon. This can result from the use of most antibiotics. However, ampicillin, clindamycin, and cephalosporins are most frequently associated. *(Kodner et al, pp. 1226–1228)*

28. **(D)** Treatment of pseudomembranous colitis involves the cessation of all present antibiotics and the replacement of fluid and electrolytes. The antibiotic of choice is metronidazole (Flagyl), which may be given IV or in PO form. If the metronidazole fails, then vancomycin is effective. The vancomycin is very expensive and has a very short shelf life, decreasing accessibility to the drug on an outpatient basis. Steroids, sulfasalazine, and colectomy are not used for treating this type of colitis. *(Kodner et al, p. 1228)*

29. **(A)** Cobblestoning results from the changes in mucosal pattern with linear ulcerations with transverse fissures. A "lead pipe" appearance radiographically is indicative of ulcerative colitis. Crohn's disease may be found anywhere in the gastrointestinal tract. It is less common in the rectal areas than ulcerative colitis. *(Kodner et al, p. 1242)*

30. **(D)** Carcinoma of the colon or rectum begins to appear 5 to 8 years after the onset of ulcerative colitis. By 10 years after onset, about 5% of patients have developed colorectal cancer; the cumulative incidence is 20% to 25% after 20 years and 30% to 40% by 30 years. If high-grade dysplasia persists on serial biopsies, the chances of finding cancer in the colon are 30% to 50%, and colectomy should be performed promptly. *(Schrock, p. 681)*

31. **(C)** The standard drugs for Crohn's colitis are steroids, sulfasalazine, immunosuppressives, and antibiotics. For ulcerative colitis, the regimen consists of sulfasalazine and corticosteroids in topical or enema form. Nasogastric suction is recommended only in severe attacks of ulcerative colitis for gastrointestinal rest as well as parenteral nu-

trition. Neither oral ampicillin or clindamycin are recommended because of the increased risk for *C. difficile* toxin. Surgery is indicated to manage specific complications, such as perforation or hemorrhage. *(Schrock, pp. 631, 681)*

32. **(B)** The current preference is to give the patient the option of a sphincter-preserving operation if the patient has adequate sphincter tone and medically can survive a long surgical procedure. This would consist of a total proctocolectomy with preservation of the anal sphincters, construction of an ileal reservoir, and anastamosis of the reservoir to the anus (ileoanal "pull-through" procedure). If the patient has poor anal tone or has other medical complications, the standard is usually total proctocolectomy and ileostomy. *(Kodner et al, pp. 1246–1248)* Abdominoperineal resection is not recommended because only the distal sigmoid, rectosigmoid, rectum, and anus is removed. *(Schrock, pp. 644–692)*

33. **(C)** Diverticular disease and angiodysplasia are the most common causes of life-threatening colonic hemorrhage. Often abdominal pain is never encountered subjectively. *(Kodner et al, pp. 1209–1210)*

34. **(D)** Mesenteric angiography is the most beneficial study in massive lower gastrointestinal bleeding that is greater than 2.0 mL/min. It accurately localizes the bleeding site and allows the use of selective intra-arterial vasoconstrictive agents. This approach will successfully stop the bleeding in more than 85% of cases in which the bleeding site is identified. A recent approach to massive gastrointestinal bleeding has been an emergent colonoscopy. The colonoscope is beneficial in visualizing the bleeding point and injecting it with vasoconstrictive agents or vasodestructive agents. Technetium-labeled red blood count is helpful in bleeding as slow as 0.5 mL/min. *(Kodner et al, pp. 1209–1210)*

35. **(D)** Carcinoma is not a complication of diverticulitis, although they may present with similar symptoms. If a carcinoma cannot be

ruled out from the patient's workup, then an elective colectomy is indicated. The remaining are all associated with diverticulitis and can necessitate surgical resection. *(Schrock, pp. 670–671)*

36. **(B)** Barium enema should not be performed when a patient has acute diverticulitis. The pressure from the barium being instilled into the colon may be enough to result in perforating a diverticulum, introducing barium into the abdominal cavity. When the patient is noted to have diverticulosis without diverticulitis, a barium enema may be performed with less risk. Currently it is recommended that during an acute phase, a water-soluble contrast agent enema under low pressure be performed if needed. This is felt to be safer because it does not allow barium into the abdominal cavity if perforation occurs. *(Schrock, p. 669)*

37. **(D)** Diabetes is not associated with anal fissure, although the inability to heal wounds is associated with diabetes. Conservative management should include stool softeners, addition of bulk to the diet, and sitz baths. If the patient fails conservative management, then a lateral internal anal sphincterotomy is indicated. *(Kodner et al, pp. 1225–1226)*

38. **(D)** Burns involving the posterior chest wall and posterior lower extremities bilaterally and the palm of the hand are calculated at 37% of total body surface. Remember the rule of nines: 9% to upper trunk, 9% to lower trunk, 9% to each leg to total 36%. The palm of one hand counts for 1%. *(Meyer and Salber, pp. 694–695)*

39. **(B)** Development of percutaneous drainage techniques of abdominal abscesses has been an important advance in the treatment of diverticulitis. CT scan or ultrasound will confirm diagnosis. This approach is preferable to laparotomy, during which abscess contents could contaminate other cavities. A transanal approach should be used if the abscess is low in the pelvis. *(Kodner et al, p. 1206)*

40. **(E)** Screening for colon carcinoma involves hemoccult study and colonoscopy. The hemoccult study or stool for blood is a very sensitive and inexpensive test that can be done by the patient at home. Colonoscopy should be done once in the fourth or fifth decade and then biannually. CEA titers may be falsely elevated in smokers and patients with systemic disease and makes the test not useful for screening purposes. *(Kodner et al, p. 1272)*

41. **(C)** Characteristically, esophageal achalasia has unsynchronized contractions of the esophagus that produces absence of peristalsis. Failure of the lower esophageal sphincter to relax makes it impossible for food to pass into the stomach. Gastroesophageal reflux is not seen in this condition, unless it results from mechanical dilation of the lower esophageal sphincter. *(Peters and DeMeester, p. 1081)*

42. **(D)** The most common antireflux procedure is the Nissen fundoplication. Requirements include increased 24-hour esophageal pH monitoring, documented mechanically defective lower esophageal sphincter tone, and adequate contractility on manometry. The other procedures are not indicated for antireflux. *(Peters and DeMeester, pp. 1068–1073)*

43. **(C)** The best initial confirming test to diagnose an esophageal motility is a barium swallow. The most cost-efficient test to start with would be the barium swallow. Once an abnormality has been found or suspected, then an esophageal manometry is felt to be appropriate. *(Peters and DeMeester, pp. 1052–1054)*

44. **(D)** Diaphragmatic hernias are a relatively common abnormality and are not always associated with symptoms. Clinical manifestations include dysphasia, postprandial fullness, volvulus, hematemesis, gastric ischemia, and recurrent pneumonia from aspiration. There is, however, no increased incidence of carcinoma either within the hernia itself or within the abdominal viscera. *(Peters and DeMeester, pp. 1106–1107)*

45. **(B)** Acute pancreatitis often is a clinical diagnosis, although elevation of the serum amylase is helpful. A more reliable indicator is total urinary amylase in 2 hours. Care must be taken not to ascribe an elevated serum amylase alone to pancreatitis, as this can occur with cholecystitis, perforated ulcer, infarcted bowel, renal failure, and mumps. Hypercalcemia often is a cause of pancreatitis, but is not primarily used as a single diagnostic lab to confirm pancreatitis. Lipase levels often are helpful if they are elevated to reveal possible early pancreatitis. *(Reber, pp. 1409–1410)*

46. **(A)** The mainstay of therapy for acute and chronic pancreatitis is supportive; repletion of fluids and electrolytes is paramount because these patients are frequently dehydrated secondary to nausea, vomiting, and thirdspacing of fluid. In addition, the gastrointestinal tract is put at rest with nasogastric suctioning to avoid stimulating the exocrine function. Analgesics are used for the pain. Surgery is not indicated unless a complication ensues, such as pseudocyst, abscess, necrosis, or hemorrhage. In addition, if gallstones are noted as the cause of the pancreatitis, the patient should be considered for a cholecystectomy to prevent recurrence. Intravenous antibiotics are not generally recommended unless a complication develops. *(Reber, p. 1411)*

47. **(E)** Mallory-Weiss syndrome is not a complication of gastroesophageal reflux. This is a condition seen after repeated forceful vomiting and is associated with bleeding. The remainder are all associated complications of gastroesophageal reflux. As a result of the distal esophagus being persistently exposed to the low pH from the stomach, esophageal ulceration with bleeding occurs and, following prolonged exposure, muscle contractures and mucosal changes such as Barrett's esophagus may appear. *(Peters and DeMeester, p. 1113)*

48. **(D)** The two most common complaints that should raise suspicions about esophageal carcinoma are dysphagia and weight loss. However, the earliest complaint seems to be dysphagia that occurs in very mild forms and then worsens with the progression of the tumor. Dysphagia is initially seen with the swallowing of solid foods, but, if undetected, will eventually progress to involve liquids and even saliva. Advanced-stage malignancies will be associated with painful swallowing and, to some extent, bleeding, although massive bleeding is not associated with esophageal malignancies. *(Peters and DeMeester, pp. 1088–1089)*

49. **(C)** The main duct emptying the pancreas is the duct of Wirsung. The minor duct is the duct of Santorini. These enter into the second part of the duodenum at the ampulla of Vater. *(Reber, p. 1418)*

50. **(A)** The development of a pancreatic pseudocyst is the most common complication of pancreatitis. It should be suspected in those patients with anorexia, weight loss, and upper abdominal pain after an episode of pancreatitis. *(Reber, p. 1418)*

51. **(D)** The advent of ERCP has made it possible to document the status of the pancreatic ducts and the presence of intraductal calcification. In the patient with chronic pancreatitis, such repeated episodes lead to deposition of calcium and eventual ductal obstruction. This is frequently the cause of pain in these patients. CT and ultrasound are helpful in evaluating the pancreas for pseudocyst or abscess. *(Reber, pp. 1413–1414)*

52. **(E)** Mature pseudocysts may also be treated nonsurgically, but these techniques are still being evaluated. External drainage may be established with a narrow-lumen catheter placed percutaneously via ultrasound or CT guidance. Successful obliteration is claimed in as many as 80 percent of cases, but if the cyst persists, surgery should be performed. Two invasive procedures are recommended if external drainage is unsuccessful. They are internal drainage with an anastomosis to the gastrointestinal tract or excision of the pseudocyst. *(Adams, p. 1419)*

53. (A) The classic triad of weight loss, diabetes, and steatorrhea should indicate severe pancreatic disease. The presence of fever would be associated with complications, such as an infected pseudocyst. Hypercalcemia can be a cause of pancreatitis associated with an abnormal parathyroid gland. Intractable pain is mostly seen in noncompliant patients with a diagnosis of alcohol-induced pancreatitis who continue to abuse alcohol. Most chronic pancreatitis cases have mild to moderate pain that can be managed well with oral narcotics. *(Reber, pp. 1414–1416)*

54. (A) Sometimes pruritis will be the only complaint a patient will have prior to the workup. Most of the time the patients will present with at least one of the following symptoms: pain-free jaundice, weight loss, epigastric pain, pruritis, or new onset of diabetes mellitus. Melanic stools are usually found in a gastrointestinal bleed and not in a pancreatic carcinoma. *(Reber, p. 1421)*

55. (D) In the standard Whipple procedure, the distal stomach, pylorus, duodenum, proximal pancreas, and gallbladder are resected. A modification of this procedure preserves the stomach and pylorus, theoretically preserving gastric function. The spleen is not involved in these procedures. *(Reber, pp. 1416–1420)*

56. (B) A "free-floating" prostate indicates a possible pelvic injury as well as a likely urethral injury. If blood is seen at the meatus, urinary catheterization should never be performed until a retrograde urethrogram has been completed. *(Schmalzreid and Guttman, p. 735)*

57. (C) An unreducible hernia in which the content of the hernia develops ischemia is said to be strangulated. *(Wantz, p. 1517)*

58. (B) A hernia through which bowel or omentum extend and then becomes edematous, usually secondary to venous congestion, is unreducible. The contents are then incarcerated. *(Wantz, p. 1517)*

59. (E) A direct hernia occurs as the result of weakened muscles in the floor of the inguinal canal. This occurs in Hesselbach's triangle, the boundaries of which are medial to the inferior epigastric artery, lateral to the rectus sheath, and superior to the inguinal ligament. *(Wantz, p. 1519)*

60. (D) The indirect hernia in males extends through the internal ring and is found within the spermatic cord and cremasteric fibers. The path of herniation is along the tunica vaginalis. This has not completely closed since descent of the testicle. These are also referred to as congenital hernias. *(Williams et al, pp. 1788–1790; Wantz, p. 1519)*

61. (A) A sliding hernia is the situation in which one wall of the hernia sac is composed of an intraperitoneal organ such as cecum or sigmoid colon. This may coexist with other forms of hernia, that is, indirect hernia. Care must be taken when resecting the hernia sac to rule out this possibility. *(Deveney, p. 717)*

62. (C) The most common type of hernia in a female from this listing is the femoral hernia. This starts off with a defect in the transversalis fascia; however, it extends under the inguinal ligament and can often grow quite large prior to its diagnosis. Overall, femoral hernias are statistically less common than inguinal hernias. Studies, unfortunately, do not reveal whether most are direct or indirect defects for the inguinal hernias. *(Deveney, p. 718)*

63. (A) Approximately 35,000 new intracranial neoplasms are diagnosed each year, half of which are metastatic from outside the central nervous system. Glioblastoma multiforme is the most common brain tumor to date. *(Edwards, p. 830)*

64. (B) This patient most likely has a ruptured disc between the L5 and S1 vertebrae, which has caused weakness in the gastrocnemius muscles and elimination of the ankle jerk, which are both controlled by the first sacral nerve root. This can also involve hypalgesia of the lateral aspect of the foot. The L5 nerve root classically causes pain along the posterolateral leg to the dorsum of the foot along with dorsiflexion weakness. *(Weinstein and Hoff, p. 854)*

65. **(A)** Ischemic orchiditis with testicular atrophy is an important, yet uncommon, complication. Bleeding, infection, recurrence, and nerve injury are potential, more common complications to groin hernioplasty. *(Wantz, pp. 1534–1536)*

66. **(A)** If a basilar skull fracture is present, a nasogastric tube should not be inserted because of the possibility of introducing the tube into the brain. *(Crumley, p. 239; Committee on Trauma, p. 170)*

67. **(C)** Melena is generally produced from upper gastrointestinal tract bleeding. The stimulatory effect of intraluminal blood increases gastrointestinal motility and will produce a rapid transit time. Melena results from the interaction of gastric acid and hemoglobin, and as little as 50 mL of blood may be enough to produce melena. Other substances, especially iron, have been known to cause black stools. Black stools can persist for up to 5 days after a significant upper gastrointestinal hemorrhage. *(Way, p. 487)*

68. **(D)** In the United States, gastric ulcers are less common than duodenal ulcerations. People between the ages of 20 and 40 are most likely to develop duodenal ulcerations due to increased gastric acid production. Gastric ulcerations occurring in people between 40 and 60 are less likely to be secondary to increased acid production. Nonsteroidal anti-inflammatory drugs are common causes of gastric ulceration. *(Way, pp. 478, 485)*

69. **(A)** Parietal cell vagotomy is vagal denervation of just the parietal cell area of the stomach. Antrectomy entails a distal half gastrectomy of the stomach with the line of gastric transection carried high on the lesser curvature to conform with the boundary of the gastrin-producing mucosa. Proximal gastrectomy removes the acid-producung cells. Truncal vagotomy resects each vagal trunk. Pyloroplasty will increase gastric emptying,

but should not significantly affect gastric acid secretion. *(Way, pp. 479–481)*

70. **(A)** Gastric acid secretion is characteristically higher than normal in patients with duodenal ulcers than in normal subjects, but only one sixth of the duodenal population has secretory levels that exceed the normal range (i.e., acid secretion in normal subjects and those with duodenal ulcer overlap considerably), so the disease cannot be explained simply as a manifestation of increased acid production. *(Way, p. 478)*

71. **(D)** Radionucleotide imaging is emerging as an effective, minimally invasive, and safe method for determining gastrointestinal bleeding. Because most gastrointestinal bleeding is not a continuous process and radionucleotide imaging can be continued for up to 24 hours, it is a useful method for determining the source of such bleeding. Radionucleotide imaging has been highly touted as a valuable tool for localizing sites of GI blood loss, with requirements of ongoing blood loss of only 0.1 mL/min reported. The accuracy and sensitivity of this imaging are as good as selective angiography, although the imaging cannot pinpoint the site of bleeding as well as does angiography. Colonoscopy is of little use in detecting the cause of massive gastrointestinal bleeding because the amount of bleeding obscures the bleeding site. A barium enema should not be performed as an early procedure because the contrast material involved will obscure subsequent angiograms. *(McFadden and Zinner, pp. 1015–1042)*

72. **(D)** The treatment of choice would be oversewing the ulcer, bilateral truncal vagotomy, and pyloroplasty. This would be the optimal choice considering the patient's age, diabetes, and active bleeding. Overall, there are multiple various treatments and the treatment of choice depends on the overall setting and the surgeon's capabilities. *(Way, pp. 479–481)*

73. **(E)** Of all the gastric malignancies, lymphomas account for approximately 2% and are mostly non-Hodgkin's lymphomas. The

treatment of choice for those with gastric lymphoma is radiotherapy. This accounts for a 5-year survival rate of approximately 50%. If outlet obstruction is present, the treatment of choice would be subtotal gastrectomy with postoperative radiotherapy. *(Way, pp. 499–500)*

74. **(E)** Gallstones greater than 2.5 cm appear to be an important determinant of cancer risk. A calcified, or "porcelain," gallbladder has been associated with a 20% incidence of gallbladder cancer. There are two basic types of gallstones, cholesterol and pigmented, resulting from alterations of the concentration of bile salts, lecithin, and cholesterol. *(Roslyn and Zinner, pp. 1376–1389)*

75. **(A)** Cholelithiasis may be present whenever conditions occur that alter the concentrations of the major elements involved in gallstone formation. Pigmented stones may occur in patients who have hematologic diseases associated with increased hemolysis. Also, hemolysis caused by mechanical trauma such as that found in a patient with aortic valve replacement results in the formation of pigmented stones. Increases in the concentration of cholesterol in the blood and bile and suppression of gallbladder emptying may be found with prolonged administration of estrogen, such as that found in the use of birth control pills. People who have undergone ileal resection of the distal third of their small intestine have an interruption in their enterohepatic circulation and a decrease of the secretion of bile salts and phospholipids, both necessary for the solubility of cholesterol. Such patients likely will develop cholelithiasis. ASCVD has never been proven to cause cholelithiasis. However, the low-fat diet postoperatively for cardiac procedures can result in a decreased function of the gallbladder, resulting in gallbladder dysfunction. *(Roslyn and Zinner, pp. 1376–1378)*

76. **(C)** The HIDA scan or technetium 99–labeled N substituted iminodiacetic acid scan uses a gamma-emitting isotope with a 6-hour half-life. These isotopes are selectively extracted by the liver and secreted into the bile. In patients with acute cholecystitis secondary to cystic duct obstruction, the isotope will fail to enter the gallbladder. This makes it the diagnostic choice for such a condition. This technique can also define obstruction of extrahepatic bile ducts, in which case the radionuclides fail to enter the intestine. These scans are associated with less toxicity than the contrast media involved in IV cholangiography. They provide adequate visualization even when bilirubin levels are as high as 10 to 20 mg/100 mL. *(Roslyn and Zinner, pp. 1378–1381; Way, p. 542, 550)*

77. **(C)** Sclerosing cholangitis appears to occur more frequently in males than in females, which is in contrast to acute cholecystitis. There have been a significant number of sclerosing cholangitis cases found to be associated with ulcerative colitis. Because it has been found that most individuals who have sclerosing cholangitis do not have stones in their gallbladder or common bile duct, this disease does not appear to be caused by irritation of the common duct due to the passage of gallstones. The cause of the disease is unknown, although it has been suggested that it may be related to viral infection. The entire extrahepatic and intrahepatic bile duct system may be involved, or the hepatic duct may be spared and the disease restricted to the common duct. The gallbladder is usually not involved. The clinical and laboratory presentation are usually that of extrahepatic jaundice. It is usually noted that the serum alkaline phosphatase level is elevated out of proportion to that of the serum bilirubin level. *(Roslyn and Zinner, pp. 1385–1386)*

78. **(E)** The solubility of cholesterol depends on the relative concentrations of conjugated bile salts, cholesterol, and phospholipids (lecithin being predominant). Cholesterol is insoluble in aqueous solution, but becomes soluble when incorporated into lecithin bile salt micelles. The ratio of the sum of the molar concentrations of bile salts plus lecithin to the molar concentration of cholesterol is termed the *lithogenous ratio*. A lowering of this ratio by either a decrease in the concentration of bile salts or lecithin or an increase in the concentration of cholesterol makes the choles-

terol less soluble and results in a more lithogenic bile. Bilirubinate, a major constituent of pigmented stones, has no effect on the solubility of other bile constituents. *(Roslyn and Zinner, pp. 1377–1378)*

79. **(B)** Cholecystokinin, which is released from the intestinal mucosa in response to food (particularly fat) and enters into the duodenum, is the primary stimulus for gallbladder emptying. Cholecystokinin also relaxes the terminal bile duct, the sphincter of Oddi, and the duodenal musculature. Vagal stimulation causes the gallbladder to contract, but the rate of gallbladder emptying is decreased following vagotomy. Sympathetic stimulation is inhibitory to the motor activity of the gallbladder, whereas secretin and hydrochloric acid have little effect on motor activity. *(Roslyn and Zinner, pp. 1370–1371)*

80. **(B)** Chenodeoxycholic acid replenishes the bile acid pool and so tends to return supersaturated bile to a more normal composition. It also has been found to decrease hepatic cholesterol synthesis. Some studies have indicated that complete dissolution of stones occurs in about 15 percent of patients and a partial response in an additional 28 percent. Chenodeoxycholic acid is less effective in dissolving large (1.5-cm) rather than small stones, and radiopaque rather than radiolucent stones. When treatment is terminated, cholelithiasis is likely to return. Side effects of this type of treatment include clinically significant hepatotoxicity. *(Roslyn and Zinner, p. 1380)*

81. **(E)** In several large series of asymptomatic patients with gallstones who were followed and who did not receive surgical treatment, symptoms developed in 50% and serious complications developed in 20%. An operative mortality of 0.7% has been reported for asymptomatic patients in contrast to a 5% mortality rate for patients with acute cholecystitis. Based on a high incidence of ultimate development of symptoms or complications and the small risk of operative mortality, it is generally felt that, unless there is a strong contraindication, the presence of cholelithia-

sis with or without symptoms is an indication for a cholecystectomy. *(Roslyn and Zinner, pp. 1378–1379)*

82. **(B)** In patients with chronic cholecystitis, ultrasonography is approximately 95% accurate for detecting gallstones and has, for the most part, replaced oral cholecystography as the initial method diagnosis. Oral cholecystography is still useful, however, to evaluate patients with typical symptoms of chronic cholecystitis who have equivocal and negative ultrasounds. HIDA scanning is most useful in the diagnosis of acute cholecystitis. CT scans can demonstrate gallstones, but this method is not appropriate for initial screening evaluations. Direct visualization of the bile duct by percutaneous transhepatic cholangiography is important in evaluating common duct obstruction. *(Roslyn and Zinner, pp. 1372–1374)*

83. **(A)** Charcot's triad, consisting of fever, jaundice, and abdominal pain, is the clinical hallmark of acute cholangitis. Initial treatment consists of fluid resuscitation and antibiotics to cover gram-negative organisms, aerobes, and enterococci. If the patient improves with these measures, cholangiographic assessment of the biliary tract is carried out to plan definitive therapy. Most cases of acute cholangitis are caused by calculus disease, although benign strictures and malignancies must be excluded. If the patient does not respond to initial nonoperative therapy, decompression of the biliary tract must be carried out. This may be done either surgically or through percutaneous techniques. *(Roslyn and Zinner, pp. 1383–1384)*

84. **(C), 85. (A), 86. (A), 87. (A).** Cholecystitis is considered to be acute or chronic, depending on the clinical presentation. The pathophysiology of both implies that the cystic duct is obstructed, usually by gallstones. In acute cholecystitis, persistent obstruction of the cystic duct leads to a chemical and bacterial inflammation of the gallbladder wall itself and potential complications are empyema, gangrene, perforation, and fistula formation. HIDA scan is considered a specific test for

acute cholecystitis because of the low rate of false-positive studies. Acute cholecystitis requires cholecystectomy, but the timing of the operation is controversial. Early cholecystectomy prevents complications and recurrent symptoms and has been shown to be as safe (in terms of morbidity and mortality) as the delayed operation that is done when symptoms resolve. Proponents of the delayed cholecystectomy have suggested that, because most episodes of acute cholecystitis resolve and because the operation may be more difficult in the case of acute inflammatory process, the operation is more appropriately carried out later. In chronic cholecystitis, intermittent cystic duct obstruction produces biliary colic. The diagnosis usually is made on the basis of symptoms and an ultrasound demonstrating cholelithiases. Chronic cholecystitis is treated by elective cholecystectomy. (Roslyn and Zinner, pp. 1378–1379)

88. (A), 89. (A), 90. (B). Ecchymosis in the mastoid region, "raccoon eyes" (periorbital ecchymosis), and hemotympanum are all indicators of a possible basilar skull fracture. A CT of the head is always indicated with these physical exam findings. Nuchal rigidity with cranial nerve palsies with motor abnormalities are indicative of a subarachnoid hemorrhage, which warrants a CT scan of the head. (Doberstein et al, pp. 539, 545)

91. (C) Metastases to the liver are most common secondary to primary colon cancer due to extensive lymphatic drainage from the colon to the liver. (Schwartz, 1994, p. 1339)

92. (D) Surgical excision is the only definitive treatment for primary hepatocellular carcinoma. Three criteria should be met before attempts at surgical resection are made. (1) The cancer should be solitary. (2) There should be no involvement of the lymph nodes, vasculature, or bile ducts. (3) There should be no distant metastases. Even with the advances in surgical techniques, anesthesia, and blood replacement, hepatic resection has reached only an acceptable level of less than 5%. Overall, only 20% to 30% of patients can undergo resection, and 5-year survival rates ap-

proach 30%. In the face of extensive cirrhosis, and with its associated morbidity and mortality, resection is contraindicated. Orthotopic liver transplantation results have not been encouraging. Radiation and/or chemotherapy have not been shown to prolong survival. (Schwartz, 1994, p. 1339)

93. (B) The protein alpha-fetoprotein (AFP) is normally present in the fetus at birth, but disappears after a few weeks. In the United States 30% of patients with primary hepatic neoplasms have AFP in their serum. If present, AFP may be used as a marker because resection of the tumor converts the test to negative. Recurrence of the same tumor would be evident by a return of AFP to the serum. The AFP may also be elevated in embryonic tumors of the ovary and testes, giving a false-positive test result. In metastatic tumors of the liver, the AFP is usually negative. (Schwartz, 1994, pp. 1337–1338)

94. (E) The etiology of portal hypertension arises from four categories of pathology: (1) increased hepatopedal flow without obstruction, such as that seen with hepatic arterial-portal venous fistulas (an infrequent cause); (2) extrahepatic outflow obstruction, as in Budd-Chiari syndrome or endophlebitis of the hepatic veins; (3) obstruction of the extrahepatic portal venous system, as in cavernomatous transformation of the portal vein (the most common etiologic factor in this category in childhood is some form of infection carried by a patent umbilical vein [neonatal omphalitis]); (4) the overwhelming majority of cases of portal hypertension are caused by intrahepatic obstruction. This category accounts for 90% of all cases. Cirrhosis (nutritional, postnecrotic, or biliary) is the most common reason for this type of postsinusoidal obstruction to portal blood flow. (Schwartz, 1994, pp. 1342–1346)

95. (E) In a patient with alcoholic cirrhosis, abstinence from alcohol is the most important factor in determining survival postshunting. A low-salt diet, control of ascites, a low-protein diet, and the use of lactulose are various therapies that are used depending on the severity of the disease. *(Schwartz, 1994, pp. 1342–1346)*

96. **(B)** Bleeding from varices that have not responded to endoscopic sclerosis in an alcoholic cirrhotic patient is the most accepted indication for surgery. Because only 30% of cirrhotic patients with varices, regardless of size, will ever bleed, choice (A) is incorrect. Emergency shunting results in an operative survival of 50% to 71% and a 7-year survival in 42% of patients. If possible, emergency shunting should be avoided. Prophylactic shunts, such as for choice (E) do not increase survival and may produce encephalopathy. If at all possible, patients with encephalopathy should not be shunted. *(Schwartz, 1994, pp. 1346–1349)*

97. **(A), 98. (C), 99. (A), 100. (A), 101. (B).** Hepatic abscesses are related to two distinct types of pathogens: *Entamoeba histolytica* and pyogenic bacteria. With pyogenic abscesses, *Escherichia coli* or other gram-negative bacteria are the most commonly isolated organisms. The most common source of these bacteria is a contiguous infection in the biliary system. Amebic abscesses are caused by *Histolytica*, and no bacteria are typically isolated from these abscesses. However, in 22% of patients, secondary infection is a complication.

Pyogenic abscesses may be solitary, multiple, and multilocular. Amebic abscesses are usually single. The right lobe of the liver is commonly involved in any abscesses of the liver because of the so-called streaming effect in the portal vein. Treatment of pyogenic abscesses consists of appropriate antibiotics plus surgical drainage. The mortality rate with a solitary pyogenic abscess is 24 percent, whereas multiple abscesses carry a 70% mortality. Undrained pyogenic abscesses have a mortality rate approaching 100%. With amebic abscesses, the treatment is conservative, consisting of the use of amebicidal drugs. Aspiration is indicated if the patient fails to respond to medication or if signs of secondary infection develop. With amebic abscesses, the mortality rate is only 7% in uncomplicated cases and 43 percent in cases where compli-

cations, such as secondary infection, develop. *(Schwartz, 1994, pp. 1326–1330)*

102. **(A)** Tenorrhaphy must be done without surface trauma along the tendon or its bed. The juncture is made end to end or by weaving one tendon with the other using nylon or wire sutures (nonabsorbable). *(Kilgore et al, p. 1171)*

103. **(B)** Malignant tumors of the small bowel are relatively infrequent. Histologically, lymphoma is the most frequent primary tumor. Survival is lowest with adenocarcinoma (20%) and higher with the other cell types (40%). Treatment of malignant small-bowel tumors is wide resection, including regional lymph nodes. This requires pancreaticoduodenectomy in duodenal lesions. With lymphomas, postoperative radiation and/or chemotherapy is indicated but has no effect with the other cell types. *(Schrock, pp. 640–642)*

104. **(C)** The cell of origin is the Kultschitzsky cell, and carcinoid tumors may arise anywhere in the gastrointestinal tract these cells occur, that is, from the stomach to the anus. The appendix is, however, the most frequently involved, followed by the ileum and rectum. Carcinoid tumors also may be found outside the gastrointestinal tract, including the bronchus and ovary. A carcinoid tumor has a tendency for multicentricity that exceeds any other neoplasm of the gastrointestinal tract. The prognosis is a function of tumor size and its site of origin, along with its histological type. *(Townsend and Thompson, pp. 1175–1177)*

105. **(B)** Meckel's diverticulum is the most frequently encountered diverticulum of the small intestine. It occurs in 2% of the population. It is a true diverticulum and is found on the antimesenteric border of the ileum about 2 feet from the ileocecal valve. Complications of Meckel's diverticulum include intestinal obstruction, which is the most common, followed by bleeding and, finally, Meckel's diverticulitis. Occasionally, Meckel's diverticulum contains ectopic gastric mucosa and can

be seen with a technetium pertechnetate scan. *(Townsend and Thompson, pp. 1179–1180)*

106. **(D)** Postoperative fever within 24 to 48 hours is secondary to atelectasis due to poor inspiration. *(Mulvihill and Pellegrini, pp. 26–27, 38)*

107. **(E)** Postoperative fever after the fifth day usually suggests a wound infection. *(Mulvihill and Pellegrini, p. 38)*

108. **(B)** Fever occurring 3 to 5 days postoperatively and poor ambulation suggest deep-vein thrombosis. *(Mulvihill and Pellegrini, pp. 37–38)*

109. **(C)** Fever occurring 3–5 days postoperatively and an indwelling catheter suggest urinary tract infection. *(Mulvihill and Pellegrini, p. 35)*

110. **(E)** With acute appendicitis, the differential diagnosis is essentially that of the acute abdomen. A diverse number of pathologies can present with a picture seemingly identical to appendicitis. In general, about 85% of the cases diagnosed preoperatively as appendicitis are positive, accounting for an acceptable 15% false-negative rate. The most common inaccurate preoperative diagnoses include mesenteric lymphadenitis; no pathology found; acute pelvic inflammatory disease; twisted ovarian cyst; and epiploic appendicitis. Diverticulitis of the sigmoid colon, particularly that portion that lies on the right side, also is included in the differential. The diagnosis of appendicitis depends on three factors: (1) the location of the inflamed appendix; (2) the sex and age of the patient; and (3) the type of appendicitis, that is, ruptured or simple. *(Schwartz, 1989a, pp. 1318–1319)*

111. **(E)** Although acute appendicitis is a diagnosis of clinical findings, radiography may be used to narrow the list of the differential diagnosis or to demonstrate complications of appendicitis. Radiographic findings consistent with, but not diagnostic of, appendicitis include distended loop(s) of small bowel in the right lower quadrant, visualization of a gas-filled appendix, and a partially filled ap-

pendix on barium enema examination. Some studies show that, with barium enema examination, the findings of a partially filled appendix, a mass effect on the medial and inferior borders of the cecum, and a mass effect or mucosal changes of terminal ileum, are pathognomonic for acute appendicitis. *(Schwartz, 1994, pp. 1308–1310)*

112. **(B)** Acute appendicitis is a surgical disease. Delaying surgery places the patient at greater risk for increased morbidity and mortality. In pregnancy, there is a fourfold increase in fetal mortality associated with appendiceal rupture. In the elderly, nonoperative treatment increases the chance of rupture and death. In patients with periappendiceal abscess formation, the treatment is controversial. Nonoperative treatment initially, in combination with antibiotic therapy, and close monitoring of the patient's clinical and laboratory course is an acceptable option in a patient with subsiding symptoms and a palpable right lower-quadrant mass. An elective appendectomy should be performed 6 weeks to 3 months later if the patient remains stable. The interval appendectomy is needed because of the high rate of recurrence. *(Schwartz, 1989a, p. 1322)*

113. **(D)** Carcinoma of the prostate is the most frequent malignant tumor in males over the age of 65. It should be noted, however, that many men die with carcinoma of the prostate and not because of it. Elevations in the serum acid phosphatase occurs from many sources, including multiple myeloma, bony tumors, benign prostatic disease, and acute urinary retention. Recent advances in transrectal ultrasound (TRUS) and prostate-specific antigen (PSA) monitoring have allowed for enhanced detection of nonpalpable tumors. The realities of clinical practice are that the combination of digital rectal examination and serum prostate-specific antigen (PSA) monitoring is the number-one effective screening protocol. Digital examination of the prostate and serum PSA are the most important methods of detecting asymptomatic prostate cancer. *(Donovan and Williams, p. 955)*

114. **(B)** Detection of the asymptomatic prostate nodule is essential to find prostate cancer in its potentially curable form. The vast majority are found on routine physical examination. More than 50% of prostatic nodules palpated on rectal examination are found to be positive for carcinoma on biopsy. The objective of treatment for asymptomatic prostate cancers should be to cure. Only surgical excision (radical prostatectomy) or radical radiation therapy can offer a cure for this disease. The 5-year survival rate in selected cases can be greater than 50%. *(Peters et al, pp. 1762–1763)*

115. **(B)** Patients usually present with a non-painful "lump" in the testis. On examination, the lesion is firm, nontender, and solid, and does not transilluminate. If a tumor is suspected, surgical exploration is indicated. Measurement by radioimmunoassay of human chorionic gonadotropin and alpha-fetoprotein markers may be useful, but surgical treatment should not be delayed. If the lesion is confined to the testis on physical examination, a scrotal surgical approach is preferred. The spermatic vessels are occluded before the testis is exteriorized for inspection to prevent tumor spread. Palpation of induration in the testis is indication for radical orchiectomy, and there is essentially no place for biopsy, as over 90% of solid lesions of the testis in this age group (average age at diagnosis is 32 years) are malignant. In patients with apparent lymphatic or pulmonary spread, the primary tumor should be resected for pathologic evaluation. *(Peters et al, p. 1764)*

116. **(D)** The differential in this patient is that of acute epididymitis versus testicular torsion. Because prompt treatment of testicular torsion is necessary to prevent testicular infarction, it may occasionally be required that the patient with acute epididymitis be explored to prevent the loss of a testis from torsion. Four hours appears to be the maximal amount of time that a testis can undergo torsion, after which irreversible damage is done. If time allows, isotopic scanning of the testis may show the characteristic absence of testicular blood flow. However, time should not be wasted in order to confirm the diagnosis. *(Peters et al, pp. 1731–1732)*

117. **(B)** Surgical therapy for urinary tract calculi has changed significantly in the last 10 years. In the past, symptomatic stone removal required an open surgical procedure. Advances in fiberoptics and the subsequent development of flexible instruments as well as small-caliber rigid endoscopes have led to the development of the subspecialty of endourology ("the closed, controlled manipulation of the entire urinary tract"). Most recently, extracorporeal shock wave lithotripsy has allowed noninvasive destruction of renal and ureteral calculi. This procedure uses high-energy shock waves transmitted through water and directly focused onto renal/ureteral stones with the aid of fluoroscopy or ultrasound. The major advantage of extracorporeal shock wave lithotripsy is the noninvasive nature of stone fragmentation, allowing the patient to pass the stone fragments without surgery. *(Peters et al, pp. 1748–1750)*

118. **(C)** The composition of urinary calculi is significant in that therapy aimed at prevention of recurrence and the etiologic abnormality may both be determined by knowing the make up of the calculi. Calcium oxalate stones are the most common urinary calculi. They account for approximately 75% of all urinary stones. Ammonium-magnesium phosphate stones make up 15% of stones and are typically found in infected urine. Uric acid stones constitute about 8% of all calculi. Finally, cystine stones represent only 1% of urinary calculi. *(Frank, p. 1748)*

119. **(B), 120. (C), 121. (A).** Joints are either fibrous or cartilaginous based on the nature of the tissue joining the bones together. A fibrous joint, such as the sutures of the skull, is made up of bones united by fibrous tissue. When bones are joined by either hyaline cartilage or fibrocartilage, they are called cartilaginous joints. The pubic symphysis and the intervertebral discs are examples of this type of joint. Synovial joints, also known as diarthrodial joints, are movable joints united by a capsule. This capsule is lined with syn-

ovium. Most joints of the extremities are synovial joints. *(Duthie and Hoaglund, p. 1981)*

122. (B), 123. (A), 124. (C), 125. (D). After the age of 35, pain after minor strains of the shoulder or spontaneous pain is common. Before attaching the diagnosis to a local condition of the shoulder, one must be certain to rule out diseases that may cause referred pain to the shoulder. Cardiac, pulmonary, and gastrointestinal pathologies may all cause referred pain to the shoulder. Pathology in the neck, including cervical arthritis and brachial plexus irritation, Pancoast's tumors, and central nervous system disease, need to be considered. Once the pathology has been located at the shoulder, knowledge of the anatomy of the shoulder makes the diagnosis easier.

Disorders of the rotator cuff, bicipital tendonitis, and subacromial bursitis are the three most common causes of primary painful shoulder disorders. The rotator cuff is made up of the common tendinous insertions of the supraspinatus, infraspinatus, teres minor, and the subscapularis muscle tendons (SITS). The rotator cuff is intimately adherent to the shoulder capsule that lies just beneath it. The rotator cuff comes in contact with the undersurface of the coracoacromial ligament when the arm is abducted past 90 degrees or is fully elevated. This may lead to mechanical irritation and subsequent degeneration.

The subacromial bursa lies between the coracoacromial ligament, the acromion, and the rotator cuff. Inflammation may occur here as a result of the mechanical irritation, causing bursitis. This typically causes unrelenting pain that is unaffected by position changes.

With supraspinatus tendonitis, the patient usually complains of low-grade shoulder pain with sudden motion or with full internal rotation and the extremes of abduction. Bicipital tendonitis presents with similar symptoms, but differentiation may be made on the basis of the anatomic location of the biceps tendon. Pain and tenderness are found over the bicipital groove. A rotator cuff tear is a physical disruption of the rotator cuff and is usually partial. Partial tears can be treated with shoulder immobilization

in a sling. Complete tears may be treated conservatively, but surgical repair often is required. *(Duthie and Hoaglund, pp. 2001–2002)*

126. (B) Peripheral nerve injuries may be categorized functionally. *Neuroapraxia* is a temporary loss of function without axonal injury. Structural damage does not occur. The foot that 'goes to sleep' after crossing the legs is an example of functional loss without pathologic change. *Axonotmesis* is the disruption of the axon with preservation of the axon sheath. Wallerian degeneration of the distal axon fragment occurs. Stretch or prolonged compression causes this functional and structural loss. Regeneration of the proximal axon occurs, but functional recovery depends on associated injuries, the amount of healthy proximal axon remaining after injury, and the age of the patient. *Neurotmesis* is the disruption of both the axon and axon sheath with corresponding loss of function. Transection of a nerve causes this phenomenon. Regeneration occurs, but function rarely returns to normal. *(Hoff and Boland, p. 1838)*

127. (C) Meniscal tears are common sports injuries and can present with effusion, a history of catching or locking, and knee pain. Patients can have joint line tenderness, limited knee motion, and a catching or 'click' associated with pain during passive extension of the knee in conjunction with manual rotation of the tibia and varus or valgus stress (MacMurray's test). At times, the clinical diagnosis is difficult. Arthrography of the knee is fairly reliable in the diagnosis of medial meniscal tears (incidence 95%), but substantially less accurate in diagnosing lateral meniscal tears (incidence 70%), owing to the distortion caused by the popliteus tendon. MRI scans, however, provide extremely accurate diagnosis of internal derangement of the knee of all types, including meniscal tears, osteochondral injuries, and anterior or posterior cruciate ligament tears. The high signal seen within the menisci also can indicate myxoid degenerative change, which is overinterpreted as a tear. Diagnostic arthoscopy provides another means of diagnosing accurately meniscal injury. Surgical arthoscopy allows repair or excision of the torn fragment simultaneously. *(Rosier, p. 1925)*

128. **(B)** Patellar pain and mild degenerative changes are very common, particularly in young females. Chondromalacia refers to the early changes of degenerative arthritis, with softening and fibrillation of the articular cartilage. The medial facet is most often involved. Chondromalacia can be related to patellar subluxation, dislocation, or chondral contusion from direct trauma. Patients complain of pain, especially with stair climbing and kneeling, which increase patellofemoral joint contact forces. Physical examination can reveal patellofemoral crepitus, pain with patellar compression, effusion, and tenderness of the patellar facets. Radiographs show patellar tilt or narrowing of the joint space, and articular cartilage degeneration and thinning are readily discernible on MRI. Evolution of chondromalacia to frank osteoarthritis is relatively unusual. *(Rosier, p. 1946)*

129. **(A)** Peripheral nerves are most sensitive to anoxia. Paralysis and anesthesia quickly develop when arterial blood flow is severely decreased. Striated muscle is almost equally sensitive and will usually become necrotic if arterial blood flow is decreased to such a degree that anesthesia and paralysis are present. Skin, bone, and tendon may survive an ischemic injury that produces irreversible, extensive muscle necrosis. *(Imparato and Riles, p. 936)*

130. **(B), 131. (A).** In acute arterial occlusion, the level of arterial obstruction may be diagnosed from the history because the exertional muscle pain occurs one joint distal to the site of occlusion. Superficial femoral artery occlusion results in calf pain. An occlusion in the external iliac artery can produce thigh pain, and aortic occlusion may be diagnosed by buttock pain. The level of occlusion often can be estimated from the color and temperature level as well as the pulse findings. The arterial pulse is absent at the site of occlusion, frequently with accentuation of the pulse immediately proximal to this point. Sensory impairment varies from hypesthesia to anes-

thesia, and motor disturbances from weakness to paralysis. *(Green and Ouriel, pp. 949–956)*

132. **(C), 133. (A).** The gangrenous digits represent occlusion of a critical digital artery. Diabetics may have a type of arterial occlusive disease that typically involves the popliteal artery and its branches down to the pedal arches. Minor trauma, unnoticed by diabetics because of their diabetic neuropathy, may progress to gangrene of the toes. Trophic ulcers, which are usually sharply demarcated, punched-out areas on the sole of the foot overlying a pressure point, are frequently found in diabetics. Palpable pedal pulses may be present. Buerger's disease is a form of chronic arterial insufficiency in which tobacco plays a major role. With its progression, superficial ulceration and gangrene will develop if arterial circulation is not improved. *(Green and Ouriel, pp. 974–975)*

134. **(D)** Peripheral artery insufficiency is predominantly a disease of the lower extremities with a classic presentation. Physical examination is of paramount importance in assessing the presence and severity of vascular disease. Acute occlusion is a dramatic event characterized by the abrupt onset of ischemia with pain, coldness, numbness, and absent pulses. Thromboangiitis obliterans (Buerger's disease) is characterized by multiple segmental occlusions of small arteries and examination shows an irregular pattern of digital ischemia. *(Krupski and Effeney, pp. 740–743)*

135. **(B)** The findings associated with acute ischemia are pulselessness, pallor, poikilothermia, pain, paralysis, and paresthesia. Paralysis and paresthesia are most important because loss of neurological function indicates a degree of tissue ischemia that will progress to gangrene unless arterial blood flow is improved. *(Green and Ouriel, pp. 929–930)*

136. **(D)** Congenital arteriovenous fistulas constitute one manifestation of a number of more commonly related abnormalities of the vascular system. The appearance may vary from a simple port wine stain to the massively hypertrophied extremity that has multiple ar-

teries, capillaries, and veins dilated and visible in and through the skin with or without abnormal arteriovenous communications. The hallmark of the complex congenital arteriovenous fistula is the palpation of a thrill and the auscultation of a bruit. The key note of treatment is conservativism. The decision to treat malformations on the surface of the body need to be based only on whether a lesion threatens to ulcerate or bleed, whether the hemihypertrophy of the extremity may lead to serious orthopedic problems, or whether the deformity is so cosmetically repulsive that the patient must have help. *(Imparato and Riles, p. 934)*

137. **(D)** The most important consideration following operation is to detect peripheral pulses, which indicate satisfactory restoration of arterial flow. If pulses cannot be detected or if previously palpable pulses disappear, an arteriogram should be performed or the site of anastomosis should be reexplored. The important principle to emphasize is that, with modern vascular techniques, traumatic injury of a normal artery can almost always be successfully repaired. Anticoagulant therapy is not recommended routinely after arterial repair, for it provides little protection from thrombus but does increase the risk of bleeding into the wound. *(Green and Ouriel, pp. 977–981)*

138. **(C)** Control of bleeding is the most urgent immediate problem and can usually be accomplished by direct digital pressure on the bleeding site or by tightly packing the wound with gauze and applying a pressure dressing. Tourniquets are best avoided for most injuries. If they are used, they must be carefully padded to avoid the risk of permanent injury to peripheral nerves. *(Shires et al, 1994, p. 176)*

139. **(C)** Compartment syndromes should be treated by decompression fasciotomy early to avoid anoxic necrosis of the muscle mass. The pulses may be normal, diminished, or absent. Its absence is a late sign and occasionally follows the loss of motor power of the muscle of the associated compartment. *(Rosier, p. 1880)*

140. **(C)** Noninvasive tests are helpful in localizing the anatomic site of obstruction in occlusive arterial disease of the lower extremities. Angiography remains the gold standard. Determination of ankle pressures—a simple and valid test—can be performed by means of a Doppler device, a strain gauge, or photo plethysmography. In patients without arterial disease, the ankle/brachial index is 1 or higher; with claudication, it is generally between 0.5 and 1; with more advanced degrees of ischemia, it is generally less than 0.5. Diabetic patients may have high indices because of calcification of the arterial wall. When doubt exists about the diagnosis of arterial occlusion, stress testing is helpful; the drop in pressure and the recovery time that result are proportional to the extent of arterial occlusive disease. Segmental pressures can help locate the level of disease. *(Green and Ouriel, p. 930)*

141. **(A)** Noninvasive studies using ultrasound, plethysmography, x-ray, and magnetic resonance imaging have been useful in confirming the diagnosis and differentiating arterial disease from other syndromes. Arteriography continues to be the most important laboratory technique. A high-quality study is essential in planning the surgical approach to reconstruction. *(Green and Ouriel, pp. 930–931)*

142. **(B), 143. (A).** Spontaneous acute arterial thrombosis occurs most commonly in the presence of an underlying stenosis due to atherosclerotic disease. Hypercoaguable states such as protein C and S deficiency may cause acute occlusion. Emboli arising from the heart constitute a majority of emboli seen. Thrombi and emboli are not interchangeable terms. *(Green and Ouriel, pp. 945–949)*

144. **(A)** Incompetent valves of the deep veins enable a long column of blood to transmit pressures of over 100 mm Hg to venules. This promotes fluid and protein loss into tissues. The perivascular fibrinous deposits interfere with normal oxygenation and metabolism of tissues. This causes the thickening and liposclerosis of the subcutaneous tissues to produce the characteristic nonpitting edema.

In patients with long-standing chronic venous insufficiency, hemosiderin deposits from the red cells are responsible for the brown pigment. (*Greenfield, p. 1005*)

145. **(A)** Abdominal aortic aneurysms are the most common of the atherosclerotic aneurysms. Men are affected more frequently than women in a ratio approximating 10 to 1. Except for traumatic and congenital malformations, almost all peripheral aneurysms result from arteriosclerosis. The majority of the peripheral aneurysms are in the popliteal artery. Infrequent sites include the femoral, carotid, and subclavian arteries. (*Green and Ouriel, pp. 933–934*)

146. **(E)** The prompt IV administration of heparin to inhibit the development of thrombi distal to the embolus is the most important therapeutic measure in the treatment of an arterial embolus. For operations on the lower extremity, local anesthesia may be used. The emboli can be removed by the insertion of a Fogarty balloon catheter through a short incision placed directly over the uppermost level of the arterial occlusion. If the embolus is localized to the incision site, the balloon catheter should be used to clear out the entire artery. An operative arteriogram should be performed to confirm the patency of the artery. A fasciotomy may help preserve limb viability if embolectomy has been delayed beyond 4 to 6 hours and increased muscle turgor was determined by palpation before operating. (*Green and Ouriel, pp. 948; Rosier, p. 1880*)

147. **(B), 148. (A).** The majority of abdominal aneurysms are atherosclerotic in nature and their pathogenesis is probably different from occlusive disease. Aneurysms result from degenerative changes in the media. Atherosclerotic occlusion results from a proliferative reaction in the media causing narrowing of the lumen. The distribution of the two processes also is different. The atherosclerotic occlusive process involves the aorta at sites of bifurcations, attachments, tapers, and curvatures. Aneurysmal disease occurs at the abdominal aorta, popliteal, carotid, femoral, iliac, and subclavian arteries. (*Green and Ouriel, pp. 926, 932*)

149. **(D), 150. (C),** In the 1940s, Leriche described the clinical characteristics of occlusion of the abdominal aorta. These are claudication, sexual impotence in the male, and absence of gangrene. The luminal narrowing may be due to fibrointimal thickening, ulceration of atherosclerotic plaques, and superimposed thrombus or embolization of portions of atherosclerotic plaques.

The progress of aortoiliac occlusive disease is slow. Symptoms of claudication appear with exercise. Sexual impotence is frequent because of decreased blood flow through the hypogastric arteries. Patients with abdominal aortic aneurysms are usually asymptomatic. They may have associated lesions, but for the most part do not complain of claudication or impotence. Occasionally, low back-pain caused by tension on the retroperitoneum by the aneurysm may be a patient's complaint. (*Green and Ouriel, pp. 926, 932*)

151. **(C), 152. (B), 153. (A).** Livedo reticularis, an unusual vasomotor condition, is characterized by a persistent mottled reddish-blue discoloration of the skin of the extremities. It is most prominent in the legs and, although it never disappears, it does worsen on exposure to cold. The pathologic feature apparently is a stenosis of the arterioles that pierce the cutis at right angles and arborize into peripheral capillaries of the skin, which accounts for the nature of the discoloration. Peripheral pulses are normal.

In erythromelalgia, the basic abnormality is an unusual sensitivity to warmth. Skin temperatures of 32°C to 36°C, which produce no effects in normal individuals, will regularly induce a painful burning sensation. The increase in temperature is usually a result of vasodilatation with increased blood flow. The exact basis for the spontaneous vasodilatation with rise in temperature and the burning sensation is not known.

Acrocyanosis is a disorder characterized by persistent, but painless, cold and cyanosis of the hands and feet. The basic pathologic condition is a slow rate of blood flow through the skin, the result of chronic arteriolar constriction that causes a high percentage of reduced hemoglobin in the blood in the capillaries and the cyanotic color. This disorder usually is found in young women who note persistent coldness and blueness of the fingers or hands for many years, worsening on exposure to cold. Peripheral pulses are normal. *(Green and Ouriel, p. 973)*

154. **(C), 155. (A), 156. (D).** Raynaud's phenomenon and Raynaud's disease have the same recurrent episodes of vasoconstriction in the upper extremities initiated by exposure to cold or emotional stress. In 10% to 15% of patients, the legs may be involved as well as the arms. Three sequential phases classically occur: pallor, cyanosis, and rubor. Raynaud's phenomenon may exist as a primary disorder, termed Raynaud's disease, or it may be a secondary manifestation of a more serious vascular disease. A critical point in the evaluation of Raynaud's disease is to determine the existence of a more severe disorder.

Buerger's disease, or thromboangiitis obliterans, is an inflammatory process involving the walls of arteries and neighboring nerve and vein that may terminate into thrombosis of the artery. Both upper and lower extremities may be affected. Heavy tobacco smoking has been almost universally associated with Buerger's disease. *(Green and Ouriel, pp. 973–975)*

157. **(A), 158. (B).** The degrees of severity of a frostbite injury have been grouped into four different types analogous to the classification of burn injury. First-degree injury consists of edema and redness of the affected part without necrosis of the skin. Formation of blisters occurs in second-degree injury. There is necrosis of the skin in a third-degree injury. In a fourth-degree injury, gangrene of the extremity develops that requires amputation. *(Green and Ouriel, p. 976)*

159. **(C)** Rapid rewarming of injured tissue, using water with a temperature in the range of

40°C to 44°C for 20 minutes is the most important aspect of treatment of frostbite. Higher temperatures are more injurious than beneficial. A frostbitten part should never be exposed to hot water, an open fire, or an oven, for the loss of sensitivity can result in thermal injury. *(Green and Ouriel, p. 976)*

160. **(A)** Buerger's disease, or thromboangiitis obliterans, is most often seen in men who smoke more than 20 cigarettes per day and are between 20 and 40 years of age. The distribution of the arterial involvement is not the same as in atherosclerotic disease. Smaller, more peripheral arteries, usually in a segmental distribution are involved, as with diabetics. *(Green and Ouriel, pp. 974–975)*

161. **(D)** The principal finding in aortoiliac occlusive disease is diminution or absence of femoral pulses, combined with absence of popliteal and pedal pulses. Diabetics most often have occlusive disease of the tibial arteries, although some also do have aortoiliac disease. Patients with Buerger's disease also may have tibial occlusive disease. The femoral and popliteal arteries in these patients should not be affected. Unless patients with abdominal aneurysm have concomitant aortoiliac occlusive disease or arterioemboli from their aneurysm, their peripheral pulses should be intact. *(Green and Ouriel, pp. 950–953)*

162. **(E)** In the diabetic, arterial occlusive disease typically involves the popliteal artery and its branches down to the pedal arches. Because of diabetic neuropathy, the patient may not be aware of minor trauma to the foot. Within hours or days of a trivial injury, a virulent necrotizing infection can appear, rapidly spreading along musculofascial planes because of the diabetic's extraordinary susceptibility to infection. *(Green and Ouriel, p. 956)*

163. **(B)** Symptomatic peripheral arterial disease occurs predominantly in males over the age of 50. Additional factors include systolic hypertension, smoking, diabetes, and hypercholesterolemia. *(Green and Ouriel, pp. 949–950)*

164. (C) The perforators adjacent to the medial malleolus often are responsible for the development of stasis ulcers at that level. When they become incompetent, the findings of perforator or deep venous disease are more serious than disease of the superficial system, which is composed of the greater and lesser saphenous veins. Primary varicosities due to valvular weakness or weakness of vein walls are associated with the superficial system, whereas secondary varicosities are present in those patients with other symptoms of deep venous disease (stasis ulcers, brawny edema, dermatitis). (*Greenfield, pp. 1005–1006*)

165. (E) The term *ischemic stroke* refers to cerebral infarction occurring as a result of impaired blood flow. Atherosclerosis is the basis of this in the vast majority of patients, but it can also occur when the lumen is occluded by emboli, hematoma, fibromuscular hyperplasia, or arteritis. Injury, trauma, or thoracic aneurysms involving the carotid artery can result in dissection and tearing of the intima. (*Imparato and Riles, p. 974*)

166. (C), 167. (A), 168. (D). The Adson's maneuver that demonstrates the obstruction of the subclavian artery by the scalenus anticus muscle is the most useful test to indicate thoracic outlet syndrome.

The Allen's test will show the integrity of the palmar arches. In patients with thoracic outlet syndrome, the radial pulse will decrease or obliterate during the Adson's maneuver, but the radial pulse should be present during the Allen's test.

The submersion test is performed for patients who complain of cold-related color and temperature changes to their upper extremities. If the submersion test is positive, patients will show classic color changes of Raynaud's phenomenon, pallor, cyanosis, and rubor.

The exercise stress test is most helpful in documenting exercise-induced claudication in patients with femoropopliteal disease. At rest, these patients may show only slightly decreased Doppler pressures and pulses. However, following exercise that produces the symptoms, the drop in pressure and recovery time is proportional to the extent of arterial occlusive disease.

The Valsalva maneuver can be used to assess venous, not peripheral, arterial disease. (*Imparato and Riles, pp. 944, 997*)

169. (C) Venous valves are the focal point of most of the pathology of venous thrombosis. The sinus in which the valve lies is where the initial thrombus forms. In addition, the loss of valvular function after recannulization of a vein produces venous insufficiency. (*Greenfield, p. 989*)

170. (B) The most common cause of secondary lymphedema is malignant disease metastatic to the lymph nodes. Surgery is another common cause. In tropical and subtropical countries, filariasis is the most common cause, producing the typical appearance of elephantiasis. (*Greenfield, p. 1011*)

171. (B) Varicella, diphtheria, tuberculosis, and rubeola are not known to cause heart disease. However, rubella occurring in the first trimester of pregnancy is one of the few infectious diseases known to cause congenital heart disease, usually patent ductus arteriosus. (*Galloway et al, 1994b, p. 779*)

172. (B) Right-to-left shunts of venous blood directly into systemic circulation, producing arterial hypoxemia and cyanosis, result from the combination of an intracardiac septal defect with obstruction to normal flow of blood into the pulmonary artery. The classic example is the tetralogy of Fallot, a combination of ventricular septal defect, malposition of the aorta, pulmonic stenosis, and right ventricular hypertrophy. (*Galloway et al, 1994b, p. 782*)

173. (A) Important principles in a pediatric intensive care unit are constant observation; monitoring of the electrocardiogram; continuous measurement of central venous, left atrial, and arterial pressure; routine measurement of blood-gas tensions and urine output; and respiratory therapy. (*Galloway et al, 1994b, p. 785*)

174. (D) Abnormalities in growth and development are among the most common signs of cardiac disease. Cyanosis may be obvious, and results simply from a decrease in cardiac output with sluggish regional blood flow through the capillary circulation. More oxygen is extracted and a greater amount of reduced hemoglobin is present. Cyanosis and clubbing, a consequence of chronic cyanosis, and polycythemia are often seen in congenital heart disease. Hepatic enlargement is the hallmark of congestive failure in children. *(Spencer, 1989a, pp. 774–776)*

175. (B), 176. (A), 177. (A), 178. (B). Cyanosis does not occur in isolated atrial and ventricular septal defects. In atrial and ventricular septal defects, the pressure in the left atrium and ventricle are greater than those in the right atrium and ventricle. The blood that is shunted is oxygenated. Pulmonary congestion occurs from an increase in pulmonary blood flow. Often a corresponding decrease in systemic blood flow occurs. With the increase in blood flow, pulmonary hypertension occurs. Patent ductus arteriosus also produces this same left-to-right shunt. Cyanotic heart diseases produce a right-to-left shunt of blood. Unoxygenated blood is in the systemic circulation producing arterial hypoxemia and cyanosis. This is due to the combination of an intracardiac septal defect with obstruction to the normal flow of blood into the pulmonary artery. The classic example of this is the tetralogy of Fallot, a combination of ventricular septal defect and pulmonic stenosis. Venous blood entering the right ventricle is then shunted directly into the aorta to produce cyanosis. In addition to the cyanosis, the malformation decreases the pulmonary blood flow and hence limits the capacity of the lungs to absorb oxygen. With transposition of the great vessels, the aorta originates from the right ventricle and the pulmonary artery from the left ventricle. As a result, venous blood returning through the vena cava to the right atrium enters the right ventricle and is then ejected directly into the aorta. Oxygenated blood returning from the lungs through the pulmonary veins to the left ventricle is then expelled through the pulmonary artery to the lungs. Cyanosis and dyspnea in the newborn are the most prominent symptoms. *(Galloway et al, 1994b, pp. 797–8, 805, 813, 824)*

179. (C) The basic noninvasive studies are the chest radiograph, electrocardiogram, and echocardiogram. The electrocardiogram is the best guide to the presence of ventricular hypertrophy. The echocardiogram has become the most valuable diagnostic test. Noninvasive two-dimensional color and Doppler echocardiography produces extremely accurate internal cardiac imaging, allowing measurement of the following: ventricular wall thickness, chamber size and configuration; shunt flow and direction; valvular location, size, and degree of regurgitant flow; and aortic or pulmonary artery size. From Doppler velocity measurement an estimate of the peak systolic gradient across a stenotic valve or coarctation is obtainable. Newer transesophageal echocardiography has increased the accuracy of this modality. Accordingly, many cases are currently treated medically or surgically based on echocardiographic studies alone. Patients with straightforward obstructive lesions, atrial septal defect, ventricular defect, or patent ductus arteriosus, or those requiring palliative emergency systemic to pulmonary shunts often are in this category. *(Galloway et al, 1994b, p. 784)*

180. (D) Coarctation of the aorta is a relatively common congenital lesion that occurs twice as frequently in males as in females. Ninety-eight percent of all aortic coarctations are located at or near the aortic isthmus (the segment of aorta adjacent to the ligamentum arteriosum or ductus arteriosus). The hemodynamic consequences of coarctation of the aorta depend on the rate of ductus arteriosus closure, the severity of obstruction, the development of collaterals, and the presence and severity of associated anomalies. There appear to be two distinct clinical presentations: patients who present in early infancy and those who present in later childhood. Infants with coarctation may have severe congestive heart failure. Over half of these infants have an associated cardiac lesion such as patent ductus arteriosus, ventricular septal defect, or endocardial cushion defect. Some infants may actually be ductus-dependent for lower-body blood flow; therefore, the ductus must be kept open with prostaglandin E until correction can be achieved. Infants with severe coarctation require immediate diagnosis and operative correction. The death rate in the first year of life without operation is approximately 75%. Operative repair in infancy can be accomplished and has approximately a 5% death rate. Many older children with coarctation are asymptomatic and well-developed. Complaints of headache, pains in the calves when running, or frequent nosebleeds are common. Most of these children have hypertension in the upper extremities, and many have electrocardiographic evidence of left ventricular hypertrophy. Essentials of diagnosis include (1) infants may have severe heart failure; children are usually asymptomatic; (2) absent or weak femoral pulses; (3) systolic pressure higher in upper extremities than in lower extremities; diastolic pressures are similar; and (4) harsh systolic murmur heard in the back. *(Verrier, pp. 388–389)*

181. **(A)** The frequent symptoms of cardiac disease are: (1) symptoms of left heart failure: dyspnea, other symptoms of pulmonary congestion; (2) symptoms of right heart failure: edema from sodium retention, hepatomegaly, ascites; (3) angina; (4) arrhythmias; (5) syncope; and (6) fatigue. With the exception of angina, these symptoms usually are *late* signs of advanced cardiac disease. The initial change in most cardiac disease is a rise in intracardiac pressure in the involved chamber subsequently followed by cardiac enlargement, usually a combination of dilatation and hypertrophy. *(Galloway et al, 1994a, p. 845)*

182. **(D)** Angina pectoris, the most common manifestation of myocardial ischemia, is demonstrated by periodic discomfort, usually substernal, typically appearing with exertion, after eating, or with extreme emotion. Characteristically these symptoms subside within 3 to 5 minutes or may be dramatically re-

lieved by sublingual nitroglycerin. In about 25 percent of patients, the symptoms are not typical and may radiate to bizarre areas, such as the teeth, the shoulder, or the epigastrium. *(Galloway et al, 1994a, p. 858)*

183. **(E)** The high percentage of coexisting disease in patients with descending thoracic aortic surgery accounts for much of the surgical morbidity and mortality. In a group of 50 patients reported by Shenaq et al, 70% had preexisting hypertension, 44% had coronary artery disease (CAD), 34% had undergone previous surgery for another aneurysm, and 8% had undergone a coronary artery bypass graft. Livesay et al noted that the three principal causes of 42 deaths in 360 patients were hemorrhage (29%), cardiac events (26%), and multiple organ failure (24%). Hemorrhagic complications were related primarily to poor quality of the aortic wall with occasional bleeding from other sources. Myocardial infarction (MI), unexpected arrhythmias, and low cardiac output (CO) were the causes of death in 3% of patients undergoing operation. Fatal stroke occurred in 1.7% of patients. Other causes of death included mesenteric infarction, acute pancreatitis, and pulmonary embolism. *(Kwitka et al, p. 764)*

184. **(C)** Extracorporeal circulation inevitably produces some trauma to the blood, primarily from exposure of blood to plastics in the oxygenator and circuits and from the use of suction to aspirate intracardiac blood. Minimizing the injury to blood during oxygenation is the basis for a membrane oxygenator rather than a bubble oxygenator. Trauma to blood from the pump itself is surprisingly small. At present, tolerance for long periods of perfusion, up to 4 to 5 hours, is surprisingly good. Overall, trauma from short-term extracorporeal circulation of up to 3 to 4 hours' duration is minimal because of the improved design of current pump oxygenators. By contrast, when the length of cardiopulmonary bypass exceeds 3 to 4 hours, the morbidity and mortality of the procedure increase significantly, with severe problems occurring after 6 hours. *(Galloway et al, 1994a, pp. 851–852)*

185. (A) In 1977, Gruntzig introduced percutaneous transluminal coronary angioplasty (PTCA) for dilating stenotic coronary arterial lesions. Successful dilation rates per stenosis currently exceed 90%; complication rates have fallen to 4%; and procedure-related myocardial infarction and death remain uncommon. Recent enthusiasm for balloon dilation has been accompanied by its increasing application to more complex forms of coronary disease and a marked increase in the number of procedures performed annually. In many centers, PTCA now is the most commonly used invasive therapy for coronary disease. Although the initial results of PTCA were considered acceptable, the major concern at present is long-term stability or revascularization. Significant restenosis occurs within the first year in up to 40% of lesions, and both symptomatic recurrence and reintervention rates have been high during follow-up. PTCA may be most useful (1) in patients with severe symptoms from low-risk obstructions (such as single-vessel and mild double-vessel disease) that do not warrant surgical intervention for prognostic reasons; and (2) in those at high risk for operation, such as patients with acute myocardial infarction, or cardiogenic shock. *(Rankin et al, pp. 364–365)*

186. (D) Early cardiac postoperative complications include bleeding, tamponade, arrhythmias, myocardial infarction, graft occlusion, coronary spasm, low cardiac output syndrome, cardiac arrest, and stroke. Other complications include delayed bleeding, postpericardiotomy syndrome with pericardial effusion, tamponade, arrhythmias, renal dysfunction, ileus, ischemic bowel, gastrointestinal hemorrhage, pneumothorax, respiratory insufficiency, pneumonia, wound infection, wound dehiscence, and, rarely, chronic cardiac dysfunction. Although the incidence of serious complication is relatively low (3% to 8%), depending on patient and operative variables, every complication can be potentially life-threatening and associated with significant morbidity. *(Galloway et al, 1994a, p. 852)*

187. (C) The cerebral anoxia following circulatory arrest produces brain injury within 3 to 4 minutes, so the diagnosis must be made and treatment begun rapidly to avoid serious brain injury. Periods of anoxia for 6 to 8 minutes may produce extensive, but reversible, brain injury, whereas longer periods regularly cause irreversible injury. When the diagnosis of ventricular fibrillation or cardiac arrest is considered, it should either be excluded within 30 to 60 seconds or treatment should be begun. *(Galloway et al, 1994a, p. 855)*

188. (C) The most common cause of mitral stenosis is still rheumatic fever associated with group A streptococcal pharyngitis. The early valvular lesions of rheumatic fever are characterized by an acute inflammatory infiltrate that gradually heals by organization with fibrous tissue. Mitral stenosis is second only to aortic stenosis in terms of mortality rate among the acquired valvular diseases. Thus, available data would support the early election of surgical therapy for this disorder. Most would agree that asymptomatic patients should be treated medically and carefully observed. In the presence of clinically or hemodynamically significant valvular obstruction, firm indications for operation include NYHA class III or IV symptoms, the onset of atrial fibrillation (independent of symptoms), worsening pulmonary hypertension, an episode of systemic embolization, and infective endocarditis. Surgical therapy should be recommended also for class II patients who are over age 40, those who have severe reduction in valve area at catheterization, and those who experience unacceptable lifestyle limitations. *(Rankin et al, pp. 368–370)*

189. (B) Aortic stenosis causes obstruction to left ventricular outflow. Resistance to left ventricular outflow produces a pressure overload on the left ventricle that compensates by the development of concentric left ventricular hypertrophy. Most patients remain asymptomatic for many years. The classic triad of symptoms includes angina pectoris, syncope, and congestive heart failure and usually denotes an aortic valve gradient greater than 50 mm Hg or a valve area less than 1.0 cm². Angina pectoris is due to the imbalance between myocardial oxygen demand and delivery caused by increased myocardial oxygen consumption, and in the 25% to 50% of patients with coronary artery disease, it is aggravated by the superimposed reduced oxygen delivery. Syncope is typically exertional and most likely related to inability of the left ventricle to increase cardiac output in the face of a fixed, high-grade obstruction. Congestive heart failure usually occurs late and is an especially ominous sign. The pulse pressure often is narrowed, with a decreased systolic arterial pressure. A harsh mid-systolic murmur is heard best at the second intercostal space and along the left sternal border. The murmur may radiate to the carotid arteries, is generally audible at the apex, and typically does not radiate into the axilla. Approximately 25% to 50% of patients also have a murmur of aortic regurgitation. *(Rankin et al, pp. 374–375)*

190. **(E)** The myocardial ischemia produced by coronary disease can produce several serious events: angina pectoris, myocardial infarction, congestive heart failure, or sudden death. Angina is the most frequent symptom, but unfortunately myocardial infarction or sudden death may appear without warning. The risk of sudden death varies with the extent of disease and the degree of impairment of ventricular function. It ranges from 2% to as high as 10%. Death apparently results from ventricular fibrillation in many cases or from myocardial infarction with acute decompensation. Myocardial infarction is the most common serious complication. *(Galloway et al, 1994a, p. 858)*

191. **(E)** Therapy for acute myocardial infarction, such as immediate administration of thrombolytic agents, both through IV and intracoronary route, has demonstrated a decrease in mortality. Angioplasty may be used in combination with intracoronary thrombolytics to reduce residual stenosis in the once-

thrombosed vessel. Patients with triple vessel disease who suffer a massive infarction should probably undergo immediate bypass, with insertion of an intra-aortic balloon pump prior to their operation. *(Spencer, 1989b, p. 888)*

192. **(D)** With proper technique and the preoperative use of dipyridamole and aspirin, patency 1 month following operation should be in the range of 90% to 95%. In the first 5 years after operation, patency decreases slowly, about 2% to 3% each year, so the 5-year patency rate is in the range of 75% to 80%. Occlusion of the graft during this time is probably due to anastomotic technique, trauma to the vein graft during harvesting, or, rarely, postoperative adhesions. *(Galloway et al, 1994a, p. 863)*

193. **(D)** In the period 5 to 10 years after operation, there is an increase of atherosclerotic disease in vein grafts and the patency rate is probably no better than 50%. For this reason, the use of the internal mammary artery has increased markedly. The 10-year patency rate is near 95%, and the internal mammary artery seems to be relatively immune to atherosclerosis. *(Galloway et al, 1994a, pp. 860–861)*

194. **(E)** In the majority of patients, the cause of chronic constrictive pericarditis is unknown, probably the end stage of an undiagnosed viral pericarditis. Tuberculosis is a rarity. In recent years, intensive radiation has become a significant cause in some series. Constrictive pericarditis may develop after an open heart operation. The pericardial cavity is obliterated by fusion of the parietal pericardium to the epicardium, forming dense scar tissue that encases and constricts the heart. Once the diagnosis has been made, pericardiectomy should be done promptly because the disease relentlessly progresses. *(Galloway et al, 1994a, p. 892)*

195. **(A)** The most common surgical trauma producing complete heart block occurs during the repair of a ventricular septal defect or an ostium primum atrial septal defect. Demand

pacemakers are now used almost exclusively. A more complex and widely used type of pacemaker is the atrial-ventricular pacemaker, or dual-chamber pacemaker, which requires electrodes in both the atrium and the ventricle. Almost all pacemakers are now externally programmable. (*Galloway et al, 1994a, p. 894*)

196. (D) Most ablative therapy for arrhythmias, either surgical or nonsurgical, is done for one of four clinical entities: (1) Wolff-Parkinson-White (WPW) syndrome with pre-excitation; (2) paroxysmal supraventricular tachycardia (PSVT) due to (a) atrioventricular (AV) node reentry or (b) concealed AV pathways; (3) sustained ventricular tachycardia; and (4) chronic atrial fibrillation. Patients with cardiac arrhythmias require EPS before treatment, and further intraoperative mapping is done at the time of surgery. Catheter ablation methods, when appropriate, can be applied in the catheterization laboratory after EPS studies are completed. (*Galloway et al, 1994a, p. 892*)

197. (C) A left ventricular aneurysm occurs when a large myocardial infarction progresses to a thinned-out transmural scar that bulges paradoxically beyond the normal cavitary contours during systole. Although aneurysms have occurred in 2% to 4% of myocardial infarctions, the incidence is probably decreasing with more aggressive infarct management. Ninety percent of aneurysms involve the anteroseptal left ventricle, and 10% are posterior. Over 50% contain mural thrombus. Surgical therapy should be considered in most cases, as prognosis with medical management is poor. Treatment consists of aneurysm resection combined with complete coronary revascularization. (*Rankin et al, p. 366*)

198. (B), 199. (A), 200. (B). The two life-threatening problems for patients with penetrating cardiac trauma are tamponade and hemorrhage. Tamponade develops rapidly as the normal pericardium can accommodate only 100 to 250 mL of blood. Small wounds, such as those from an icepick or knife, often produce tamponade because the laceration in the pericardium is small. Bullets or large knives threaten immediate death from exsanguination as blood can be expelled through the pericardial laceration into the pleural cavity. The treatment should be control of the hemorrhage through emergency thoracotomy. The key to tamponade is to consider the diagnosis in any patient with hypotension and a penetrating thoracic wound and performing a pericardial aspiration. Blunt cardiac trauma usually results from automobile accidents when the steering wheel impacts against the chest. The direct injury may be a cardiac contusion. The contusion varies from simple subepicardial hemorrhage to a full-thickness myocardial contusion. The clinical picture is that of pericarditis with a pericardial effusion and chest pain. (*Galloway et al, 1994a, pp. 887–888*)

REFERENCES

Adams JT. Pancreas. In Schwartz SI et al (eds). *Principles of Surgery*, 6th ed. New York: McGraw-Hill; 1994: 1401–1432.

Bland KI, Copeland EM. Breast. In Schwartz SI et al (eds). *Principles of Surgery*, 6th ed. New York: McGraw-Hill; 1994: 531–594.

Clark OH. Thyroid and parathyroid. In Way LW (ed), *Current Surgical Diagnosis and Treatment*, 10th ed. Norwalk, CT: Appleton & Lange; 1994: 274–292.

Committee on Trauma, ACS. *Thoracic Trauma*. Chicago, IL: American College of Surgeons; 1993.

Crumley RL. Maxillofacial and Neck Trauma. In Ho MT, Saunders CE (eds), *Current Emergency Diagnosis and Treatment*, 5th ed. Englewood Cliffs, NJ: Prentice-Hall; 1990: 228–244.

Deveney KE. Hernias and other lesions of the abdominal wall. In Way LW (ed), *Current Surgerical Diagnosis and Treatment*, 10th ed. Norwalk, CT: Appleton & Lange; 1994: 712–724.

Doberstein C, Rodts G, McBride D. Neurosurgical Critical Care. In Bogard FS, Sue DY (eds). *Current Critical Care Diagnosis and Treatment*, 1st ed. Norwalk, CT: Appleton & Lange; 1994: 539–554.

Donovan JF, Williams RD. Urology. In Way LW (ed), *Current Surgical Diagnosis & Treatment*, 10th ed. Norwalk, CT: Appleton & Lange; 1994: 907–973.

Duthie RB, Hoaglund FT. Orthopaedics. In Schwartz SI et al (eds), *Principles of Surgery*, 5th ed. New York: McGraw-Hill; 1989: 1879–2020.

Edwards MS. Brain Tumors. In Way LW (ed), *Current Surgical Diagnosis and Treatment*, 10th ed. Norwalk, CT: Appleton & Lange; 1994: 829–834.

Frank IN. Urology. In Schwartz SI et al (eds), *Principles of Surgery*, 5th ed. New York: McGraw-Hill; 1989: 1729–1780.

Galloway AC, Colvin SB, Grossi EA, Spencer FC. Acquired heart disease. In Schwartz SI et al (eds), *Principles of Surgery*, 6th ed. New York: McGraw-Hill; 1994a: 845–902.

Galloway AC, Colvin SB, Spencer FC. Congenital heart disease. In Schwartz SI et al (eds), *Principles of Surgery*, 6th ed. New York: McGraw-Hill; 1994b: 779–844.

Green RM, Ouriel K. Peripheral arterial disease. In Schwartz SI et al (eds), *Principles of Surgery*, 6th ed. New York: McGraw-Hill; 1994: 925–988.

Greenfield LJ. Venous and lymphatic disease. In Schwartz SI et al (eds), *Principles of Surgery*, 6th ed. New York: McGraw-Hill; 1994: 989–1014.

Hoff JT, Boland MF. Neurosurgery. In Schwartz SI et al (eds), *Principles of Surgery*, 6th ed. New York: McGraw-Hill; 1994: 1831–1860.

Imparato AM, Riles TS. Peripheral arterial disease. In Schwartz SI et al (eds), *Principles of Surgery*, 5th ed. New York: McGraw-Hill; 1989: 933–1010.

Kaplan EL. Thyroid and parathyroid. In Schwartz SI et al (eds), *Principles of Surgery*, 6th ed. New York: McGraw-Hill; 1994: 1611–1680.

Kilgore ES, Graham III WP, Markinson RE. Hand Surgery. In Way LW (ed), *Current Surgical Diagnosis and Treatment*, 10th ed. Norwalk, CT: Appleton & Lange; 1994: 1165–1189.

Kodner IJ, Fry RD, Fleshman JW, Birnbaum EH. Colon, rectum, and anus. In Schwartz SI et al (eds), *Principles of Surgery*, 6th ed. New York: McGraw-Hill; 1994: 1191–1306.

Krupski WC, Effeney DJ. Arteries. In Way LW (ed), *Current Surgical Diagnosis and Treatment*, 10th ed. Norwalk, CT: Appleton & Lange; 1994: 739–771.

Kwitka G, Roseberg JN, Nugent M. Thoracic aortic disease. In Kaplan JA (ed), *Cardiac Anesthesia*, 3rd ed. Philadelphia: Saunders; 1993: 758–780

McFadden DW, Zinner MJ. Manifestations of gastrointestinal disease. In Schwartz SI et al (eds), *Principles of Surgery*, 6th ed. New York: McGraw-Hill; 1994: 1015–1042.

Meyer AA, Salber P. *Current Emergency Diagnosis and Treatment*, 4th ed. Norwalk, CT: Appleton & Lange; 1992: 694–695.

Mulvilhill SJ, Pellegrini CA. Postoperative Complications. In Way LW (ed), *Current Surgical Diagnosis and Treatment*, 10th ed. Norwalk, CT: Appleton & Lange; 1994: 24–39.

Peters JH, DeMeester TR. Esophagus and diaphragmatic hernia. In Schwartz SI et al (eds), *Principles of Surgery*, 6th ed. New York: McGraw-Hill; 1994: 1043–1122.

Peters PC, Boone TB, Frank IN, McConnel JD, Preminger GM. Urology. In Schwartz SI et al (eds), *Principles of Surgery*, 6th ed. New York: McGraw-Hill; 1994: 1725–1792.

Rankin JS, Hennein HA, Keith FM. The Heart: I. Acquired Diseases. In Way LW (ed), *Current Surgical Diagnosis and Treatment*, 10th ed. Norwalk, CT: Appleton & Lange; 1994: 358–382.

Reber HA. Pancreas. In Schwartz SI et al (eds), *Principles of Surgery*, 6th ed. New York: McGraw-Hill; 1994: 1401–1432.

Rosier RN. Orthopaedics. In Schwartz SI et al (eds), *Principles of Surgery*, 6th ed. New York: McGraw-Hill; 1994: 1861–1966.

Roslyn JJ, Zinner MJ. Gallbladder and extrahepatic biliary system. In Schwartz SI et al (eds), *Principles of Surgery*, 6th ed. New York: McGraw-Hill; 1994: 1367–1400.

Schamlzreid T, Guttman D. Critical Care. In Bogard FS, Sue DY (eds), *Current Critical Care Diagnosis and Treatment*, 1st ed. Norwalk, CT: Appleton & Lange; 1994: 731–740.

Schrock TR. Small intestine. In Way LW (ed), *Current Surgical Diagnosis and Treatment*, 10th ed. Norwalk, CT: Appleton & Lange; 1994: 615–643.

Schwartz SI. Appendix. In Schwartz SI et al (eds), *Principles of Surgery*, 6th ed. New York: McGraw-Hill; 1994: 1307–1318.

Schwartz SI. Hemostasis, surgical bleeding and transfusion. In Schwartz SI et al (eds), *Principles of Surgery*, 6th ed. New York: McGraw-Hill; 1994: 95–118.

Schwartz SI. Liver. In Schwartz SI et al (eds), *Principles of Surgery*, 6th ed. New York: McGraw-Hill; 1994: 1319–1366.

Shires GT III, Canizaro PC, Carrico CJ. Shock. In Schwartz SI et al (eds), *Principles of Surgery*, 5th ed. New York: McGraw-Hill; 1989: 137–180.

Shires GT, Thal ER, Jones RC, et al. Trauma. In Schwartz SI et al (eds), *Principles of Surgery*, 6th ed. New York: McGraw-Hill; 1994: 175–224.

Spencer FC. Congenital heart disease. In Schwartz SI et al (eds), *Principles of Surgery*, 5th ed. New York: McGraw-Hill; 1989a: 771–842.

Spencer FC. Acquired heart disease. In Schwartz SI et al (eds), *Principles of Surgery*, 5th ed. New York: McGraw-Hill; 1989b: 843–908.

Townsend CM Jr, Thompson JC. Small intestine. In Schwartz SI et al (eds), *Principles of Surgery*, 6th ed. New York: McGraw-Hill; 1994: 1153–1190.

Verrier ED. The Heart: II. Congenital Diseases. In Way LW (ed), *Current Surgical Diagnosis and Treatment*, 10th ed. Norwalk, CT: Appleton & Lange; 1994: 383–410.

Wantz GE. Abdominal wall hernias. In Schwartz SI et al (eds), *Principles of Surgery*, 6th ed. New York: McGraw-Hill; 1994: 1517–1544.

Way LW. Biliary tract. In Way LW (ed), *Current Surgical Diagnosis and Treatment*, 10th ed. Norwalk, CT: Appleton & Lange; 1994: 537–566.

Weinstein PR, Hoff JT. Intervertebral disk disease. In Way LW (ed), *Current Surgical Diagnosis and Treatment*, 10th ed. Norwalk, CT: Appleton & Lange; 1994: 851–856.

Williams PL et al eds, *Gray's Anatomy: The Anatomical Basis of Medicine and Surgery*. 38th ed. New York: Churchill Livingstone; 1995: 1788–1790.

CHAPTER 3

Pediatrics
Questions

Marsha R. Mayo-Adams, PA-C

DIRECTIONS: (Questions 1 through 3): Each of the numbered items or incomplete statements in this section is followed by answers or by completions of the statement. Select the ONE lettered answer or completion that is BEST in each case.

Questions 1 through 3

1. All of the following would be included in the differential diagnosis of a child with chronic diarrhea (more than 14 days) EXCEPT?

    (A) giardiasis
    (B) celiac disease
    (C) lymphangiectasia
    (D) rotavirus
    (E) AIDS

2. The most common malignancy of childhood is acute lymphoblastic leukemia (ALL). Which of the following is NOT true in relationship to this disease?

    (A) It occurs more frequently in patients with chromosomal abnormalities.
    (B) Anemia, thrombocytopenia, and neutropenia are common at presentation.
    (C) Prognosis is worse for patients with onset in a child older than 2 years.
    (D) The disease is heterogenous, requiring different treatment regimens.
    (E) Hypereosinophilia may be present at diagnosis and is considered reactive.

3. When evaluating a child for attention deficit hyperactivity disorder (ADHD), all of the following statements are considered true EXCEPT

    (A) During preschool years, most children continue to have short attention spans.
    (B) Situational inattention may result when a young child is faced with developmentally inappropriate expectations.
    (C) Most children with learning disorders also demonstrate impaired attention.
    (D) Estimates suggest that 8% to 10% of school-age children fulfill the diagnostic criteria for ADHD.
    (E) Inattention and hyperactivity often are associated with primary neurological disorders.

DIRECTIONS (Questions 4 through 17): Each group of items in the following section consists of lettered headings followed by a set of numbered words or phrases. For each numbered word or phrase, select the ONE lettered heading that is most closely associated with it. Each lettered heading may be selected once, more than once, or not at all.

Questions 4 through 7

For each cardiac lesion, select the commonly associated physical findings.

(A) decreased, delayed or absent femoral pulses

(B) bounding pulses with hyperdynamic precordium, in premature infants with murmur, if any

(C) wide, fixed split second heart sound

(D) evidence of gross congestive failure without a systolic murmur

(E) holosystolic murmur along the lower left sternal border not heard in the first days of life

4. Secundum atrial septal defect

5. Ventricular septal defect

6. Persistent ductus arteriosus

7. Coarctation of aorta

Questions 8 through 11

Dermatological diseases are common in pediatric patients. Match the diagnosis with the most appropriate statement.

(A) characterized by a pattern of inheritance that can be autosomal dominant or recessive

(B) will subside after the first few months of life

(C) slow but spontaneous involution

(D) a staphylococcal infection

(E) may involve the diaper area

8. Neonatal pustular melanosis

9. Strawberry hemangiomas

10. Seborrheic dermatitis

11. Epidermolysis bullosa

Questions 12 through 15

For each age group, select the most common orthopedic problem.

(A) subluxation of radial head

(B) scoliosis

(C) fracture of clavicle

(D) Legg–Calvé–Perthes disease

(E) slipped capital femoral epiphysis

12. Adolescent female

13. Newborn

14. Male, age 5–9 years

15. 1 to 4 years

Questions 16 and 17

(A) involves the dorsa of the toes and distal aspect of the foot

(B) seen in prepubertal children

(C) both

(D) neither

16. Allergic contact dermatitis

17. Tinea pedis

DIRECTIONS (Questions 18 through 23): Each of the numbered items or incomplete statements in this section is followed by answers or by completions of the statement. Select the ONE lettered answer or completion that is BEST in each case.

Questions 18 through 23

18. An 8-year-old female presents with evidence of polyarthritis. The chart shows that she had a documented beta-streptococcus infection 20 days previously. The differential diagnosis includes rheumatic fever. What additional finding would permit you to make the diagnosis of rheumatic fever based on clinical examination (modified Jones criteria)?

(A) fever

(B) arthralgia

(C) acute pharyngitis

(D) carditis

(E) erythema multiforme

19. Which of the following is true regarding adolescent gynecomastia?

(A) Gynecomastia begins in Tanner stage II–III and normally disappears in 1 to 2 years.

(B) The underlying mass may be fixed and there may be skin dimpling.

(C) Gynecomastia is due to excess fatty tissue in an obese patient.

(D) Gynecomastia is not a painful condition.

(E) Surgical intervention in not a consideration in treating gynecomastia.

20. The most common vasculitis in childhood is Henoch–Schönlein purpura (HSP). All the following are true about this condition EXCEPT

(A) Colicky abdominal pain may be present.

(B) A protein-losing enteropathy secondary to intestinal involvement is part of the spectrum of this disease.

(C) Most children with HSP have renal involvement.

(D) Platelet counts are abnormal, as are coagulation studies.

(E) Joint, ankle, and knee pain are associated with HSP.

21. The most common thrombocytopenia of childhood is idiopathic thrombocytopenia purpura. To substantiate the diagnosis, which laboratory test would you order?

(A) clot retraction

(B) bleeding time

(C) platelet count

(D) manual differential

(E) ANA test

22. A 4-month-old presents with generalized malaise, fever, hyperirritability, a bulging fontanelle, and positive Kernig's and Brudzinski's signs. A lumbar puncture reveals elevated lymphocytes, normal protein concentration, and normal glucose concentration. This clinical picture is most suggestive of

(A) bacterial meningitis

(B) mycotic meningitis

(C) viral meningitis

(D) infectious mononucleosis

(E) Lyme borreliosis

23. A young patient is brought into the emergency room after an automobile accident. His skin is cold, clammy, and pale, and his neck veins are flat. You notice signs of trauma to the right upper quadrant of the abdomen. What type of shock is this patient likely to have?

(A) cardiogenic shock

(B) hypovolemic shock

(C) simple shock

(D) vasogenic shock

(E) terminal shock

DIRECTIONS (Questions 24 through 33): Each group of items in the following section consists of lettered headings followed by a set of numbered words or phrases. For each numbered word or phrase, select the ONE lettered heading that is most closely associated with it. Each lettered heading may be selected once, more than once, or not at all.

Questions 24 through 33

(A) rubella

(B) erythema infectiousum

(C) infectious mononucleosis/Epstein–Barr virus

(D) varicella

(E) measles

24. The oral mucosa may be erythematous, and Forscheimer spots may be present on the soft palate.

25. This virus has the ability to remain latent in sensory ganglia and may reappear at times of physical stress as a rash following a dermatome pattern.

26. Infection with this parvovirus leads to its "slapped cheek" appearance.

27. This diagnosis should be suspected in a child or adolescent with a prolonged illness that includes fever, lymphadenopathy, and fatigue.

28. Maternal congenital infection during the first 4 months of gestation may lead to growth retardation, cardiac, ocular, and hearing abnormalities.

29. Complications of this infection can include neutropenia, thrombocytopenia, pneumonia, and in rare cases, splenic rupture.

30. This viral rash is classically described as widely scattered macules and papules that rapidly progress to vesicles.

31. Koplik spots are a pathognomonic manifestation of this disease.

32. Complications of this viral infection most commonly include secondary bacterial skin infections.

33. The characteristic course of this viral disease consists of fever, cough, rhinitis, conjunctivitis, diarrhea, and vomiting. The maculopapular rash begins on the forehead and then spreads to the rest of the body.

DIRECTIONS (Questions 34 through 37): Match the following types of poisonings with their antidote.

Questions 34 through 37

    (A) methylene blue
    (B) oxygen
    (C) atropine sulfate
    (D) naloxone
    (E) syrup of ipecac

34. Carbon monoxide

35. Methemoglobin (nitrates)

36. Narcotics

37. Organophosphates

DIRECTIONS (Questions 38 through 42): Each of the numbered items or incomplete statements in this section is followed by answers or by completions of the statement. Select the ONE lettered answer or completion that is BEST in each case.

Questions 38 through 42

38. The most dangerous inflicted injury in terms of morbidity and mortality is

    (A) a skull fracture
    (B) an intra-abdominal injury
    (C) a subdural hematoma
    (D) a subgaleal hematoma
    (E) multiple fractures of the extremities

39. Radiological characteristics of inflicted injuries include all of the following EXCEPT

    (A) spiral fractures
    (B) multiple fractures in different stages of healing
    (C) symmetrical fractures
    (D) fractures of the scapula or sternum
    (E) evidence of subperiostial bleeding

40. The diagnosis of childhood sexual molestation is most frequently made by

    (A) the child's emotional distress and fearfulness of a physical examination
    (B) the child's detailed explicit account of his or her experience
    (C) physical evidence of perineal trauma; that is, redness, swelling, discharge, abrasions
    (D) laboratory evidence of gonorrhea in cultures of the mouth, anal area, or vaginal discharge
    (E) parental complaints of recent onset of sexualized behaviors, including masturbation and explicit vocabulary

41. Clinical experience indicates that most infants with polycythemia

    (A) are in respiratory distress
    (B) develop convulsions
    (C) exhibit priaprism
    (D) are asymptomatic
    (E) develop necrotizing enterocolitis

42. All of the following are true with regard to hyaline membrane disease (HMD) EXCEPT

    (A) Symptoms usually develop within minutes of birth.
    (B) The infant with HMD is almost always premature.
    (C) The unventilated infant may require an increasing oxygen requirement over 24 to 48 hours.
    (D) Chest x-rays show bilateral lung infiltrates.
    (E) Current prevention includes surfactant replacement before 1 to 2 hours.

DIRECTIONS (Questions 43 through 54): Each group of items in this section consists of lettered headings followed by a set of numbered words or phrases. For each numbered word or phrase, select the ONE lettered heading that is most closely associated with it. Each lettered heading may be selected once, more than once, or not at all.

Questions 43 through 46

From statistical reviews of reported cases of childhood maltreatment, the abuser is

    (A) in 1% of the cases
    (B) in 4 % of the cases
    (C) in 5 % of the cases
    (D) in 25% of the cases
    (E) in 90% of the cases

43. A related caretaker of the child

44. A sibling of the victim

45. An unrelated babysitter

46. A male friend of the mother

Questions 47 through 54

    (A) group A streptococcal infection(s)
    (B) group B streptocococcal infection(s)
    (C) pneumococcal infection(s)
    (D) staphylococcal infection(s)
    (E) meningococcal infection(s)

47. This infection presents with fever, malaise, and an exudative pharyngitis with petechiae on the soft palate.

48. This bacteria can produce an enterotoxin that causes severe vomiting and diarrhea 2 to 6 hours after ingestion.

49. This infectious agent is the most common cause of otitis media in children.

50. This infectious agent is the most common cause of neonatal sepsis.

51. A skin infection with this bacteria often causes honey-crusted lesions around the nasal and oral orifices.

52. Rheumatic fever can result following this infection.

53. Patients with this type of infection may present as acutely ill, and with a high fever, irritability, and a petechial rash.

54. A pneumonia from this type of infection may classically present with the onset of shaking chills and rust-colored sputum.

DIRECTIONS (Questions 55 through 74): Each of the following numbered items or incomplete statements in this section is followed by answers or by completions of the statement. Select the ONE lettered answer or completion that is the BEST in each case.

Questions 55 through 74

55. True polycythemia in children can be caused by

    (A) cyanotic congenital heart disease
    (B) placental dysfunction
    (C) hemoglobinopathies
    (D) all of the above
    (E) none of the above

56. Factors known to affect neonatal bilirubin levels include

(A) genetics
(B) infant feeding practices
(C) ethnic factors
(D) all of the above
(E) none of the above

57. A 4-month-old infant born to a mother infected with HIV

(A) has a 90% chance of developing AIDS
(B) cannot definitely be diagnosed with AIDS until 15 months of age
(C) may be ELISA positive for HIV because of a transplacental antibody
(D) if diagnosed with AIDS, will most certainly live only 2 to 4 years
(E) cannot contract HIV through breast feeding

58. Which of the following infants should be given the varicella-zoster immune globin?

(A) an infant whose mother develops varicella 1 day after delivery
(B) a 1-day-old infant whose 2-year-old brother develops varicella
(C) a 1-month-old infant who is exposed to varicella
(D) a 1-month-old infant who develops varicella
(E) none of the above

59. The Jones criteria for diagnosis of rheumatic fever includes all of the following as major criteria EXCEPT

(A) carditis
(B) polyarthritis
(C) Sydenham's chorea
(D) erythema chronicum migrans
(E) subcutaneous nodules

60. All of the following are true of infant colic EXCEPT

(A) Colicky crying can occur at any time of the day.
(B) Colic is more common in males than females.
(C) Colic begins in the first month of life, usually the first week.
(D) Colic is sometimes believed to be related to swallowed air.
(E) Colic is not thought to be related to mother anxiety.

61. All of the following are true regarding cryptorchidism EXCEPT

(A) It is more common in premature than full-term infants.
(B) It is more commonly unilateral than bilateral.
(C) It is frequently associated with fragile X syndrome.
(D) It may be easily confused with retractile testes in childhood.
(E) It predisposes to testicular cancer.

62. All the following are true regarding sports participation by teens EXCEPT

(A) Epiphyseal injuries, although uncommon, can cause variation in growth.
(B) The cardiac abnormality most associated with sudden death is hypertrophic cardiomyopathy.
(C) Children with Down syndrome should not be allowed to participate in contact sports until an x-ray evaluation of the neck has been completed.
(D) Isometric exercise should be encouraged for teens with mildly elevated blood pressure.
(E) Swimming is an activity with low likelihood of inducing bronchospasm in an asthmatic.

63. All the following statements concerning adolescent suicide are true EXCEPT

    (A) The method of suicide most commonly used by teenagers is a firearm.
    (B) Leaving a suicide note suggests premeditation and should be considered a sign of serious intent.
    (C) Male adolescents lead female adolescents in the incidence of suicide attempts, but females outnumber males in completed suicides.
    (D) It is difficult to assess the seriousness of intent by the actual potency or medical lethality of the method.
    (E) Adolescents are more prone to following a suicide "trend" among groups of their peers and may attempt group suicides.

64. Anorexia nervosa patients are characterized by all of the following EXCEPT

    (A) They were model children before their illness.
    (B) They exhibit signs of excessive physical activity.
    (C) They are preoccupied with food preparation.
    (D) One percent are males.
    (E) There often is a coexisting diagnosis of depression/anxiety or obsessive/compulsive disorder.

65. Down syndrome involves all the following EXCEPT

    (A) incidence in the general population of 1 in 600 to 800 births
    (B) the presence of an extra number 18 chromosome
    (C) increased frequency of congenital heart disease
    (D) an association with advanced maternal age
    (E) varying degrees of mental retardation

66. The following statements regarding the DPT immunization are correct EXCEPT

    (A) The diphtheria portion of the DPT is a toxoid.
    (B) The vaccine should be administered at 2, 4, 6, and 15 months.
    (C) Typical mild to moderate reactions include low-grade fever, pain and erythema at the injection site, and mild irritability.
    (D) The most severe reactions have been attributed to the tetanus portion of the immunization.
    (E) The risk of reaction to the immunization is far less than the risk of mortality/morbidity from the actual illnesses.

67. Multiple white papules approximately 1 to 2 mm in diameter scattered over the forehead, nose, and cheeks are present in up to 40% of newborns. These papules are called

    (A) sebaceous gland hyperplasia
    (B) erythema toxicum
    (C) acne neonatorum
    (D) milia
    (E) systemic neonate candidiasis

68. In Native Americans, Asian, and African American infants, a blue/black macule usually found located over the buttocks or lumbrosacral area is called a

    (A) blue nevus
    (B) café au lait lesion
    (C) nevus of ota
    (D) congenital melanocytic nevi
    (E) mongolian spot

69. Associated risk factors for young children developing otitis media include all of the following EXCEPT

    (A) frequent upper-respiratory infections
    (B) more horizontally placed eustachian tubes
    (C) lack of up-to-date immunizations
    (D) enrollment in a day-care setting
    (E) exposure to cigarette smoke

70. A 5-year-old child presents at the ER with a 5-hour history of sudden onset of severe sore throat, fever, difficulty breathing, and drooling. Which of the following diagnoses is most likely?

    (A) acute laryngotracheobronchitis
    (B) pharyngitis
    (C) bronchiolitis
    (D) laryngotracheomalacia
    (E) epiglottitis

71. A 10-day-old male infant presents to the office with poor weight gain, dehydration, and a history of projectile vomiting. You should suspect

    (A) intussusception
    (B) pyloric stenosis
    (C) peptic ulcer disease
    (D) colic
    (E) formula intolerance

72. An adolescent male presents to your office with low-grade fever, fatigue, jaundice, and liver tenderness after returning from a family camping trip where he swam in a river. The most likely diagnosis is

    (A) hepatitis A
    (B) hepatitis B
    (C) hepatitis C
    (D) infectious mononucleosis
    (E) giardiasis

73. A 10-year-old presents to your office with vomiting and progressive CNS depression. Upon examination you find that he is recovering from the chicken pox. Your clinical suspicion should be high for

    (A) Guillain–Barré syndrome
    (B) Reye's syndrome
    (C) hepatitis C
    (D) all of the above
    (E) none of the above

74. A 4-month-old infant presents to your office with decreased nursing, increased spitting, and white patches in the mouth. This indicates

    (A) herpangina
    (B) stomatitis
    (C) candidiasis
    (D) streptococcal pharyngitis
    (E) teething

DIRECTIONS (Questions 75 through 100): Each group of items in the section consists of lettered headings followed by a set of numbered words or phrases. Select the ONE lettered heading that is most closely associated with it. Each lettered heading may be selected once, more than once, or not at all.

Questions 75 through 84

The average child should be able to do the following tasks by which of the listed ages?

    (A) 3 months
    (B) 6 months
    (C) 12 months
    (D) 18 months
    (E) 24 months

75. Feed self with spoon

76. Produce spontaneous and responsive smiling

77. Roll over

78. Walk independently

79. Feed self with finger foods

80. Recognize named objects

81. Follow two-step commands

82. Utter wordlike vocalizations

83. Use intelligible single words to express needs

84. Mouth and shake objects

Questions 85 through 89

    (A) tender, swollen tibial tuberosity in an adolescent
    (B) painful, typically symmetrical, swollen joints

(C) pain and crepitus

(D) obese child with progressive pain and limp

(E) incomplete tearing of a ligament with associated pain and swelling

85. Osteoarthritis

86. Mild or moderate sprain

87. Osgood–Schlatter disease

88. Slipped capital femoral epiphysis

89. Juvenile rheumatoid arthritis

Questions 90 through 94

(A) Marfan's syndrome

(B) torticollis

(C) talipes equinovirus

(D) scoliosis

90. A syndrome characterized by unusually long fingers and toes

91. A deformity characterized by a chin rotated to the opposite side of the affected sternocleidomastoid muscle

92. A lateral curvature of the spine

93. Idiopathic disease found more frequently in adolescent females

94. Joint complex is subluxed medially and plantarward

Questions 95 through 100

(A) trisomy 18

(B) trisomy 21

(C) Turner's syndrome

(D) Ehler–Danlos syndrome

(E) osteogenesis imperfecta

95. Hypermobility of joints and hyperelasticity of skin

96. Webbing of the neck, absence of secondary sex characteristics, coarctation of the aorta

97. Upslanting palpebral fissures, flat nasal bridge, large protruding tongue

98. Blue sclera and excessive bone fragility

99. Epicanthal folds, simian lines, and facial grimace with crying

100. High nasal bridge, overriding fingers, nail hypoplasia, small facies with prominent occiput

Answers and Explanations

1. **(D)** The differential diagnosis includes *G. lamblia,* milk protein allergy, AIDS, ulcerative colitis, pseudomembraneous colitis, acrodermatitis enteropathica, primary immunodeficiency syndromes, disaccharide deficiencies, celiac disease, irritable bowel syndrome, ganglioneuroma or other vasoactive-secretion tumors, intestinal lymphangiectasia, immunoproliferative small intestinal disease, and congenital chloride- or sodium-losing diarrhea. Many of these can be distinguished on the basis of history, physicial, or screening laboratory examinations. Viral gastroenteritis that include the rotavirus are often severe but typically self-limited illnesses, lasting from 2 to 7 days. *(Behrman et al, pp. 979–980; Jenson and Baltimore, pp. 1114–1121)*

2. **(C)** Lymphoid leukemias occur more often than expected in patients with immunodeficiencies, chromosomal abnormalities, and ataxia telangiectasia. On initial examination most patients have anemia and thrombocytopenia, although as many as 25% may have platelet counts less than 3,000/mm and about 20% will have counts less than 50,000/mm. Hypereosinophilia may be present at diagnosis as well and is considered to be reactive in nature. The treatment of ALL varies with the clinical risk features. Unfavorable prognostic features include onset before 2 years or after 10 years of age, with a white cell count over 100,000/mm or a mediastinal mass. *(Rudolph et al, pp. 1271–1272)*

3. **(D)** The disorder termed attention deficit hyperactivity disorder is a subject of great debate. When considering this diagnosis, one should take into account behaviors that are related to normal development, variations in every child's temperament, situational inattention, any psychiatric comorbidity. It is estimated to affect 2% to 4% of school age children. ADHD is characterized by short attention span, impulsivity, and overactivity. *(Rudolph et al, pp. 115–118)*

4. **(C)** The characteristic finding of atrial septal defect is wide, fixed splitting of the second heart sound. *(Oski et al, pp. 1418–1423)*

5. **(E)** The murmur of a ventricular septal defect is not present in the immediate newborn period until pulmonary vascular resistance falls. It is a high-pitched harsh holosystolic murmur well localized along the left sternal border. *(Oski et al, pp. 1426–1428)*

6. **(B)** The classical auscultatory finding of a patent ductus arteriosus is a continuous machine-like murmur localized under the left clavicle. It should be suspected in any premature infant with hyperdynamic precordium and bounding pulses even in absence of a significant murmur. *(Oski et al, p. 358)*

7. **(A)** Below the coarctation there is a narrowed pulse pressure with decreased systolic and diastolic pressure. There may be a

tactile sensation of delay between radial and femoral pulses, though the pulse discrepancy may not be apparent in the infant because the widely patent ductus serves as a route of flow to the descending aorta. *(Oski et al, pp. 1438–1442)*

8. **(B)** This is a recently described condition that presents with clusters of easily ruptured vesicopustules on the forehead, neck, and lower back. The lesions have a rim of scale after they rupture and the base may be hyperpigmented. The melanosis gradually subsides over the first few months of life. *(Crapo et al, p. 501; Hoekelman, p. 468)*

9. **(C)** Strawberry hemangiomas are raised from the skin. At birth they may be identified as macular areas or erythema. These hemangiomas grow during the first months of life and eventually involute spontaneously without scarring. Therapy is not advised in the great majority of cases. Occasionally, the location will necessitate earlier treatment. *(Avery and First, p. 1149; Crapo et al, p. 502; Hoekelman, p. 469)*

10. **(E)** Seborrheic dermatitis may be identified in the axillae, neck folds, scalp, and diaper area. The presence of greasy-appearing plaques that are adherent suggests the diagnosis. It is an inflammmatory disorder of the sebaceous glands. For severe and persistent lesions, and particularly for lesions in the diaper area, 1% hydrocortisone cream is helpful. *(Crapo et al, pp. 503–504)*

11. **(A)** Epidermolysis bullosa can be either autosomal dominant or autosomal recessive in inheritance. The recessive form is the most severe and can be fatal. The dominant form can range from being a nuisance to a moderate medical problem. Emollients to decrease friction and the prevention of bacterial infection of the blisters are important steps in managing this disease. *(Crapo et al, p. 503)*

12. **(B)** Idiopathic scoliosis is more common in adolescent females than in males. There appears to be a pattern of inheritance that is multifactoral and an autosomal dominant genetic pattern with variable penetrance. *(Behrman et al, pp. 1713–1714)*

13. **(C)** The most common fracture in the newborn is that of the clavicle, which occurs during labor and delivery. In treating this fracture, immobilization is unnecessary. Pinning the total sleeve to the shirt and gentle handling will reduce the discomfort. *(Behrman et al, p. 457)*

14. **(D)** Legg–Calvé–Perthes disease (avascular necrosis of the femoral head) is more common in males than females. It occurs in children from 3 to 11 with the most common age range being 5 to 9. *(Behrman et al, pp. 1706–1709)*

15. **(A)** Subluxation of the radial head (nursemaid elbow) is a very common injury that occurs in children between 1 and 4 years of age. The child presents with refusal to move the arm and holds it slightly flexed at the elbow and pronated at the forearm. The lesion is a tear in the annular ligament at its attachment on the radius. *(Behrman et al, pp. 1710–1711)*

16. **(C)** Allergic contact dermatitis in children, often caused by a reaction to shoe dyes, rubber, and other chemicals, involves the dorsum of the toes and the distal foot. The lesions are erythematous, scaly, and vesicular and are seen in prepubertal children. *(Polin et al, p. 38; Crapo et al, pp. 490–491)*

17. **(D)** Tinea pedis presents as interdigital maceration, scaling, and fissures. The scaling occurs primarily on the instep or weightbearing surface. Pruritus is a common symptom. Secondary bacterial infection is common. It is rarely seen before puberty. *(Polin et al, p. 38; Crapo et al, pp. 490–491)*

18. **(D)** The diagnosis of rheumatic fever is based on clinical grounds. The modified Jones criteria are classic for diagnosis. Two major manifestations or one major and two minor manifestations strongly suggest rheumatic fever. The major criteria are polyarthritis, carditis, erythema marginatum, subcu-

taneous nodules, and Sydenham's chorea. The minor manifestations are fever, arthralgia, previous rheumatic fever or rheumatic heart disease, an elevated sedimentation rate or C-reactive protein, and a prolonged P-R interval. *(Behrman et al, pp. 642–643)*

19. **(A)** Gynecomastia begins in Tanner stage II–III and disappears in 1 to 2 years. The underlying mass is mobile and there is no skin dimpling that would suggest a cancerous mass. The tissue is breast tissue, not fatty tissue secondary to obesity. Tenderness is a common symptom, as is irritation by clothing, which is relieved by wearing undershirts. Surgical intervention is not a common consideration; however, there are those males who have persistent breast tissue beyond the usual time for resolution and who are having significant psychologic problems with this disorder. Hence, surgery is considered, recommended, and successful. *(Kempe et al, p. 245)*

20. **(D)** Colicky abdominal pain is a common presenting symptom but not invariably present. The edema experienced by these patients is thought to be related to a protein-losing enteropathy secondary to the intestinal involvement in the disease. Most children have renal involvement in HSP. Not all patients have hematuria, but renal biopsy confirms the presence of renal disease in all patients. Platelet counts and coagulation studies are normal. Joint, ankle, and knee pain may be the presenting complaint. *(Hoekelman, pp. 276–277)*

21. **(C)** In idiopathic thrombocytopenic purpura (ITP), the platelet count is reduced to below 20,000/mm (some authors say less than 50,000/mm). Clot retraction, bleeding time, and the tourniquet test depend on platelet function and are abnormal in ITP. The white blood cell count is normal and anemia is usually not present. Although the differential smear may show decreased platelets, the working diagnosis is made by a platelet count and confirmed by bone examination. In adolescents, systemic lupus erythematosus is a consideration in the differential diagnosis

of thrombocytopenic purpura. This would make the ANA test appropriate for ruling out that disease, but would not substantiate the diagnosis of ITP. *(Behrman et al, pp. 1281–1283)*

22. **(C)** The cellular response in most cases of acute viral meningitis is predominately mononuclear cells, and with bacterial meningitis the differential classically shows a predominance of polymorphonuclear cells. Glucose is an important indicator of severe brain involvement. It is equally important in the differential diagnosis of bacterial meningitis and a more chronic infection such as tuberculosis. The CSF protein level increases in most cases of bacterial meningitis and ranges between 100 and 500 mg/dL. In viral meningitis the protein level usually ranges from 50 to 150 mg/dL. It is very uncommon for infectious mononucleosis to advance to the point of central nervous system symptoms. *(Jenson et al, pp. 792–796)*

23. **(B)** Hypovolemic shock occurs after a reduction in blood volume caused by factors that include hemorrhage (internal or external); plasma loss via burns, sepsis, nephrotic syndrome; fluid shift due to third spacing; fluid and electrolyte loss; or fluid shift due to endocrine conditions such as diabetes mellitus, diabetes insipidus, hypothyroidism, and adrenal insufficiency. Cardiogenic shock stems from a dysfunction of the heart that may result from myocardial insufficiency or mechanical obstruction to the flow of blood into and out of the heart. Distributive or vasogenic shock is due to decreased intravascular volume secondary to leaky capillaries resulting from conditions such as septic shock, anaphylaxis, or barbiturate intoxication. Clinically, the patient's skin is warm, dry, and flushed initially. Terminal shock is irreversible damage to the heart and brain due to altered metabolism and tissue perfusion. *(Barkin, pp. 50–51, Schmitt, pp. 591–596, 608–611)*

24. **(A), 25. (D), 26. (B), 27. (C), 28. (A), 29. (C), 30. (D), 31. (E) 32. (D), 33. (E).** Rubella is a moderately contagious virus that is transmitted through direct person-to-person contact or via contaminated respiratory secretions. Forscheimer spots are present in 50% to 75% of cases. Rubella causes a characteristic syndrome or congenital abnormalities in infants born alive to mothers who have had gestational rubella. The syndrome may include growth retardation, cardiac, ocular, and hearing abnormalities.

Erythema infectiosum (Fifth disease) is a viral exanthem recently found to be caused by human parvovirus. This disease occurs commonly in the winter and spring, and children and young adolescents are most frequently affected. A mild, nonspecific prodromal illness may precede the development of skin lesions. The exanthem begins on the face, where erythema and edema give the cheeks a characteristic "slapped cheek" appearance. Within several days, an erythematous, macular eruption develops on the trunk, buttocks, and extremities. Lesions in the involved area coalesce into a lacy reticular pattern.

Infectious mononucleosis is a viral illness of worldwide distribution caused by the Epstein-Barr virus. The disease begins with fever and malaise. Pharyngitis and lymphadenopathy commonly develop and may be accompanied by hepatosplenomegaly and jaundice. This infection should be suspected in the child or adolescent who has a prolonged illness with fatigue, fever, and lymphadenopathy. Rare complications include splenic rupture, aplastic anemia, and pneumonia.

Varicella zoster, or chickenpox is an extremely common childhood viral illness. After an incubation period of 10 to 20 days, small erythematous macules erupt on the scalp, face, and trunk. Vesicles develop within 24 hours and evolve over 1 to 2 days. Mild constitutional symptoms, including a low-grade fever, headache, and malaise, may be present, but children are not usually seriously ill. The most common complication of varicella is secondary bacterial skin infection. Rarely, the varicella may become purpuric, and progression of purpura fulminans has been reported.

Measles (rubeola) before widespread immunization was a common disease, primarily affecting children between 5 and 9 years of age. Koplik spots have long been considered pathognomonic of the diagnosis of measles. The cutaneous lesions of measles are preceded for 3 to 5 days by a prodrome consisting of fever, cough, rhinitis, conjunctivitis, diarrhea, and vomiting. Cervical lymphadenopathy may be present. The exanthem, consisting initially of discrete, red macules and papules, begins on the forehead and spreads over several days to involve the face, trunk, and extremities. (Jenson et al, pp. 572–574, 663–678)

34. **(B) 35. (A), 36. (D), 37. (C).** Carbon monoxide has an affinity for hemoglobin approximately 250 times that of oxygen. Thus, at a carbon monoxide air concentration of only 0.1% (1,000 parts per million), about one half of hemoglobin binding sites are occupied by the toxin. The half-life of the carboxyhemoglobin complex is 4 to 5 hours in room air, but can be shortened to about 40 minutes by administration of 100% oxygen.

Methemoglobinemia is an oxidized form of hemoglobin that is incapable of carrying oxygen. It may be formed by a variety of oxidizing agents, including nitrate-containing well water, as well as many medications, dyes, and industrial chemicals. Methemoglobin is incapable of carrying oxygen, and its presence produces a functional anemia. It also may interfere with oxygen delivery at the tissues by causing a leftward shift in the oxygen–hemoglobin dissociation curve. Methylene blue is a specific antidote and is the treatment of choice for significant methemoglobinemia.

Narcotic overdose in children and newborns can cause significant respiratory depression. Administration of naloxone, a competitive antagonist, should be performed intravenously to restore ventilation, antagonize coma, and reverse hypotension.

Organophosphates and carbamate insecticides are widely used for control of vector-borne disease; in food production, transport, and storage; and for domestic insect control.

These compounds can be found throughout the world in urban, suburban, and rural environments. Pediatric exposures to these insecticides account for more than 8,000 events/year in the United States alone. Atropine effectively counteracts all muscarinic and some of the central nervous system (CNS) effects of excessive acetylcholine. Atropine alone may be sufficient therapy in carbamate poisoning or in mild to moderate organophosphate poisonings when there are no significant CNS signs, muscular effects, or respiratory insufficiencies. *(Rudolph et al, pp. 817–843)*

38. **(C)** A subdural hematoma is the most dangerous inflicted injury, often causing death or serious neurological sequelae (ie, seizures, blindness, and/or mental retardation). Subdurals may be associated with skull fractures, but fractures will heal. Intra-abdominal injuries are the second most common cause of death in battered children. Because the abdominal wall is flexible, the force of a blow to the abdomen is usually absorbed by the internal organs, thus causing a ruptured liver or spleen, tears of the small intestine, or intramural hematomas. Subgaleal hematomas, although unsightly, usually resolve within a month, leaving no residual. Extremity fractures, if properly treated, heal without deformity or residual deficit in function. *(Behrman et al, p. 80)*

39. **(C)** Bone trauma is found in 10% to 20% of physically abused children. Inflicted fractures of the shaft of bones are usually spiral rather than transverse, and spiral fractures of the femur prior to the age of walking are usually inflicted. Multiple bony injuries at different stages of healing imply repeated assaults and are diagnostic of nonaccidental trauma. Fractures of the scapula or sternum are so unusual that they should arouse suspicion of inflicted injury. Many inflicted injuries result from pulling on an extremity. This force tears the periosteum from the bone, thus causing subperiostial bleeding. By 4 to 6 weeks after the injury, calcification occurs. Rare bone diseases, such as scurvy and syphilis may radiologically resemble nonaccidental bone trauma, but the bony changes are symmetrical. *(Behrman et al, p. 80)*

40. **(B)** Most frequently, children do not disclose sexual molestation for a long time. Therefore, at the time they present to the health care provider they are not having acute emotional distress. Also, because of the delay in disclosure, physical findings are usually absent. Positive cultures for gonorrhea are confirmatory evidence of sexual activity, but in and of themselves do not make a diagnosis. Parental assessments of a child's emotional state and behavioral changes also are supportive of the diagnosis. The diagnosis most often rests on the graphic history offered by the victim. This can include descriptions of sexual behaviors not commensurate with a child's development or experience level. *(Behrman et al, p. 82)*

41. **(D)** Most polycythemic infants are asymptomatic. Common early symptoms include plethora, cyanosis, lethargy, hypotonia, poor suck and feeding, and tremulousness. Serious complications include cardiorespiratory disease, seizures, peripheral gangrene, necrotizing enterocolitis, renal failure, and priaprism. *(Taeusch et al, pp. 822–823; Rudolph et al, pp. 252–255)*

42. **(D)** Symptoms of HMD occur after the onset of breathing. The incidence is 60% at 29 weeks' gestation and declines with maturation near zero by 39 weeks. The unventilated infant frequently requires 40% to 50% oxygen after birth but then develops an increasing oxygen requirement over 24 to 48 hours reaching as high as 100%. Chest x-rays show diffuse, fine granular densities. The appearance may be more marked at the lung bases than at the apices, and lung volume is ultimately decreased.

Current prevention includes prevention of premature birth, antenatal treatment of women with premature labor with glucocorticoid hormones and surfactant replacement, either prophylactically for small premature infants at risk for HMD or treatment of infants with established HMD. *(Taeusch et al, pp. 498–504; Rudolph et al, pp. 1598–1605)*

43. (E) 44. (A) 45. (B) 46. (C). The abuser is a related caretaker in 90% of the cases, a male friend of the mother in 5%, an unrelated babysitter in 4%, and a sibling in 1%. These statistics are apt to change as do social conditions: that is, currently, women are more likely to be involved in abuse, but this difference disappears in families in which the mothers work and fathers are the primary caretakers. There also is a trend for increased reporting of abuse in daycare settings. *(Behrman et al, p. 79; Rudolph et al, p. 571)*

47. (A) 48. (D), 49. (C), 50. (B), 51. (D), 52. (A), 53. (E), 54. (C). Group A beta-hemolytic streptococcus can present in many varied forms. An acute pharyngitis typically presents with fever, malaise, exudate on tonsils, palatal petechiae, and severe pain with swallowing. Untreated or prolonged infections can lead to rheumatic fever.

Staphylococcal infections are common in children and range from mild furuncle to very severe disseminated septicemia and toxic shock syndrome. Besides having the ability to cause both toxic and invasive disease, the staphylococci often are difficult to treat because of antibiotic resistance and formation of sequestered sites of infection. When ingested, typically food is seeded with *Staphylococcus aureus* and then allowed to incubate at room temperature, during which time one of the seven types of enterotoxins is formed. Shortly after ingestion, the preformed toxin acts on intestinal receptors to cause vomiting and diarrhea. Staph is greatly implicated in bullous impetigo.

The meningococcus is a normal commensal organism of the human upper respiratory tract. Colonization only infrequently leads to disseminated disease, yet the meningococcus remains a significant pathogen worldwide. The spectrum of invasive meningococcal disease also varies, but the most common presentation is meningococcemia with or without meningitis. Initially symptoms may include fever, pharyngitis, arthralgias, and myalgias but progress rapidly to meningitis and/or generalized sepsis with a hemorrhagic rash. The dominant features on examination include a toxic-appearing febrile patient with rash and signs of meningeal irritation.

The pneumococcus *(Streptococcus pneumoniae)* is a normal inhabitant of the upper respiratory tract of many children who are asymptomatic carriers of this organism. It is also a very important pathogen, a causative agent of otitis media (OM), sinusitis, and pneumonia. Less frequently it is responsible for bacteremia and meningitis. With pneumococcal pneumonia, the classic presenting signs are onset of shaking chills, fever, cough, and rust-colored sputum. Studies have shown that otitis media is caused more frequently by *S. pneumonia* than any other bacteria.

Neonatal sepsis (sepsis neonatorum) refers to the clinical condition associated with serious bacterial infections, especially bacteremia in infants during their first 4 weeks of life. The two most commonly isolated organisms in neonates with sepsis are group B beta hemolytic streptococci and *Escherichia coli*, accounting for 23% to 54% of all infections. *(Rudolph et al, pp. 536, 583–584, 601–602, 604–606)*

55. (D) Polycythemia beyond the immediate neonatal period is seen with arterial hypoxia due to cyanotic heart disease or pulmonary disorders. It can be caused by renal, hepatic, or cellular tumors or by hemoglobinopathies with increased oxygen affinity. *(Taeusch et al, pp. 822–823, Rudolph et al, pp. 252–255)*

56. (D) Genetic (parents' and infant's blood types) and ethnic factors are known to affect neonatal bilirubin levels. With Rh and ABO incompatibility, hemolysis of infant blood cells and subsequent release of bilirubin occurs. Serum bilirubin values appear to be significantly higher in apparently normal Chinese, Japanese, Korean, and American Indian babies. Some perinatal events associated with increased bilirubin include delayed cord clamping and traumatic delivery. Surveys indicate that somewhere between 1 in 50 and 1 in 200 breastfed infants will develop hyperbilirubinemia. This is usually of late onset (after the third day). Kernicterus has never been reported with breastfeeding jaundice. Temporary cessation of breastfeeding should be performed only if bilirubin levels have approached 20 mg/dL or when such interruption is crucial in establishing an etiology. *(Taeusch et al, pp. 754–757; Rudolph et al, pp. 1133, 1193–1200)*

57. **(B)** In children younger than 15 months of age, HIV seropositivity may be due to the passive transmission of maternal antibody in the perinatal period. Diagnosis of AIDS disease in younger children must be confirmed by a positive viral culture, a positive antigen, or indirect abnormalities, or a decreased T/T ratio. Of infants born to HIV infected mothers, 30% will acquire HIV infection. *(Jenson et al, pp. 578–581)*

58. **(A)** Varicella zoster immune globin (VZIG) should be given to a newborn infant of a mother who had chickenpox within 5 days before delivery or within 48 hours after delivery. VZIG does not modify established varicella. A newborn exposed to at sibling with varicella is not considered to be at high risk for complicated varicella because transplacental maternal antibody will usually protect the infant. *(Report of the Committee of Infectious Diseases, pp. 442–444; Gerber et al, pp. 153–155; Jenson and Baltimore, pp. 1416–1421)*

59. **(D)** The following are the major manifestations of rheumatic fever: carditis, polyarthritis, chorea, erythema marginatum, and subcutaneous nodules. Erythema chronicum migrans (now more commonly known as simply erythema migrans) is the first clinical manifestation of *Borrelia burgdorferi*, or Lyme disease. Described as an annular rash that first appears at the site of the tick bite and gradually expands and becomes larger in diameter, it can occur anywhere on the body, most commonly at the axillae, periumbilical, thighs, and groin. Erythema marginatum lesions begin as small, pink, or red macules that may be slightly raised. Over time, these lesions expand centrifugally, leading to areas with clear centers surrounded by distinct, pink, serpiginous, or circular margins most

often found on the trunk, but never on the face. *(Rudolph and Baltimore, pp. 429–431, 643–645)*

60. **(B)** Colic is not predominant in either sex. Its rate of occurrence is equal in both males and females. Colic crying may occur at any time of the day, although it frequently occurs at the same time each day. The cause of colic is not known, but it is felt to be associated with hunger and with swallowed air that passes into the intestines. While mother anxiety can increase the reporting of colic symptoms, even anxious parents are accurate in their reporting of quality and quantity of crying. Most colic resolves by age 3 months. However, 30% of babies with colic will have symptoms up to 4 months of age. In the absence of infant or parental illness, the outcome, including mother–infant interaction, is excellent. *(Behrman et al, pp. 128–129; Rudolph et al, pp. 98–100)*

61. **(C)** In fragile X syndrome the testes are large. Fragile X syndrome also is associated with mental retardation. Cryptorchid testes are associated with many congenital and chromosomal abnormalities. *(Behrman et al, pp. 295, 1378)*

62. **(D)** Isometric exercises such as weight lifting should be discouraged in adolescents with hypertension, as this form of exercise produces a marked increase in both systolic and diastolic pressures. Severe fractures involving the epiphysis may result in growth disturbance if not properly treated. Hypertrophic cardiomyopathy is characterized by a massive ventricular septum. It can occur at any age and in some instances is transmitted in an autosomal dominant pattern. Many children are asymptomatic and are evaluated only because of heart murmur, but even those children are at risk for sudden death. As many as 10% to 20% of children with Down syndrome have atlantoaxial instability, and children with this diagnosis should have cervical x-ray prior to their participation in sports. Activities such as swimming, which generally does not induce bronchospasm, should be encouraged for asth-

matics. *(Behrman et al, pp. 587–592, 1210–1211, 1721–1725)*

63. **(C)** Any mention of suicide ideation should be treated as a real threat to the child's safety until proven otherwise. Fifty percent of completed suicides follow previous attempts or threats. Adolescent females will attempt suicide twice as often as adolescent males but males are twice as successful as females. Firearms are the most common method of suicide followed by hanging, jumping, carbon monoxide, and self-poisoning. Suicide attempters most often will try self-poisoning followed by cutting their wrists.

Determining if a child is at risk for suicide requires asking specific questions, such as: "Have you thought of hurting yourself?" "Have you ever wished you were dead?" "Have you planned a way to kill yourself?" Indications of suicidal thoughts will require a psychiatric evaluation to determine whether the patient is a risk to his or her own personal safety. It is crucial to obtain a "no suicide agreement," in which the patient promises not to harm himself or herself or agrees to tell a parent or provider whether he or she is feeling suicidal. Suicidal behavior has become increasingly common, and studies have shown that an increase in suicide and suicidal gestures often is noted in communities where adolescent suicide has recently occurred. *(Rudolph et al, pp. 40–42, 172–173)*

64. **(D)** Anorexic patients show excessive physical activity, deny hunger, and yet are preoccupied with food preparation and academic success. Most parents will describe their anorexic child as model children before the illness. Of the children affected, 5% to 10% will be male, many of whom have gender identity issues. *(Behrman et al, p. 533; Rudolph et al, pp. 40–43)*

65. **(B)** Down syndrome is due to the presence of an extra number 21 chromosome and is the most frequently occurring chromosomal abnormality. Some of the characteristics include low nasal bridge, upward slanted palpebral fissures on the face, simian creases on the palms, and increased frequency (30% to 50%) of congenital heart disease. Down syndrome is associated with increased maternal age, although the exact etiology is unclear. Mental retardation is a universal feature of Down syndrome, although the range of IQ scores is wide.

66. **(D)** The DPT is composed of diphtheria toxoid, tetanus toxoid, and inactivated whole *Bordetella pertussis* cells. The vaccination is recommended to be given at ages 2, 4, 6, and 15 months with a booster given between ages 4 and 6 years. Contraindications to DPT are previous severe reactions to DPT, including encephalopathy within 7 days of administration of previous dose of DPT; fever of >40°C within 48 hours after vaccination with a prior dose of DPT; collapse or shock-like state within 48 hours of prior dose of DPT; seizures within 3 days of receiving a prior dose of DPT; persistent, inconsolable crying lasting >3 hours within 48 hours of receiving a prior DPT vaccination. The most severe reactions occur with the pertussis portion of the vaccine. Common side effects to the vaccination include pain and swelling at the site of the injection. Systemic reactions include low to moderate fever, fretfulness, drowsiness, vomiting, and anorexia. *(Rudolph et al, pp. 31–33)*

67. **(D)** Milia are tiny inclusion cysts derived from follicular or ductal epithelia that are most common on the face of full-term newborns but may be seen on other areas. These 1 to 2-mm white papules express a cheesy-white material when lanced. Acne neonatorum is characterized by appearance at 3 to 4 weeks of comedones, papules, pustules on the face, especially the cheeks and forehead. Erythema toxicum is characterized by appearance at 24 to 48 hours to a few weeks old of erythematous macules, papules, and pustules which occur on the buttocks, torso, and proximal extremities. It is not seen on the palms and soles. Sebaceous gland hyperplasia is not typically seen in newborns, and sys-

temic neonate candidiasis is characterized by erythema and fine papules that evolve into pustules and can appear anywhere on the body but are not commonly seen in 40% of newborns. *(Rudolph et al, pp. 883–887)*

68. **(E)** Mongolian spots (dermal melanosis) are very common in darkly pigmented races and occur in 80% to 90% of Asian and African American newborns. They are described as a poorly defined blue-gray discoloration that is present at birth. The most frequent location is the skin overlying the buttocks and sacrococcygeal region, but other areas maybe involved. Mongolian spots are caused by the persistence of migrating melanocytes within the lower dermis. These lesions often disappear by age 2, although mongolian spots on the extremities may not. Café au lait spots are sharply defined evenly pigmented macules that may occur on any part of the skin surface. Blue nevus is a dome-shaped blue to black nodule of 0.3 to 1.0 cm. Blue nevi may rarely be present at birth, but more commonly arise during childhood or adolescence. Congenital melanocytic nevi are present in 1% to 2% of newborns. These lesions vary in size from those less than 1 mm to lesions that cover large areas of skin. These lesions can be flat, verrucous, or nodular. A nevus of ota is a unilateral, mottled, blue to brown discoloration involving the periorbital skin and forehead. *(Rudolph et al, pp. 884, 902)*

69. **(C)** Because of the large number of infectious agents that contribute to the occurrence of acute otitis media, immunization is not a practical consideration to control middle-ear infection. The other factors listed are well-known contributors to increased risk for developing infections, especially in otitis-prone children. *(Jenson et al, pp. 923–933)*

70. **(E)** Epiglottitis is a cellulitis of the supraglottic structures and is typically caused by *Haemophilis influenzae* type B. This illness progresses rapidly, usually occurs in a child older than 2, and presents with a history of rapid onset of fever, sore throat, and muffled voice. Stridor and respiratory distress may follow, and drooling or pooling of secretions is noted in 70% of the patients. Acute laryngotracheobronchitis, or croup, is a very common infection occurring seasonally with peaks in fall and early winter. It presents with nasal congestion and irritation followed by Coryza, sore throat, and cough. Fever develops within 24 hours of symptoms and is usually mild. A hoarse or barky cough is classic. Bronchiolitis is classically seen in winter months and presents initially with cough, coryza, and rhinorrhea. It then progresses within a few days to noisy raspy breathing and wheezing. Symptoms usually resolve within 5 days. A small number of infants will require hospitalization and only with supportive treatment will improve. Laryngotracheomalacia results from instability of the trachea due to pliable or soft tracheal cartilage. The signs include wheezing, stridor, and respiratory distress that may worsen with administration of inhaled bronchodilators. Symptoms usually lessen with time, and in most patients no specific therapy is indicated. *(Jenson et al, pp. 951–970; Rudolph et al, p. 1582)*

71. **(B)** Pyloric stenosis classically will present with the following history: commonly firstborn male, gradual onset on projectile vomiting after 3 weeks of age. However, 20% will be symptomatic from birth. These infants may present with weight loss or poor weight gain. Careful history taking will differentiate between failure to thrive and pyloric stenosis. Intussusception, which occurs when one portion of the bowel invaginates or telescopes into the lumen of adjoining bowel, is common among children age 2 months to 5 years and presents with pain, vomiting, and blood in the stools. One classic description is "currant-jelly stools." Children with chronic inflammatory bowel disease present with diarrhea, rectal bleeding, pain, anorexia, and weight loss. Their age is typically between 2 and 14. *(Rudolph et al, pp. 411, 1068, 1070, 1092–1099)*

72. **(A)** Hepatitis A infection is transmitted by the fecal–oral route. Usually by oral ingestion of shellfish, water, or food contaminated by

sewage. Signs and symptoms are usually mild and nonspecific. Hepatitis A is highly contagious, and epidemics may arise from a common source of virus. Hepatitis B and C are transmitted only by parenteral means, sexually, or perinatally. Infectious mononucleosis symptoms include fever, sore throat, fatigue, malaise, and lymphadenopathy. Giardiasis causes acute and chronic diarrhea associated with intestinal malabsorption. *(Jenson and Baltimore, pp. 568, 1114–1115, 1169–1171)*

73. **(B)** Reye–Johnson syndrome typically follows an illness with influenza type B viral infections, but will often follow varicella. Most commonly seen in children age 6 to 12 years. Often the history reveals that the child was recovering from an illness when vomiting, anorexia, and listlessness reoccur. Mild cognitive changes may follow, or it may develop further to delirium followed by light coma with decorticate posturing. The deeper the coma, the greater the child is at risk for serious neurological sequelae and/or death. There is an association of Reye–Johnson syndrome with salicylate ingestion. Encephalitis, or encephalopathy, is a broad term used to describe a disturbance of consciousness ranging from mild confusion to deep coma. Reye–Johnson syndrome is one of the types of acute encephalopathy.

Hepatitis C is a viral illness contracted only parentally, sexually, or perinatally, and symptoms, although serious, are not that severe. Cerebal palsy is a static encephalopathy and refers to a state of chronic cerebral dysfunction.

Guillain–Barré syndrome is an acute inflammatory demyelinating polyradiculoneuropathy that begins with a rapidly evolving weakness of the legs, followed by involvement of the arms. This illness can go on to hamper cranial nerve function and respiratory compromise due to intercostal muscle weakness. *(Rudolph et al, pp. 1885–1890, 1892–1896, 1970–1972, 1997)*

74. **(C)** Oral candidiasis or thrush, typically presents with discrete white, curd-like patches and plaques on the buccal mucosa, tongue, gums, and palate. They are difficult to remove and are located on an erythematous base. They can be very painful and interfere with nursing.

Herpangina can be caused by any of several coxsackievirus or echo virus types and usually present with painful vesicles on an erythematous base and may be accompanied by fever, headache, and pharyngitis and dysphagia.

Herpes simplex virus stomatitis involves the gingiva and vermilion border with extensive involvement and rapid progression from macules to papules within 24 hours. Lesions are tender, very friable, and typically heal within 1 to 2 weeks.

Streptococcal pharyngitis may cause decreased nursing and white patches on the tonsils. However, this is not typically seen in infants, and the white patches or exudate are not seen on the buccal mucosa, tongue, gums, or palate. Teething may cause decreased nursing and mild fever, but is not associated with white patches in the mouth. *(Jenson and Baltimore, pp. 675, 679, 901–902)*

75. **(D) 76. (A), 77. (B), 78. (D), 79. (C), 80. (D), 81. (E), 82. (C), 83. (D), 84. (B).** There are average normal developmental gains for every age group, and although it is important to monitor every child's developmental progress; every child is different and develops at his or her own pace. By 3 months an infant should be smiling both responsively and spontaneously. By 6 months an infant should be able to roll over, grasp objects, and bring them to the mouth. At 1 year infants should be able to feed themselves with finger foods and make word-like vocalizations. At 18 months toddlers should be able to feed themselves with a spoon (spilling some), walk independently and use single intelligible words to express self. The average 2-year-old should be able to follow two-step commands. *(Rudolph et al, pp. 3–44)*

85. **(C)** **86.** **(E)** **87.** **(A)** **88.** **(D)** **89.** **(B).** Osteoarthritis is manifested when the physical examination of the patellofemoral compartment of the knee joint yields pain and crepitus. A mild or moderate sprain is diagnosed by incomplete tearing of a ligament as opposed to a strain that involves the tendon. Tearing of a tendon can cause instability in a joint. Osgood–Schlatter disease is a painful inflammatory disorder of the proximal tibial physis at the point of insertion of the patellar tendon on the tibia. A slipped capital femoral epiphysis occurs when the epiphysis falls posteriorly and medially. This can occur suddenly or gradually and is a problem of late childhood or adolescence. It commonly affects boys twice as often as girls, and the classic patient is an overweight, hypogonadal boy with skeletal maturity lagging behind chronologic age. Juvenile rheumatoid arthritis is described as the persistence of objective inflammatory findings in one or more joints for 6 or more weeks. The joint involvement is classically symmetrical but can occur unilaterally. *(Bates, pp. 450–451; Rudolph et al, pp. 479, 2129, 2145–2154)*

90. **(A),** **91.** **(B),** **92.** **(D),** **93.** **(D),** **94.** **(C).** Marfan's syndrome is an inherited disorder of connective tissue that involves the skin, skeleton, aorta, heart, and eyes. Unusually long limbs and spider fingers and toes are a portion of the skeletal manifestations that can be observed.

Torticollis presents with a tightened sternocleidomastoid muscle on one side, and the chin is rotated toward that side. Patients will often present with no complaints, just the head held to one side or history of inconsolable crying. This may also be noted at birth.

Scoliosis is a curvature of the spine measuring 10 degrees or more in the frontal plane. The idiopathic form is detected more often in adolescent females and there is no apparent etiology. The congenital form is caused by failure of formation or fusion of ossific nuclei of the vertebrae in utero.

Clubfoot, or congenital talipes equinovirus is a deformity that occurs in utero and includes deformity of the forefoot, hindfoot, and ankle. This can occur unilaterally or bilaterally and is typically an extreme plantar flexion of the ankle and medial angulation of the foot. *(Rudolph et al, pp. 392–394, 2134, 2143–2145, 2153–2155)*

95. **(D),** **96.(C),** **97.** **(B),** **98.** **(E),** **99.** **(B),** **100.** **(A).** Ehlers–Danlos syndrome includes a group of syndromes of connective tissue disorders that include a variety of the following features; hyperextensible skin, hypermobile joints, dystrophic scarring, and easy bruisability.

Turner's syndrome is a form of gonadal dysgenesis. The most common features include: atypical facies, broad chest, low hairline, webbed neck, coarctation of the aorta, hypertension, and absence of secondary sex characteristics.

Trisomy 21 or Down syndrome is the most common malformation-mental retardation syndrome in humans. Among its physical features are upslanting palpebral fissures, flat nasal bridge, large protruding tongue, epicanthal folds, simian lines, and facial grimace with crying.

Osteogenesis imperfecta is commonly described as belonging to a group of genetic skeletal dysplasias. Its features include excessive bone fragility and blue sclera. Hearing loss develops later in life.

Trisomy 18 has a distinct form of malformation including: high nasal bridge, short palpebral fissures, micrognathia, small mouth, overriding fingers and hypoplastic nails. *(Rudolph et al, pp. 208–213, 297, 405, 394, 387, 1782–1783)*

REFERENCES

Avery ME. First, LR (eds), *Pediatric Medicine,* 1st ed. Baltimore MD: Williams & Williams; 1989.

Barkin RM. *Emergency Pediatrics,* 3rd ed. St. Louis, MO: Mosby; 1990.

Bates B. *A Guide to Physical Examination and History Taking,* 5th ed. Philadelphia: Lippincott; 1991.

Behrman RE, et al (eds). *Nelson Textbook of Pediatrics,* 14th ed. Philadelphia: Saunders; 1992.

Crapo JD, Hamilton MA, Edgman S (eds). *Medicine and Pediatrics in One Book.* St. Louis, MO: Mosby; 1988.

Gerber MA, Randolph MD, DeMae K, et al. *Failure of once-daily penicillin V therapy for streptococcal pharyngitis.* Am J Dis Child. 1989; 143: 153–155.

Hoekelman RA, et al. *Primary Pediatric Care,* 2nd ed. St. Louis, MO: Mosby; 1992.

Jenson HB, Baltimore RS. *Pediatric Infectious Diseases.* Norwalk, CT: Appleton & Lange; 1995.

Kempe CH, et al (eds). *Current Pediatric Diagnosis and Treatment,* 10th ed. Norwalk, CT: Appleton & Lange; 1991.

Oski A, et al (eds). *Principles and practice of pediatrics.* Philadelphia: Lippincott; 1990.

Polin RA, Ditmar MF. *Pediatrics Secrets.* St. Louis, MO: Mosby; 1989.

Report of the Committee of Infectious Diseases (The Red Book), 21st ed. Elk Grove Village, IL: American Academy of Pediatrics; 1989.

Rudolph AM, Hoffman JIE, Rudolph CD. *Rudolph's Pediatrics,* 20th ed. Norwalk, CT: Appleton & Lange; 1991.

Schmitt BD. *Your Child's Health.* Toronto: Bantam; 1991.

Taeusch HW, Ballard RA, Avery ME. *Schaffer and Avery's Diseases of the Newborn,* 6th ed. Philadelphia: Saunders; 1992.

CHAPTER 4

Emergency Medicine
Questions

Scott B. Harp, EMT-P, PA-C

DIRECTIONS (Questions 1 through 3): Each of the numbered items or incomplete statements in this section is followed by answers or by completions of the statement. Select the ONE lettered answer or completion that is BEST in each case.

Questions 1 through 3

1. The most common form of shock in the initial phase of multisystem trauma is

    (A) hypovolemic shock
    (B) septic shock
    (C) neurogenic shock
    (D) cardiogenic shock
    (E) burn shock

2. Using the rule-of-nines, calculate the body surface area (BSA) involvement of an adult with a circumferential burn injury involving the left leg and right arm.

    (A) 9%
    (B) 18%
    (C) 27%
    (D) 36%
    (E) 70%

3. Alcohol is involved in what percent of fatal single vehicle accidents?

    (A) 10%
    (B) 20%
    (C) 40%

    (D) 60%
    (E) 100%

DIRECTIONS (Questions 4 through 7): Each group of items in this section consists of lettered headings followed by a set of numbered words or phrases. For each numbered word or phrase, select the ONE lettered heading that is most closely associated with it. Each lettered heading may be selected once, more than once, or not at all.

Questions 4 through 7

Match the type of shock with its characteristic physical findings.

    (A) hypotension without tachycardia, peripheral vasodilation
    (B) hypotension, tachycardia, distended neck veins
    (C) near normal blood pressure, tachycardia, wide pulse pressure
    (D) tachycardia, peripheral vasoconstriction, narrow pulse pressure
    (E) tachycardia, edema due to loss of plasma volume

4. Hypovolemic shock

5. Septic shock

6. Cardiogenic shock

7. Neurogenic shock

DIRECTIONS (Questions 8 through 14): Each of the numbered items or incomplete statements in this section is followed by answers or by completions of the statement. Select the ONE lettered answer or completion that is BEST in each case.

Questions 8 through 14

8. Potentially lethal chest trauma includes all of the following EXCEPT

    (A) pneumothorax
    (B) hemothorax
    (C) open chest wound
    (D) cardiac tamponade

9. All of the following are indicated for the treatment of corneal ulceration EXCEPT

    (A) topical antibiotic treatment
    (B) topical cycloplegics
    (C) prompt ophthalmology referral
    (D) topical steroids

10. Common causes of hypovolemic shock in the trauma patient include all of the following EXCEPT

    (A) femur fractures
    (B) pelvic fractures
    (C) hemothorax
    (D) closed head injury

11. Compartment syndromes often result from crush injuries or fractures of an extremity. Reliable early signs and symptoms include all of the following EXCEPT

    (A) pulselessness and decreased capillary refill
    (B) decreased sensation of nerves transversing the involved compartment
    (C) tense swelling of the compartment
    (D) pain increased by passive stretching of the compartment

12. Emergency care of the major burn patient includes all of the following EXCEPT

    (A) administration of IV fluids
    (B) supplemental oxygen therapy

    (C) prophylactic IV antibiotics
    (D) analgesia

13. Which one of the following radiographic findings would be considered the most reliable finding suggestive of aortic transection?

    (A) obliteration of aortic knob
    (B) widened mediastinum
    (C) presence of pleural cap
    (D) deviation of trachea to the right
    (E) multiple rib fractures

14. Treatment of flail chest injuries includes which one of the following?

    (A) positioning the patient on the affected side
    (B) positioning the patient away from the affected side
    (C) placing sandbags on the flail segment
    (D) intubating and performing positive pressure ventilation in patients with respiratory distress
    (E) performing chest decompression

DIRECTIONS (Questions 15 through 17): Each group of items in this section consists of lettered headings followed by a set of numbered words or phrases. For each numbered word or phrase, select the ONE lettered heading that is most closely associated with it. Each lettered heading may be selected once, more than once, or not at all.

Questions 15 through 17

Match the following diagnosis with the corresponding physical finding.

    (A) an infection localized to the finger tuft
    (B) an infection localized around the nail fold
    (C) an infection over the hair-bearing regions of the hand and arm

15. Paronychia

16. Felon

17. Carbuncle

DIRECTIONS (Questions 18 through 26): Each of the numbered items or incomplete statements in this section is followed by answers or by completions of the statement. Select the ONE lettered answer or completion that is BEST in each case.

Questions 18 through 26

18. Which spinal nerve supplies sensation to only the middle finger?

    (A) C5
    (B) C6
    (C) C7
    (D) C8
    (E) T1

19. Sensation to the skin of the legs and feet is derived from lumbar and sacral nerves. Which spinal nerve supplies sensation to the lateral aspect of the foot?

    (A) L3
    (B) L4
    (C) L5
    (D) S1
    (E) S2

20. Which one of the following sexually transmitted diseases could be described as a painful ulcerative lesion?

    (A) chancroid
    (B) lymphogranuloma venereum
    (C) granuloma inguinala
    (D) condyloma acuminata
    (E) syphilis

21. Radiographic findings suggestive of small-bowel obstruction include which of the following?

    (A) large amount of gas within the large bowel
    (B) free intraperitoneal air seen best under the diaphragm on the upright abdominal film
    (C) dilated loops of small-bowel proximal to the affected area
    (D) haustral markings that do not cross the entire lumen

22. A 35-year-old male presents to the ER with a 2-hour history of severe epigastric pain. He reports the sudden onset of this discomfort. The patient denies vomiting. He reports a long history of intermittent abdominal pain relieved by antacids. The patient is lying on the stretcher, avoiding all movement. The abdomen is diffusely tender with muscular rigidity and guarding. The most likely diagnosis is

    (A) acute cholecystitis
    (B) perforated duodenal ulcer
    (C) acute appendicitis
    (D) acute diverticulitis
    (E) cholelithiasis

23. Which of the following is NOT a common cause of small-bowel obstruction?

    (A) mesenteric lymphadenopathy
    (B) intussusception
    (C) abdominal wall or internal hernias
    (D) adhesions from previous abdominal surgeries

24. Which of the following medications is recommended as first-line therapy when treating the severely hyperkalemic patient with significant ECG changes?

    (A) sodium bicarbonate
    (B) insulin and $D_{50}W$
    (C) calcium gluconate
    (D) nebulized albuterol
    (E) sodium polystyrene sulfonate

25. Which of the following would NOT be included when treating the patient with acute abdominal pain?

    (A) nasogastric suctioning
    (B) serial physical exams
    (C) adequate anesthesia
    (D) intravascular volume replacement

26. Murphy's sign is best described as

    (A) referred pain from the abdomen to the shoulder or scapula
    (B) rebound tenderness often seen in peritonitis
    (C) pain with palpation of the right upper quadrant upon deep inspiration, pain causes patient to halt inspiratory effort
    (D) abdominal pain elicited by gently rocking the pelvis
    (E) a fetal position assumed by the patient with abdominal pain

DIRECTIONS (Questions 27 through 30): Each group of items in this section consists of lettered headings followed by a set of numbered words or phrases. For each numbered word or phrase, select the ONE lettered heading that is most closely associated with it. Each lettered heading may be selected once, more than once, or not at all.

Questions 27 through 30

Match the following pain patterns and location with the most likely diagnosis.

    (A) sudden, severe midepigastric pain that progresses to diffuse abdominal discomfort
    (B) sudden, severe right upper-quadrant pain with radiation to the right scapular and shoulder region
    (C) severe epigastric pain with radiation to the back
    (D) vague midabdominal pain that localizes to the right lower quadrant

27. Perforated duodenal ulcer

28. Acute cholecystitis

29. Appendicitis

30. Acute pancreatitis

DIRECTIONS (Questions 31 through 37): Each of the numbered items or incomplete statements in this section is followed by answers or by completions of the statement. Select the ONE lettered answer or completion that is BEST in each case.

Questions 31 through 37

31. A 65-year-old white male presents to the ER with a 6-hour complaint of progressive pain at the right lower extremity. Upon further questioning, he mentions that over the past 6 months he has noticed that after walking approximately one block, the right leg "gives out." His past medical history is significant for hypertension, diabetes type II, and a 25-pack-year history of cigarette smoking. Examination reveals a cool right foot. He has a palpable right femoral pulse with unobtainable pulses at the popliteal, dorsalis pedis, and posterior tibial points. There is no pedal edema and the motor-sensory function at the foot is intact. Which of the following is the most likely cause?

    (A) arterial embolization
    (B) deep venous thrombosis
    (C) arterial thrombosis
    (D) thrombophlebitis
    (E) spinal stenosis

32. A 60-year-old male presents to the ER with hematemesis. Past medical history is significant for cirrhosis. Physical examination is significant for disorientation, ascites, and splenomegaly. The most likely diagnosis is

    (A) upper gastrointestinal (UGI) bleeding secondary to perforated duodenal ulcer
    (B) UGI bleeding secondary to erosive gastritis
    (C) UGI bleeding secondary to Mallory–Weiss tears
    (D) UGI bleeding secondary to gastroesophageal varices
    (E) UGI bleeding secondary to Boerhaave syndrome

33. Proper treatment of soft-tissue abscesses in an otherwise healthy individual consists of which of the following?

    (A) application of hot packs
    (B) observation and close follow-up
    (C) administration of broad-spectrum antibiotics

(D) incision, drainage, and local wound care

(E) application of topical antibiotics

34. Which of the following statements is true regarding pilonidal abscesses?

(A) They arise from fistulous communications with the rectosigmoid colon.

(B) They commonly have a chronic waxing and waning course.

(C) They require chronic antibiotic therapy for definitive treatment.

(D) Frank abscess formation can be readily appreciated over the presacral area.

35. Which of the following is considered to be a contraindication for excision of a sebaceous cyst?

(A) recurrent infections

(B) acute inflammation

(C) increasing size

(D) head or neck location

36. Which of the following best describes a boutonniere deformity?

(A) loss of extension in the distal phalangeal joint

(B) hyperextended distal interphalangeal (DIP) joint and flexed proximal interphalangeal (PIP) joint

(C) flexion of DIP joint

(D) lateral displacement at the PIP joint

37. Proper first aid care following a suspected venomous snake bite includes all of the following EXCEPT

(A) rapid transportation to the nearest hospital

(B) immobilization of the affected extremity

(C) application of a constricting band, proximal to the wound to impede lymphatic drainage

(D) application of ice to the affected area

(E) positioning the affected area below the level of the heart

DIRECTIONS (Questions 38 through 41): Each group of items in this section consists of lettered headings followed by a set of numbered words or phrases. For each numbered word or phrase, select the ONE lettered heading that is most closely associated with it. Each lettered heading may be selected once, more than once, or not at all.

Questions 38 through 41

Match the following kidney, ureter, and bladder (KUB) radiographic findings with the most likely corresponding abdominal process.

(A) free air beneath the diaphragm

(B) loss of psoas shadow

(C) dilated loops of small bowel with air fluid levels

(D) lower rib fractures

(E) essentially normal KUB

38. Small-bowel obstruction

39. Retroperitoneal abscess

40. Duodenal ulcer perforation

41. Hemoperitoneum

DIRECTIONS (Questions 42 through 55): Each of the numbered items or incomplete statements in this section is followed by answers or by completions of the statement. Select the ONE lettered answer or completion that is BEST in each case.

Questions 42 through 55

42. The most common cause of large-bowel obstruction in the adult is which of the following?

(A) diverticulitis

(B) abdominal wall hernias

(C) carcinoma

(D) sigmoid volvulus

(E) adhesions

43. Which of the following is the most important aspect of managing epistaxis?

    (A) immediate insertion of anterior packing
    (B) compression of the mobile portion of the nose
    (C) localizing the site of bleeding
    (D) immediate insertion of posterior packing
    (E) place patient in a supine position

44. Which of the following is a common finding in the patient with acute diverticulitis?

    (A) severe abdominal tenderness
    (B) left flank pain
    (C) frank bleeding
    (D) left lower-quadrant pain
    (E) chronic diarrhea

45. During the initial assessment and resuscitation of the patient with multiple blunt trauma, all of the following roentgenograms should be obtained EXCEPT

    (A) cervical spine
    (B) anterior-posterior (AP) chest
    (C) anterior-posterior (AP) pelvis
    (D) skull x-rays

46. Early signs and symptoms suggestive of inhalation injury in the burn patient includes all of the following EXCEPT

    (A) singed nasal hair
    (B) carbonaceous sputum
    (C) darkened oral or nasal mucosa
    (D) patchy infiltrates on chest radiograph

47. Burn shock is best described as

    (A) hypovolemia due to loss of plasma volume into the extravascular spaces
    (B) hypovolemia due to widespread thermal lysis of blood vessels
    (C) cardiogenic shock due to myocardial depression
    (D) hypovolemia due to bleeding from the burn wound
    (E) heart failure due to renal failure and volume overload

48. Which one of the following medications is used to treat an acute dystonic reaction?

    (A) Haldol
    (B) Cogentin
    (C) Prolixin
    (D) Navane
    (E) Thorazine

49. Which one of the following is recommended for treating a chemical burn caused by hydrofluoric acid?

    (A) dressings soaked with iced calcium gluconate solution after irrigation with water
    (B) copious irrigation with water followed by polyethylene glycol solution
    (C) application of copper sulfate solution
    (D) copious irrigation with water followed by sodium bicarbonate solution

50. The most effective method of providing anesthesia for repair of finger lacerations, fractured phalanx, or abscess drainage is

    (A) topical anesthetics
    (B) bier block
    (C) digital block
    (D) intramuscular analgesia
    (E) ice packs

51. Which of the following is the correct term used to describe the dermatologic manifestations of Lyme disease?

    (A) erysipelas
    (B) pityriasis rosea
    (C) erythema multiforme
    (D) erythema migrans

52. The most commonly fractured bone is the

    (A) distal tibia
    (B) clavicle
    (C) distal radius
    (D) rib
    (E) mandible

53. The best method of restoring adequate intravascular volume in the hypovolemic patient is

(A) central venous lines, namely, subclavian or jugular lines

(B) saphenous vein cutdowns

(C) large peripheral IVs

(D) fluid boluses via the infusion part of pulmonary artery catheters

(E) administration of antidiuretic hormone

54. General principles of chest tube insertion include all of the following EXCEPT

(A) inserting the chest tube no lower than the 5th intercostal space

(B) placing the tube under the inferior aspect of the rib

(C) inserting the chest tube between the anterior to midaxillary line

(D) after puncturing the pleura, placing a gloved finger through the pleura to check for adhesed lung

55. Which one of the following medications is contraindicated when treating a suspected tricyclic antidepressant (TCA) overdose?

(A) diazepam

(B) sodium bicarbonate

(C) lidocaine

(D) phenytoin

(E) procainamide

DIRECTIONS (Questions 56 through 63): Each group of items in this section consists of lettered headings followed by a set of numbered words or phrases. For each numbered word or phrase, select the ONE lettered heading that is most closely associated with it. Each lettered heading may be selected once, more than once, or not at all.

Questions 56 through 59

Match the following types of fractures with their common complications.

(A) femoral shaft fractures

(B) femoral neck fractures

(C) open tibial fractures

(D) supracondylar humeral fracture

(E) scapular fractures

56. Osteomyelitis

57. Volkmann's ischemic contracture

58. Avascular necrosis

59. Fat emboli syndrome

Questions 60 through 63

Match the following cord syndromes with their clinical characteristics.

(A) anterior cord syndrome

(B) Brown–Sequard syndrome

(C) nerve root syndrome

(D) complete cord syndrome

(E) disc herniations

60. Flaccid paralysis below cord lesion

61. Complete paralysis, loss of pain perception with preservation of light touch, proprioception, and temperature sensation

62. Hemisection of the cord resulting in loss of proprioception, vibration, and light touch on the side of the lesion, loss of pain and temperature on the contralateral side

63. Typically occurs as a cervical injury with motor deficits that are more severe than sensory deficit

DIRECTIONS (Questions 64 through 76): Each of the numbered items or incomplete statements in this section is followed by answers or by completions of the statement. Select the ONE lettered answer or completion that is BEST in each case.

Questions 64 through 76

64. Clinical signs of lumbar disc herniation include all of the following EXCEPT

(A) hyperreflexia of deep-tendon reflexes

(B) sciatic pain with straight leg raising

(C) muscle weakness

(D) low-back pain made worse by Valsalva

65. A 65-year-old male presents to the ER with anorexia, malaise, shaking, chills, and watery diarrhea. Chest x-ray demonstrates small alveolar infiltrates. Sputum samples are somewhat watery with Gram stains demonstrating a few polymorphonuclear leukocytes and no predominant bacterial species. Temperature is 103°F. The most likely diagnosis is

    (A) *Klebsiella pneumoniae*
    (B) Lyme disease
    (C) Legionnaire's disease
    (D) mycoplasma pneumonia
    (E) viral meningitis

66. Each of the following signs could be present in a patient with meningitis EXCEPT

    (A) Brudzinski's sign
    (B) Kernig's sign
    (C) purpura
    (D) petechiae
    (E) Chvostek's sign

67. A 30-year-old white male presents to the urgent treatment center with a complaint of a 4-week persistent cough. He has no past medical history. He has a 15-pack-year history of cigarette smoking. Which of the following would be the most likely diagnosis?

    (A) postnasal drip
    (B) gastroesophageal reflux
    (C) tumor
    (D) chronic bronchitis
    (E) bronchiectasis

68. A 45-year-old black female presents to the ER with a 3-day complaint of abdominal pain, nausea, and vomiting. She has a medical history of insulin-dependent diabetes. Lab values show a glucose level of 550, plasma ketone level is markedly positive, a pH on arterial blood gases of 7.21, pCO_2 of 25, pO_2 of 70, and an HCO_3 of 10. Initial treatment of this patient should include all of the following EXCEPT

    (A) intravenous regular insulin
    (B) aggressive administration of isotonic intravenous fluid
    (C) intravenous administration of $NaHCO_3$
    (D) low-flow oxygen per nasal cannula

69. The most common precipitating factor in the development of diabetic ketoacidosis is

    (A) omission of daily insulin
    (B) misuse of oral hyperglycemia medications
    (C) pancreatitis
    (D) infection
    (E) inappropriately high doses of insulin

70. A 25-year-old white male presents to the ER with a chief complaint of a "rapid heart beat." Upon examination, you note him to be very anxious and diaphoretic. His pulse rate is 120 with a blood pressure of 190/100 and a respiratory rate of 28. His pupils are 6 mm bilaterally and light reactive. Upon questioning, he readily admits to substance abuse over the past 3 days. Which of the following would most likely be positive on a urine drug screen?

    (A) benzodiazepines
    (B) opiates
    (C) barbiturates
    (D) cocaine
    (E) marijuana

71. A male multisystem trauma patient is found to have a "free-floating" prostate on rectal exam and blood is noted at the urinary meatus. The initial step in evaluating these findings is

    (A) intravenous pyelogram
    (B) pelvic CT scan
    (C) retrograde urethrogram
    (D) insertion of a Foley catheter to obtain a urine sample
    (E) insertion of suprapubic catheter

72. The proper rate and sequence of ventilation and chest compression in one-person CPR is

(A) one ventilation per 15 compressions at a rate of 80 to 100 compressions per minute

(B) two ventilations per 7 compressions at a rate of 80 to 100 compressions per minute

(C) one ventilation per 7 compressions at a rate of 80 to 100 compressions per minute

(D) two ventilations per 15 compressions at a rate of 80 to 100 compressions per minute

(E) three ventilations per 15 compressions at a rate of 80 to 100 compressions per minute

73. Which of the following is NOT true regarding the Heimlich maneuver?

(A) Airway obstruction can be relieved by subdiaphragmatic compression forcing an artificial cough.

(B) Proper hand position is in the midline of the abdomen below the xiphoid process and above the umbilicus.

(C) Each thrust should be separate and distinct.

(D) Proper hand position is in the midline atop the xiphoid process.

(E) This maneuver is performed only on the choking patient who is unable to speak.

74. Which of the following is NOT characteristic of an achilles tendon rupture?

(A) loss of dorsiflexion

(B) acute onset of severe lower-calf pain

(C) loss of plantar flexion

(D) common in males aged 40 to 50

75. A young athlete comes to the ER with complaints of a dull ache in the upper third of the calf. The pain was mild at first but over the last week has increased, with pain present at rest. Initial radiography is negative. This history suggests

(A) ruptured Achilles tendon

(B) lower-extremity fascial hernia

(C) shin splints

(D) Osgood–Schlatter disease

(E) fibular stress fracture

76. Which of the following statements is NOT correct regarding pediatric fractures?

(A) The most common site of fractures in children is at the epiphyseal plate.

(B) Salter type II fractures, which involve a metaphysis fracture and epiphyseal plate slip, usually require open reduction and are at risk for bone growth arrest.

(C) The strongest element of a child's bone is the periosteum.

(D) Metaphyseal fracture alignment is, as a rule, less important in children than in adults.

DIRECTIONS (Questions 77 through 80): Each group of items in this section consists of lettered headings followed by a set of numbered words or phrases. For each numbered word or phrase, select the ONE lettered heading that is most closely associated with it. Each lettered heading may be selected once, more than once, or not at all.

Questions 77 through 80

Match the following fractures and dislocations with their anatomical description.

(A) comminuted
(B) subluxation
(C) compression
(D) diastasis
(E) avulsion

77. Disruption of the interosseous membrane connecting two joints

78. Caused by impaction of one bone upon another

79. Disruption of a joint with partial contact remaining between the two bones that make up the joint

80. Any fracture where there are more than two segments

Answers and Explanations

1. **(A)** The most common form of shock in the initial stages of multisystem trauma is hypovolemic shock from hemorrhage. Neurogenic shock can occur from spinal injuries that result in a loss of peripheral vascular sympathetic tone. Cardiogenic shock can occur with severe chest trauma and is characterized by shock that is unresponsive to fluid resuscitation accompanied by high central venous pressures. Septic shock occurs as a result of bacterial infection, usually late in the trauma patient's hospital course. *(Committee on Trauma, ACS, pp. 62–64)*

2. **(C)** The "rule-of-nines" is a method for calculating the BSA involvement of burn injuries. The system divides various parts of the body into multiples of nine (Fig. 4–1). Bear in mind that the full BSA value for an extremity is assigned only for circumferential injuries. For example, if only the anterior surface of the arm were involved, this would constitute 4.5% BSA. BSA for various body parts varies in adults and children. *(Moylan, p. 448)*

3. **(D)** Alcohol is involved in more than half of all drownings, fires, falls, pedestrian injuries, assaults, and suicides. The use of alcohol is one of the major predisposing factors to an individual sustaining a traumatic injury. *(Waller, pp. 307–347)*

4. **(D)** Hypovolemic shock produces peripheral vasoconstriction as central organ systems are preferentially perfused. Tachycardia results from an effort to maintain

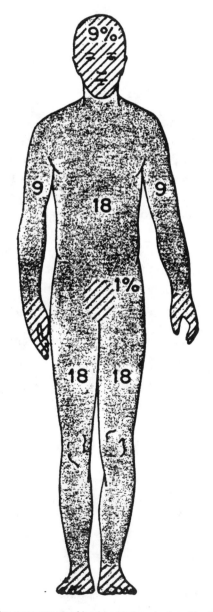

Fig. 4–1. The percentage of body area is calculated by the rule-of-nines.

adequate perfusion. A narrow pulse pressure is often noted. (*Committee on Trauma, ACS, pp. 62–64*)

5. **(C)** Septic shock produces a hyperdynamic cardiac output with a wide pulse pressure, near-normal blood pressure, and tachycardia. This frequently results from gram-negative septicemia secondary to exotoxin release. (*Committee on Trauma, ACS, pp. 62–64*)

6. **(B)** Cardiogenic shock results from cardiac failure; distention of the neck veins is a classic characteristic. Hypotension and tachycardia are common findings. Cardiogenic shock can arise from infarctions occurring at the time of the traumatic event, cardiac contusions, and direct cardiac injury. (*Committee on Trauma, ACS, pp. 62–64*)

7. **(A)** Neurogenic shock occurs when spinal trauma causes a loss of peripheral vascular sympathetic tone, resulting in vasodilation with hypotension and bradycardia. Isolated head injuries do not cause shock in the adult. Infants and small children can lose sufficient intravascular volume with a head injury for hypovolemic shock to occur. (*Committee on Trauma, ACS, pp. 62–64*)

8. **(A)** Hemothorax can result in significant blood loss and hypoxemia. Open chest wounds can cause equilibration between atmospheric and intrathoracic pressure, thus resulting in impaired gas exchange. Cardiac tamponade commonly results from penetrating chest injuries. Even small amounts of blood trapped within the pericardium can restrict cardiac filling. Pneumothorax is usually well tolerated by the healthy adult. (*Committee on Trauma, ACS, pp. 94–95*)

9. **(D)** Immediate institution of aggressive topical antibiotic treatment is indicated, as well as topical cycloplegics, to help reduce inflammation and pain. Also prompt ophthalmology referral is recommended. Both topical steroids and bandaging of the eye are contraindicated in this condition. (*Rakel, p. 72*)

10. **(D)** Isolated head injury in adults does not cause hypovolemic shock. For symptomatic hypovolemia to occur, an adult must lose up to 35% of total blood volume. The cranial vault cannot accommodate this amount of volume. Pelvic and femur fractures are often associated with significant bleeding that can often be unappreciated due to the expandibility of surrounding soft tissues. Hemothorax can cause significant blood volume loss. (*Committee on Trauma, ACS, p. 136*)

11. **(A)** Compartment syndromes develop from an increase in pressure within fascial planes, causing local ischemia. Decreased sensation from nerve compression and local pain, as well as tense swelling and weakness, are early signs and symptoms. Pulselessness and decreased capillary refill are late signs associated with compartment syndromes. (*Committee on Trauma, ACS, pp. 227–228*)

12. **(C)** Major burn patients requires volume resuscitation to combat burn shock. Both supplemental oxygen and analgesia are routinely used. Prophylactic antibiotics are not indicated in the early postburn period. (*Committee on Trauma, ACS, p. 253*)

13. **(B)** Aortic rupture results from stresses caused by unequal rates of horizontal deceleration. These stresses are greatest at fixation points of the arch, such as the great vessels. Most aortic tears occur at the isthmus. Definitive diagnosis is achieved by aortography. A widened mediastinum is considered to be the most reliable finding on a chest x-ray. (*Committee on Trauma, ACS, p. 132*)

14. **(D)** Flail chest occurs when multiple contiguous ribs are fractured, resulting in a free-floating segment of chest wall. Normal respiratory motion of the chest is impaired. The main pathophysiological event is contusion of the lung beneath the bony injury. Sandbags do nothing to address this problem. Positioning the patient onto the affected side is impractical in the multiple-injury patient. In patients with respiratory distress secondary to flail chest and contusion of the underlying

lung, intubation and positive pressure ventilation are indicated. Chest decompression is
indicated for the treatment of a tension pneumothorax. (*Committee on Trauma, ACS, p. 15*)

15. **(B)** Paronychia is an inflammatory involvement of the nail fold on the ulnar or radial
side of the involved digit. It typically presents as a well-localized abscess around the
nail fold. (*Simon and Koenigsknecht, p. 372*)

16. **(A)** Felon is an infection localized to the finger tuft. It is commonly referred to as a pulp
space infection of the distal phalangeal area.
(*Simon and Koenigsknecht, p. 372*)

17. **(C)** Carbuncle is a common infection occurring over the hair-bearing regions of the
hand and arm. (*Simon and Koenigsknecht, p. 371*)

18. **(C)** C5 supplies sensation to the lateral aspect of the arm. C6 supplies sensation to the
lateral forearm, thumb, and index finger. C7
supplies the middle finger (Fig. 4–2). C8 supplies ring and little finger, medial palm. (*Galli
et al, p. 73*)

19. **(D)** (See Fig. 4–3). The L3 dermatome covers
the anterior thigh. The L4 dermatome covers
the medial aspect of the leg. The L5 dermatome covers the lateral leg and dorsum of
the foot while the S1 dermatome involves the
lateral aspect of the foot. (*Hoppenfeld, p. 230*)

20. **(A)** Lymphogranuloma venereum, syphilis,
and granuloma inguinala are all described as
having painless ulcerative lesions. Condyloma acuminata also is characteristically
painless, but it is described as a papilloma-

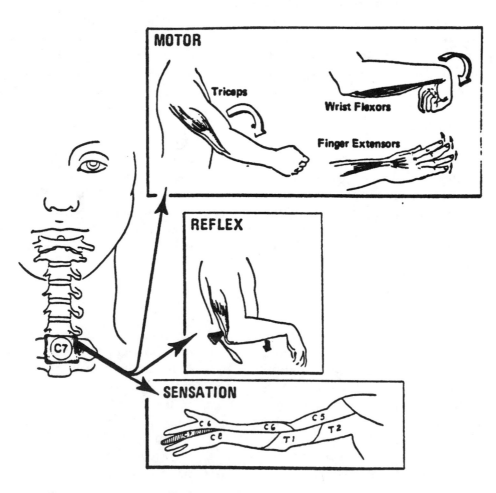

Fig. 4–2. The C7 neurologic level.

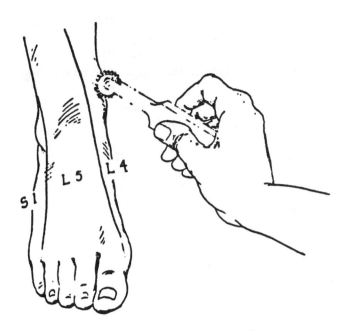

Fig. 4–3. Sensation of the foot.

tous pedunculated-type lesion. Chancroid is classically described as a painful ulcerative lesion. (*Hacker and Moore, pp. 378–385*)

21. **(C)** The abdominal radiograph of a small-bowel obstruction will often reveal air fluid levels within distended loops of small bowel, proximal to the point of obstruction. Free air denotes perforation of the stomach, small or large bowel. Minimal gas will be found in the large bowel, or distal to the point of obstruction. Haustral markings of the small bowel will cross the entire lumen. (*Mettler, pp. 204–205*)

22. **(B)** The sudden onset of abdominal pain and signs of peritonitis occurring in a patient with a history of dyspepsia are keys to the differential diagnosis. Acute cholecystitis often is accompanied by nausea and vomiting; patients are also quite restless in the early stages. Appendicitis begins with rather dull pain that gradually worsens. Patients with acute diverticulitis often give a history of episodic left lower-quadrant pain. The pain occurs rather suddenly but is usually localized to the left lower quadrant. (*Diethelm and Stanley, pp. 736–755*)

23. **(A)** Intra-abdominal adhesions and abdominal hernias are the most common causes of small-bowel obstruction. In children, intussusception is frequently encountered. Mesenteric lymphadenopathy would not, in and of itself, cause the bowel to obstruct. (*Diethelm and Stanley, pp. 736–755*)

24. **(C)** Calcium gluconate will antagonize the cardiac and neuromuscular effects of hyperkalemia within minutes of intravenous administration of a 10% calcium gluconate solution. The remainder of medications listed also are used to decrease the serum potassium level, but do not rapidly antagonize the life-threatening cardiac effects. Administration of intravenous $D_{50}W$ simultaneously with regular insulin will cause the serum potassium level to decrease as a result of intracellular shift. Sodium bicarbonate administration will increase the pH, thereby causing a transcellular shift of potassium from extracellular fluid (ECF) to intracellular fluid (ICF). Nebulized albuterol also has been recently used for hyperkalemic patients on dialysis to promote ECF to ICF flux of potassium. Sodium polystyrene sulfonate (Kayexalate), a cation exchange resin, is commonly used to treat the hyperkalemic patient. (*Bosker et al, pp. 376–378*)

25. **(C)** Nasogastric suctioning acts as both a treatment and diagnostic maneuver in the patient with acute abdominal pain. Nasogastric suctioning relieves gastric dilatation and helps lessen the likelihood of aspiration. Suctioned material can be examined for occult blood. Serial abdominal exams provide a wealth of data regarding the progression or regression of an abdominal process. Many abdominal diseases cause significant third-space volume losses, necessitating careful attention to intravascular volume status. Providing a patient with analgesia prior to the establishment of a definitive diagnosis is extremely dangerous, as it renders further serial exams and patient reports meaningless. (*Diethelm and Stanley, pp. 736–755*)

26. **(C)** Murphy's sign is caused by the descent of the liver and gallbladder during deep inspiration coming into contact with the examiner's fingers during right subcostal palpation. If the gallbladder is inflamed, pain will be produced, halting the inspiratory effort. This is pathognomonic for cholecystitis. *(Diethelm and Stanley, pp. 736–755)*

27. **(A)** Perforated duodenal ulcer pain begins suddenly, located in the midepigastric region. As peritonitis progresses, generalized abdominal pain is noted. This can cause a rigid or "board-like" abdomen on exam. There may be "free air" noted on plain radiographs of the upright abdomen. *(Diethelm and Stanley, pp. 736–755)*

28. **(B)** Acute cholecystitis often begins suddenly with rapidly increasing pain. Pain is referred to the right shoulder and scapular area as subdiaphragmatic irritation triggers the phrenic nerve. Nonvisualization of radionucleotide in the gallbladder during HIDA scan is diagnostic. *(Diethelm and Stanley, pp. 736–755)*

29. **(D)** Appendicitis has rather vague and variable initial symptoms. However, over time, pain usually localizes to the right lower quadrant. Anorexia or even aversion to food is frequently seen. Fever of greater than 101°F is uncommon. *(Diethelm and Stanley, pp. 736–755)*

30. **(C)** In acute pancreatitis, patients usually complain of the rapid onset of deep unrelenting midepigastric pain with radiation to the back. Patients may often give a history of intermittent dull epigastric pain. Alcoholism and cholelithiasis are the most frequent causes. *(Diethelm and Stanley, pp. 736–755)*

31. **(C)** The patient with arterial thrombosis will commonly have a history of limiting claudication. The patient with arterial embolization will rarely have a clear-cut history of limiting claudication and will often present with a history of "sudden pain" at the affected extremity. Both deep venous thrombosis and thrombophlebitis do not primarily present with pulselessness. *(Rutherford, pp. 654, 1781)*

32. **(D)** Bleeding from gastroesophageal varices is a result of portal hypertension due to a relative or absolute obstruction of splenic blood flow. Cirrhosis resulting from acute alcoholic hepatitis is a common cause of portal hypertension. Cirrhosis is commonly associated with variceal bleeding, encephalopathy, and ascites. Splenomegaly is a common finding. Emergency endoscopy should be performed on all patients with UGI bleeding, as other causes of bleeding may be present. *(Olthoff et al, pp. 636–668)*

33. **(D)** Definitive care of soft-tissue abscesses is achieved through incision and drainage. Antibiotics in the healthy individual are unnecessary. Packing gauze should be placed into the wound to permit drainage and prevent premature closure of the skin edges. *(Warren, pp. 591–609)*

34. **(B)** Pilonidal abscesses are presacral soft-tissue infections, usually chronic in nature. These do not communicate with the rectosigmoid. It is often easy to overlook the subtle appearance of these abscesses in the perisacral area. As multiple septations occur within the abscess cavity, wide excision is required for resolution. *(Warren, pp. 591–609)*

35. **(B)** Sebaceous cysts that are acutely inflamed require incision and drainage, followed by excision after the acute inflammation has resolved. Sebaceous cysts that are increasing in size, recurrently infected, or malodorous are all indications for excision. Sebaceous cysts result from obstructed secretory glands. Definitive treatment requires excision of the cyst capsule. *(Rakel, p. 975)*

36. **(B)** Boutonniere deformity results after an avulsion or laceration of the central extensor mechanism resulting in a flexion deformity at the PIP joint and hyperextension at the DIP joint. This deformity usually manifests itself insidiously as a result of gradual stretching of the injured hood. *(Simon and Koenigsknecht, p. 367; Hoppenfeld, p. 87)*

37. **(D)** Proper care of a suspected poisonous snake bite includes rapid transportation to the nearest hospital, immobilization of the wound, positioning below the level of the heart, and application of a constricting band proximal to the wound to impede lymphatic drainage. Ice should not be applied. *(Ho and Saunders, p. 720)*

38. **(C)** Dilated small bowel with air-fluid levels is indicative of small-bowel obstruction. The dilation is seen proximal to the point of obstruction with decompressed bowel distal to the lesion. *(Diethelm and Stanley, pp. 736–755)*

39. **(B)** The psoas muscle is a posterior retroperitoneal structure. This paired set of muscles is usually easily discerned on plain abdominal radiographs. Loss of this shadow may be indicative of a mass effect obscuring the psoas outline. *(Diethelm and Stanley, pp. 736–755)*

40. **(A)** Free intra-abdominal air is indicative of perforation of a hollow viscus, that is, the small or large bowel or stomach. It is best seen in an upright film where air will accumulate under the diaphragm. *(Diethelm and Stanley, pp. 736–755)*

41. **(D)** Hemoperitoneum is a difficult diagnosis to make based on a plain x-ray alone. Associated injuries such as lower rib fractures indicate that the patient's abdomen has been subjected to great force. Such findings would lead the clinician to strongly suspect liver or spleen injuries. *(Diethelm and Stanley, pp. 736–755)*

42. **(C)** Carcinoma of the colon is the most common cause of large-bowel obstruction in the adult. Diverticulitis can also cause large-bowel obstruction, and patients often give a history of intermittent left lower-quadrant pain. Sigmoid volvulus is a less common cause of large-bowel obstruction. It is seen most often in elderly persons with poor bowel habits and chronic constipation. *(Diethelm and Stanley, pp. 736–755)*

43. **(C)** The most important aspect of managing epistaxis is localizing the site of bleeding. Once the site of bleeding has been identified,

then the proper therapy can be initiated. *(Rakel, p. 55)*

44. **(D)** Left lower-quadrant abdominal pain is a common finding in the patient with acute diverticulitis. Severe abdominal pain and frank bleeding are uncommon findings. Left flank pain is more indicative of renal disease. *(Rakel, p. 350)*

45. **(D)** Cervical spine, AP chest, and AP pelvis x-rays should be obtained while still in the resuscitation area after all life-threatening injuries are identified and treated. Then complete films should be obtained. *(Committee on Trauma, ACS, p. 27)*

46. **(D)** Singed nasal hair, carbonaceous sputum, darkened oral or nasal mucous membranes, and history of burns in an enclosed space are highly suggestive for the presence of inhalation injury. Bronchoscopy is used for definitive diagnosis. Even with the most severe inhalation injury, early chest x-rays appear normal. *(Herndon et al, p. 157)*

47. **(A)** Burn shock results from increased capillary permeability that permits the loss of plasma volume and macromolecules from the intravascular to the extravascular spaces. This transmigration of fluid leads to extensive edema formation and hypovolemia. Formulas for aggressive fluid resuscitation are designed to combat this phenomenon. All burn patients with injuries to greater than 20% BSA are at risk for significant plasma volume loss. *(Demling, p. 189)*

48. **(B)** Acute dystonia is one of the most common side affects of antipsychotic medications. Haldol, prolixin, navane, and thorazine are all antipsychotic agents. Cogentin is the medication used to treat an acute dystonic reaction. *(Tintinalli et al, p. 1081)*

49. **(A)** The recommended initial treatment for chemical burns caused by hydrofluoric acid is copious irrigation with water followed by calcium gluconate solution (10%). Polyethylene glycol is used for treating burns caused by phenol. Copper sulfate (3%) solution can

be used for burns caused by phosphorus. As a general rule, one should not attempt to neutralize the burn with a weak reciprocal chemical. *(Ho and Saunders, p. 699)*

50. **(C)** Digital blocks are accomplished by the injection of local anesthesia (without epinephrine) into nerves on the lateral and medial aspects of the digit. Bier block is the IV introduction of anesthesia into the limb that is occluded by an inflated BP cuff. This method is useful in soft tissue procedures on the hand and forearm. Topical anesthetics and intramuscular analgesia are ineffective in providing proper patient comfort. *(Simmon and Brenner, 1987a, p. 108)*

51. **(D)** Erythema migrans is commonly referred to as a "bull's eye" type lesion seen approximately 1 week after a bite by an *Ixodes* tick. This lesion is found on approximately 75% of patients with Lyme disease. Erysipelas is a specific type of superficial cellulitis. Pityriasis rosea is classically described as beginning with a "herald patch" and associated with a self-limiting illness. Erythema multiforme presents with painful, burning patches and is typically a self-limiting condition. *(Rakel, pp. 880–881)*

52. **(B)** The most commonly fractured bone is the clavicle. Overall clavicular fractures account for 5% of all fractures in all age groups. These fractures are usually treated with a figure-of-eight clavicular wrap. *(Simmon and Brenner, 1987b, p. 218)*

53. **(C)** Flow through a catheter is adversely affected by its length. Long indwelling central venous lines such as subclavian, jugular, or pulmonary artery catheters do not have the flow characteristics necessary for volume resuscitation. These types of lines are time-consuming to place and carry with them significant morbidity. The proper method of volume replacement is via two or more short-length, large-bore peripheral IVs. *(Committee on Trauma, ACS, p. 16)*

54. **(B)** Chest tubes should be placed no lower than the 5th intercostal space to avoid injury to the diaphragm. Placement of the tube medial to the anterior axillary line increases the risk of lacerating the internal mammary vessels. The tube should be placed over the rib to avoid the intercostal neurovascular bundle. After puncturing the pleura, a gloved finger should be placed to avoid injury to other organs and to clear adhesions. *(Committee on Trauma, ACS, p. 108)*

55. **(E)** Either lidocaine or phenytoin are recommended for treating ventricular arrhythmias secondary to TCA overdose. Diazepam should be used to treat both ventricular arrhythmias and hypotension. Quinidine-like drugs (i.e., procainamide) are contraindicated because they have been shown to worsen cardiotoxicity. *(Ho and Saunders, p. 765)*

56. **(C)** Osteomyelitis is infection of the bone, which often becomes chronic. Destruction of bone often is the consequence of this condition. This is most often the result of an open or "compound" fracture. This complication can be prevented by meticulous wound care designed to remove all foreign and devitalized material. *(Adams, p. 54)*

57. **(D)** Volkmann's ischemic contracture results from brachial artery injury in the setting of supracondylar humeral fracture. Ischemic damage to the flexor muscles of the forearm result in a flexion contraction of the hand and wrist. Other injuries that result in compartment syndromes may yield the same ischemic injury. *(Adams, p. 143)*

58. **(B)** Avascular necrosis is bony necrosis secondary to insufficient blood supply. It usually occurs in a fracture near the articular surface of a bone, especially if the terminal fragment is devoid of soft-tissue attachments. This may occur following fracture of the femoral neck. Other common sites include navicular, scaphoid, and talar fractures. *(Adams, p. 60)*

59. **(A)** Fat emboli syndrome is an uncommon, but serious, complication of long bone fractures, mainly at the femur or tibia. It usually

occurs 2 days following injury and is characterized by alterations in mental status and/or respiratory insufficiency. Patients will often demonstrate a petechial rash. The etiology remains unclear; however, it is postulated that fat globules or released fatty acids play a role. (Adams, p. 54)

60. **(D)** Complete cord syndrome is characterized by complete flaccid paralysis and loss of all sensation below the level of injury. Deep tendon reflexes are absent. Injuries to the C1–C4 level result in respiratory arrest due to the respiratory muscle paralysis. (Galli et al, pp. 12–19)

61. **(A)** Anterior cord syndromes occur most commonly in hyperflexion injuries of the cervical spine. Clinically, there is immediate, complete paralysis and loss of sensation below the lesion. Light touch, proprioception, and vibratory sense are spared, as they are controlled through the intact dorsal columns. These patients have a much better prognosis for recovery than do those with complete cord lesions. (Galli et al, pp. 12–19)

62. **(B)** Brown–Sequard syndrome results from functional or anatomic hemisection of the spinal cord. The consequence is loss of proprioception, vibration, and light touch on the ipsilateral side of the injury and loss of pain and proprioception on the contralateral side. (Galli et al, pp. 12–19)

63. **(C)** Nerve root syndrome commonly occurs in the cervical region and results from isolated nerve root injuries. Unilateral facet dislocations and disc herniations are the most common causes. (Galli et al, pp. 12–19)

64. **(A)** Lumbar disc herniation results from herniation of the central nucleus pulposus causing nerve root compression with sciatica and lower-extremity symptoms. The pain of lumbar disc herniation is worsened by coughing, sneezing, and the Valsalva maneuver. It is associated with flattening of the lumbar curve and muscle spasm. Nerve root compression, most commonly L4–L5 or L5–S1, often results

in muscle weakness and neurological deficits. Deep-tendon reflexes are commonly reduced. (Galli et al, p. 256)

65. **(C)** Legionnaire's disease is suggested by the presence of a constellation of symptoms, including fever, respiratory symptoms, toxemia, constitutional symptoms, diarrhea, and a typically nonproductive cough.

Mycoplasma pneumonia accounts for 25% of all community-acquired pneumonia. Symptoms include upper- and lower-respiratory tract complaints, fever, cough, and headaches. The treatment of choice is erythromycin.

Klebsiella pneumoniae is seen most commonly in immunosuppressed individuals as a necrotizing lobar pneumonia. The entity is frequently associated with lung abscess and empyema. *Klebsiella* often has a rapid onset associated with pleuritic chest pain, shortness of breath, and rigors.

Lyme disease is a tick-borne illness characterized by malaise, fatigue, fever, myalgia, lymphadenopathy, and malar rash. (Zwanger, p. 257; Pavikrishnan, p. 253)

66. **(E)** Purpura and petechiae are classical clinical findings. Brudzinski's sign and Kernig's sign are special maneuvers used to detect meningeal signs. Chvostek's sign is associated with hypocalcemia and tetanus in newborns and children. (Rakel, p. 1063; Bates, p. 533–534)

67. **(D)** Chronic cough is the fifth most common reason for clinic visits. It is traditionally defined as a cough present for more than 3 weeks. The most common cause of cough in a smoker is chronic bronchitis. Postnasal drip, gastroesophageal reflux, and asthma also should be considered in the differential diagnosis. Tumor is a less common cause of chronic cough in this age group. (Rakel, p. 98)

68. **(C)** Patients in diabetic ketoacidosis most often present with nausea, vomiting, abdominal pain, and anorexia. Because of severe volume depletion, aggressive fluid administration is begun immediately. An initial loading dose of regular insulin 0.15–0.3 units/kg

is given by rapid intravenous injection once the diagnosis has been made. Administration of NaHCO₃ has not been shown to improve recovery. Mild to moderate acidosis (pH >7.2) can be quickly corrected with administration of fluid/insulin and should not be treated with NaHCO₃. *(Ho and Saunders, p. 448; Rakel, p. 632)*

69. **(D)** The most common precipitating factor in diabetic ketoacidosis is infection. All ketoacidotic patients must be thoroughly screened for the presence of an occult infectious process. Stressors, such as infection, cause the production of counterregulatory hormones such as glucagon, catecholamines, and cortisol. Stress hormone production, and their resultant anti-insulin effect, in conjunction with a relatively insufficient supply of insulin, set the stage for the development of ketoacidosis. *(Ragland, pp. 490–491)*

70. **(D)** Signs of stimulant overdose (cocaine) include hyperactivity, diaphoresis, dilated pupils, tachycardia, and hypertension. Signs of overdose with benzodiazepines and barbiturates are hypotension, respiratory depression, and dysarthria. The same signs also are present in an opiate overdose, along with bradycardia and miotic pupils. *(Rakel, pp. 1137–1138)*

71. **(C)** A "high-riding" or "free-floating" prostate on rectal exam, or blood at the urinary meatus is indicative of urethral injury. Intravenous pyelograms or pelvic CT scans are less than optimal imaging modalities to assess this entity. Insertion of a Foley catheter is contraindicated, as a partial urethral tear may be completed. Retrograde urethrograms should be performed to assess the integrity of the urethra prior to catheterization. *(Ahlering et al, p. 663)*

72. **(D)** The proper sequence of one-person CPR as proposed by the American Heart Association is 15 compressions alternating with 2 ventilations. Two-person CPR is performed using five compressions to one ventilation. *(Albarran-Sotelo et al, p. 47)*

73. **(D)** The Heimlich maneuver is performed with the rescuer either kneeling astride the recumbent victim or standing behind the upright victim. Sharp, abdominal thrusts designed to quickly raise intra-abdominal pressure are applied. Care is taken to maintain hand placement below the xiphoid process to lessen the risk of rib fracture. The Heimlich maneuver is performed only on the choking patient who cannot speak. *(Albarran-Sotelo et al, p. 58; Ho and Saunders, p. 11)*

74. **(A)** The most common site of Achilles tendon rupture is approximately 2 inches above the point of calcaneal attachment. This injury is common among sedentary men aged 40 to 50 years, but is also seen in athletes. Patients will often complain of agonizing lower-calf pain and demonstrate an inability to plantar flex the foot. Partial tears are often misdiagnosed as some plantar flexion is preserved. *(Simon and Koenigsknecht, p. 407)*

75. **(E)** The fibula is the most common site of stress fractures. It is commonly seen in young athletes, military recruits, and dancers. Early radiographs are often negative, but in 10 to 14 days a fine transverse line will often be seen, tracing the fracture site. The entity is commonly misdiagnosed as shin splints, which are more often characterized by pain on the anteriomedial surface of the distal leg. Fascial hernias are easily diagnosed by the presence of a reducible mass when the muscle is relaxed. Osgood–Schlatter disease is a painful condition of the tibial tuberosity seen in adolescents. *(Simon and Koenigsknecht, p. 392)*

76. **(B)** Children's bones are more porous than adults'. The periosteum is the strongest element, and the epiphyseal plate the weakest. The epiphysis is the "growth plate" of young bones. Salter classification III and IV fractures have a high risk of growth arrest. As a general rule metaphyseal fractures in children require less alignment than those in adults (Fig. 4–4). *(Simon and Koenigsknecht, p. 19)*

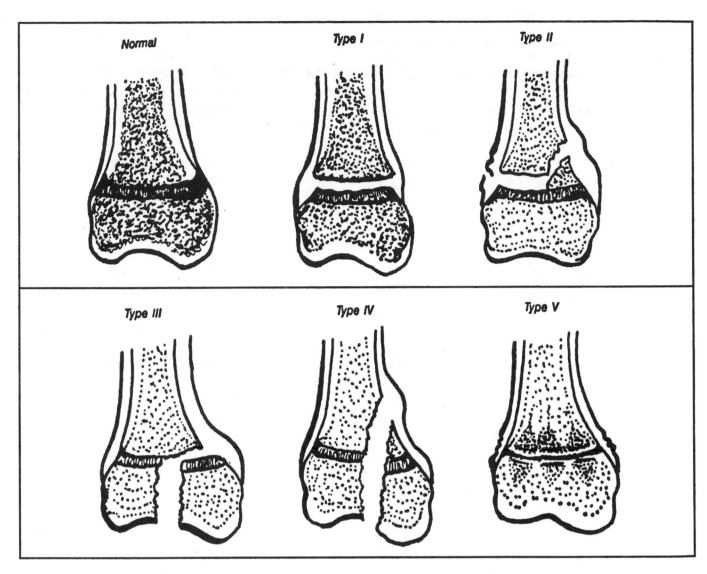

Fig. 4–4. The Salter–Harris classification system used in epiphyseal injuries.

77. **(D)** Diastasis is a disruption of the interosseous membrane of a joint. This presents as a joint injury with edema and tenderness, as in a superior ankle dislocation. *(Simon and Koenigsknecht, pp. 4–5, 402)*

78. **(C)** Compression fractures occur as a result of axial loading of one bone upon another. Most commonly seen in the spinal vertebrae of the elderly with complaints of pain and occasionally radicular nerve pain. *(Simon and Koenigsknecht, pp. 4–5)*

79. **(B)** Subluxation involves a partial dislocation of a joint in that there is continued contact of the bones. The clinical presentation is similar to a dislocation. *(Simon and Koenigsknecht, pp. 4–5)*

80. **(A)** Comminuted fracture by definition implies more than two bone fragments. Variation of this is the butterfly fracture, where a v-shaped fragment is seen, or a segmented fracture, where there are two transverse fractures with a piece or segment of bone between. *(Simon and Koenigsknecht, pp. 2–3)*

REFERENCES

Adams JC. Complications of fractures. In Adams JC, *Outline of Fractures*. Edinburgh: Churchill Livingstone; 1992.

Ahlering T, Weintraub P, Weinburg A, Skinner D. Urologic surgery and trauma. In Civetta E (ed), *Critical Care*. London: Lippincott; 1992.

Albarran-Sotelo R, Flint L, Kelly K (eds). *Instructor's Manual for Basic Life Support*. Washington, DC: American Heart Association; 1987.

Bates B. *A Guide to Physical Examination and History Taking*. Philadelphia: Lippincott; 1995.

Bosker G, Talon D, Goldman H, Albrich M. *The Manual of Emergency Medicine Therapeutics*. St. Louis, MO: Mosby-Yearbook; 1995.

Committee on Trauma. *Advanced Trauma Life Support*. Chicago: ACS; 1993.

Demling R. Fluid resuscitation. In Bostwick JA (ed), *The Art and Science of Burn Care*. Rockville, MD: Aspen; 1987.

Diethelm AG, Stanley RJ. The acute abdomen. In Sabiston DS (ed), *Textbook in Surgery*. Philadelphia: Saunders; 1991: 736–755.

Galli RL, Spraite DW, Simon RR. *Emergency Orthopedics of the Spine*. Norwalk, CT: Appleton & Lange; 1989.

Hacker N, Moore J. *Essentials of Obstetrics and Gynecology*. Philadelphia: Saunders; 1992.

Herndon DJ, Thompson PB, Brown M, Traber DL. Diagnosis, pathophysiology and treatment of inhalation injury. In Boswick JA (ed), *The Art and Science of Burn Care*. Rockville, MD: Aspen; 1987.

Ho MT, Saunders CE. *Current Emergency Diagnosis and Treatment*. Norwalk, CT: Appleton & Lange; 1992.

Hopppenfeld S. *Physical Examination of the Spine and Extremities*. New York: Appleton-Century-Crofts; 1976.

Mettler FA. *Essentials of Radiology*. Philadelphia: Saunders; 1996.

Moylan JA. Burn injury. In Moylan JA (ed), *Trauma Surgery*. Philadelphia: Lippincott; 1992: 17.2–17.16.

Olthoff KM, Brown SL, Busuttil RW. Portal hypertension. In Moore W (ed), *Vascular Surgery: A Comprehensive Review*. New York: Grune & Stratton; 1991: 636–668.

Pavikrishnan KP. Viral and mycoplasma pneumonias in adults. In Crome JE, Ruiz RL (eds), *Emergency Medicine, A Comprehensive Study Guide*. New York: McGraw-Hill; 1988.

Ragland G. Diabetic ketoacidosis in adults. In Krome JE, Ruiz RL (eds), *Emergency Medicine, A Comprehensive Study Guide*. New York: McGraw-Hill; 1988.

Rakel R. *Saunders Manual of Medical Practice*. Philadelphia: Saunders; 1996.

Rutherford R. *Vascular Surgery*. Philadelphia: Saunders; 1995.

Simmon RR, Brenner BE. Anesthesia and regional blocks. In Simmon RR, Brenner BE (eds), *Emergency Procedures and Techniques*. Baltimore, MD: Williams & Wilkins; 1987a.

Simmon RR, Brenner BE. Orthopedic procedures. In Simmon RR, Brenner BE (eds), *Emergency Procedures and Techniques*. Baltimore, MD: Williams & Wilkins; 1987b.

Simon R, Koenigsknecht SJ. *Emergency Orthopedics: The Extremities*. Norwalk, CT: Appleton & Lange; 1995.

Tintinalli J, Krome R, Ruiz E. *Emergency Medicine, A Comprehensive Study Guide*. New York: McGraw-Hill; 1992.

Waller JA. Alcohol and unintentional injury. In Kissin B, Begleiter H (eds), *The Biology of Alcoholism*, vol. 4. New York: Plenum; 1976.

Warren T. Incision and drainage of cutaneous abscesses and soft tissue infections. In Roberts JR (ed), *Clinical Procedures in Emergency Medicine*. Philadelphia: Saunders; 1991: 591–609.

Zwanger M. Legionnaire's disease. In Krome JE, Ruiz RL (eds), *Emergency Medicine, A Comprehensive Study Guide*. New York: McGraw-Hill; 1988.

CHAPTER 5

Internal Medicine: HIV-AIDS
Questions

Rebecca Lovell Scott, PhD, PA-C

DIRECTIONS (Questions 1 through 8): Each group of items in this section consists of lettered headings followed by a set of numbered words or phrases. For each numbered word or phrase, select the ONE lettered heading that is most closely associated with it. Each lettered heading may be selected once, more than once, or not at all.

Questions 1 through 4

For each disease process, select the drug of choice with which it is treated.

    (A) amphotericin B
    (B) ganciclovir
    (C) trimethoprim-sulfamethoxazole (Bactrim/Septra)
    (D) acyclovir
    (E) pyrimethamine and sulfadiazine

1. *Pneumocystis carinii* pneumonia (PCP)

2. Toxoplasmic encephalitis

3. Cryptococcal meningitis

4. Cytomegalovirus (CMV) chorioretinitis

Questions 5 through 8

    (A) cryptococcal meningitis
    (B) toxoplasmic encephalitis
    (C) both
    (D) neither

5. Computerized tomography (CT) of the head is usually normal.

6. Presenting symptoms are headache, fever, and altered sensorium.

7. Cerebrospinal fluid (CSF) may show normal protein and glucose as well as absence of pleocytosis.

8. Chronic suppressive therapy is required to prevent recurrences.

DIRECTIONS (Questions 9 through 25): Each of the numbered items or incomplete statements in this section is followed by answers or by completions of the statement. Select the ONE lettered answer or completion that is BEST in each case.

Questions 9 through 25

9. All the following statements about patterns of HIV infection in the United States are true EXCEPT

    (A) The cumulative incidence of AIDS cases is disproportionately higher in African-Americans and Hispanics than in whites.
    (B) Recent rates of reported AIDS cases are highest in the Northeast and lowest in the Midwest.

(C) The percentage of reported AIDS cases in women has gradually decreased over time.

(D) The highest risk of HIV infection in pediatric patients occurs in children born to women who themselves are at risk for HIV infection.

(E) In the South, the proportions of cases of AIDS resulting from heterosexual transmission among adolescents and young adults (ages 13–29 years) is higher in towns and rural areas than in towns and rural areas in other parts of the country.

10. Which one of the following tests is used initially to evaluate the presence of HIV infection in a patient?

(A) HIV antibody status by ELISA

(B) HIV serum p24 antigen status

(C) HIV antibody status by Western blot

(D) T-lymphocyte subset studies

(E) in vitro culture of HIV from patient's blood

11. HIV-infected patients are at increased risk for all the following central nervous system (CNS) diseases EXCEPT

(A) progressive multifocal leukoencephalopathy (PML)

(B) primary CNS lymphoma

(C) cryptococcoma

(D) bacterial meningitis

(E) TB meningitis

12. Which one of the following statements is true about pediatric HIV infection?

(A) A positive HIV antibody status in a neonate reflects the presence of HIV infection.

(B) Symptoms of HIV infection are often seen in the first 6 weeks of life.

(C) Chronic lymphocytic infiltrative pneumonia (LIP) and chronic parotid enlargement are commonly seen in children.

(D) Kaposi's sarcoma is frequently diagnosed in children but is difficult to treat.

(E) Neurological involvement, principally progressive encephalopathy, has been described in 10% to 20% of pediatric AIDS cases.

13. Which of the following would be LEAST appropriate in the evaluation of an HIV-infected patient with profuse diarrhea?

(A) routine stool evaluations

(B) sigmoidoscopy/colonoscopy with biopsy

(C) stool for acid-fast bacteria (AFB)

(D) barium enema

(E) blood cultures for CMV (cytomegalovirus) and MAC (*Mycobacterium avium complex*)

14. All of the following are true of didanosine (ddI) and zalcitabine (ddC) EXCEPT

(A) Both are nucleoside analog reverse transcriptase inhibitors.

(B) Peripheral neuropathy is a common adverse effect for both.

(C) Both are alternative antiretroviral agents to zidovudine in the event of development of intolerance or disease progression.

(D) Dosing for both medications is twice a day.

(E) Pancreatitis is more common in ddI users than in ddC users.

15. Which of the following statements is TRUE about esophagitis in the HIV-infected patient?

(A) The diagnosis of *Candida* esophagitis is frequently made on the characteristic presentation of odynophagia, dysphagia, feeling of obstruction, and substernal chest pain.

(B) *Candida* esophagitis can only be distinguished from herpes virus or cytomegalovirus (CMV) esophagitis by endoscopy.

(C) Diagnosis of CMV is made by culture of biopsy specimens.

(D) Epstein–Barr virus is a common cause of esophageal ulcers in HIV-infected patients.

(E) The most common infection caused by Herpes simplex virus in the HIV-infected patient is esophagitis.

16. Administration of zidovudine in HIV-infected patients is often associated with anemia and neutropenia, myopathy, headache and nausea, and
(A) pancreatitis
(B) peripheral neuropathy
(C) hyperuricemia
(D) urticaria
(E) bluish discoloration of the nail beds

17. The incidence of new HIV infection in groups at recognized risk between 1985 and the present has shown
(A) a decline in the percent of men who have sex with men
(B) an increase in the percent of hemophiliacs
(C) a decrease in the percent of IV drug users
(D) elimination of the category of persons with no known risk factor
(E) a decrease in the percent of heterosexuals

18. Which of the following clinical conditions were included in the expanded Centers for Disease Control and Prevention surveillance case definition effective January 1, 1993, that had not been included prior to 1993?
(A) invasive cervical cancer
(B) Kaposi's sarcoma
(C) *Pneumocystis carinii* pneumonia
(D) syphilis
(E) unexplained diarrhea

19. All of the following statements about *Mycobacterium avium* complex (MAC) infection are true EXCEPT

(A) It often infects the bone marrow, causing pancytopenia.
(B) It can be present in any organ in the body.
(C) It often produces symptoms of chronic fever, diaphoresis, and weight loss.
(D) It usually occurs in patients with mildly depressed CD4 counts.
(E) It is a multiresistant organism whose therapy involves new, broad-spectrum antibiotics.

20. Medications acceptable for prophylaxis of *Pneumocystis carinii* pneumonia (PCP) include trimethoprim-sulfamethoxazole, aerosolized pentamidine, and
(A) Dapsone
(B) ciprofloxacin
(C) ethambutol
(D) clarithromycin
(E) rifampin

21. Neurological syndromes seen in HIV-infected patients
(A) affect only the central nervous system
(B) rarely represent opportunistic infection of the nervous system
(C) are sometimes difficult to distinguish from the neurotoxic effects of drugs used to treat AIDS
(D) present essentially the same way they do in non-HIV–infected patients
(E) are mostly caused by invasion of the tissue by HIV-1

22. The risk of HIV transmission
(A) for homosexual men decreases for those who practice receptive anal intercourse
(B) for blood recipients decreased dramatically in 1985 when routine screening of blood for HIV antibodies became available
(C) for sexual active persons remains the same in the presence of sexually transmitted diseases other than HIV/AIDS

(D) for blood recipients decreases if blood is donated by a family member

(E) for condom users is significantly decreased with the use of nonoxynol-9

23. The risk of HIV transmission to health care workers

(A) is greatly reduced when universal precautions are implemented

(B) is higher than the risk of hepatitis B virus (HBV) transmission

(C) is approximately 1 in 100 following a single needlestick exposure to blood from an HIV-infected patient

(D) has been documented from exposure to body fluids other than blood, such as feces, sputum, urine, or vomitus

(E) is greatly reduced with use of prophylactic zidovudine administration following an accidental exposure

24. Which of the following statements regarding viral infections in AIDS patients is true?

(A) Isolation of cytomegalovirus (CMV) from the lung is uncommon and warrants initiation of antiviral treatment.

(B) Administration of antiviral treatment for active herpes simplex virus (HSV) infection has shown risk of serious complications and no reduction in morbidity.

(C) In treatment of mucocutaneous HSV, topical acyclovir reduces the formation of new lesions as well as the risk of dissemination.

(D) Disseminated varicella zoster virus (VZV) infection warrants hospitalization and treatment with high-dose IV acyclovir.

(E) Varicella pneumonia typically presents with mild symptoms and may be treated with oral acyclovir.

25. AIDS-associated Kaposi's sarcoma

(A) may present in the lung as nodular infiltrates

(B) is seen primarily in IV drug users

(C) rarely responds to alpha-interferon administration

(D) when treated with radiotherapy is associated with a high response rate and an improved prognosis

(E) presents with relatively indolent cutaneous lesions

Answers and Explanations

1. **(C)** Trimethoprim/sulfamethoxazole is the drug of choice in treating *P. carinii* pneumonia (PCP); dosing is based on the trimethoprim component at 15 to 20 mg/kg/day intravenously in divided doses for 21 days. Trimethoprim/sulfamethoxazole is associated with a high frequency of adverse reactions that include rash, leukopenia, thrombocytopenia, nausea, vomiting, or nephritis. If patients have a history of intolerance to sulfonamides or trimethoprim, oral or intravenous clindamycin (1,800 to 2,400 mg/day) and oral primaquine (15 mg primaquine base per day) is effective. Some patients may experience rash, diarrhea, leukopenia, and mild methemoglobinemia on this regimen. G6PD-deficient patients should avoid primaquine. In mild cases of PCP where the patient is not acutely ill and is able to take oral medications, TMP/SMX can be given orally, or Dapsone 100 mg daily and TMP 15–20 mg/kg in divided doses, both orally, can be given to sulfonamide-allergic patients. As Dapsone may cause hemolytic anemia, particularly in G6PD-deficient patients, this must be ruled out prior to its usage. In severe cases of PCP, where the patient is acutely ill with a PO_2 <70 mm Hg, early treatment with prednisone has been demonstrated to decrease the rate of occurrence of respiratory failure and death. Prednisone should be started orally at a dose of 40 mg twice a day for 5 days, then 40 mg daily for 5 days, then 20 mg daily for the remaining 11 days of the anti-PCP treatment. Other less effective treatments include atovaquone 750 mg orally three times a day with fatty foods to improve absorption and trimetrexate, a folate antagonist, as a daily intravenous infusion of 45 mg/m² over 60 to 90 minutes. (*Bartlett and Feinberg, p. 233; Bozzette et al, pp. 1451–1457; Noble, p. 937*)

2. **(E)** Standard treatment of an acute episode of toxoplasmic encephalitis is the combination of pyrimethamine at a 200-mg loading dose, then 50 to 100 mg daily orally and sulfadiazine at 4 to 6 g daily in divided doses orally. This combination blocks folic acid metabolism of the proliferative form of *Toxoplasma gondii* and is synergistic against the organism. Corticosteroids often are indicated to manage increased intracranial pressure from mass effect. Associated with this treatment is a high frequency of toxic side effects, most commonly bone marrow suppression and rash. Folinic acid should be added to the therapy at doses of 10 to 30 mg daily in an effort to prevent bone marrow suppression. In the event of severe toxicity, sulfadiazine should be discontinued, as it is more often responsible for the toxicity. Clindamycin has been recognized to be an effective drug for the treatment of toxoplasmosis and may be used as a second-line agent with pyrimethamine. The recommended dosage is 2,400 to 4,800 mg/day intravenously in divided doses depending on the patient's clinical status and tolerance of the medication. The toxic effects include nausea, vomiting, diarrhea, neutropenia, rash, and pseudomembranous colitis. Recently, three new macrolide/

azolide antibiotics (clarithromycin, azithromycin, and roxithromycin) have been found to be effective alternative treatments for toxoplasmosis. *(Bartlett and Feinberg, p. 233; Luft and Remington, pp. 211–222; Noble, p. 941)*

3. **(A)** Standard treatment for cryptococcal meningitis is amphotericin B at 0.5 to 0.8 mg/kg per day IV. The side effects of amphotericin B commonly include high fever, rigors, nausea, vomiting, hypotension, and renal dysfunction. Cerebrospinal fluid (CSF) cultures should become sterile during initial therapy, and CSF cryptococcal antigen titers usually fall with therapy. 5-Flucytosine (5-FC), another antifungal agent, may prove useful when added to amphotericin B in patients with severe cryptococcal disease at a dose of 150 mg/kg daily in divided doses. Fluconazole, an oral triazole antifungal agent, may be an alternative treatment for patients with mild cryptococcal disease. However, patients with altered mental status, a CSF cryptococcal antigen titer of greater than 1:1024, and a CSF white cell count less than 20 cells/mm^3 have a higher mortality rate with fluconazole treatment. Because most deaths occur early in the treatment, an alternative may be amphotericin B for 2 weeks, followed by fluconazole. *(Bartlett and Feinberg, p. 233; Noble, pp. 941–942; Saag et al, pp. 83–94)*

4. **(B)** Ganciclovir is the recommended treatment of CMV chorioretinitis. Initial treatment consists of 5 mg/kg intravenously bid for 14 to 21 days with duration of "induction therapy" depending on the degree of response determined by follow-up ophthalmologic exams. Maintenance treatment 5 to 7 days a week at 6 mg/kg once daily is required to prevent recurrence of lesions, as it has been shown that with cessation of therapy, retinal lesions usually recur. The toxicity of ganciclovir includes bone marrow suppression (particularly neutropenia and thrombocytopenia), rash, headache, confusion, nausea, and vomiting, and may be the limiting factor in determining dose and duration of maintenance treatment. Because both ganciclovir and zidovudine (AZT) are myelosuppressive,

patients treated with ganciclovir may not be able to tolerate the full recommended dose of zidovudine. Foscarnet, another antiviral agent, is an alternate drug used in the treatment of CMV chorioretinitis. The induction dose is 60 mg/kg intravenously every 8 hours for 14 to 21 days, with a maintenance dose of 90 to 120 mg/kg IV daily. The primary toxicity of foscarnet is renal with one third of patients experiencing a decrease in renal function requiring adjustment in dose or interruption of therapy. However, full doses of zidovudine can be used with foscarnet. *(Drew, pp. 495–501; Studies of Ocular Complications of AIDS Research Group, in Collaboration with the AIDS Clinical Trials Group, pp. 213–220)*

5. **(A)** A CT of the head is usually normal in cryptococcal meningitis, although in rare circumstances, a ring-enhancing lesion can be demonstrated if a cyptococcoma is present. Diagnosis of cryptococcal meningitis requires isolation of *Cryptococcus neoformans* from CSF. A head CT has become indispensable for diagnosis and management of patients with toxoplasmic encephalitis. The study most often reveals multiple hypodense, ring-enhancing lesions more frequently seen in the basal ganglia and corticomedullary junction. Double-dose contrast gives maximal enhancement of lesions and is, therefore, preferable to single-dose studies. Magnetic resonance imaging (MRI) is more sensitive and may demonstrate lesions not picked up by CT scan, but there are no findings pathognomonic for toxoplasmosis. Definitive diagnosis is made by demonstration of *T. gondii* cysts or tachyzoites in brain tissue obtained by biopsy. This procedure is recommended for patients with presumptive toxoplasmic encephalitis based on head CT or MRI who have not responded to empiric therapy within 3 to 4 weeks. *(Grant and Armstrong, pp. 457–459; Luft and Remington, pp. 211–222)*

6. **(C)** Clinical presentation of toxoplasmic encephalitis, the most common CNS infection in AIDS patients, includes fever and headache in more than one half of patients, altered mental status, focal neurological deficits, and seizures. Hemiparesis is the

most common focal finding, but patients may also present with ataxia, visual field loss, and cranial nerve palsies. Less commonly, toxoplasma may involve retina, lung, heart, abdomen, and testes. Cryptococcal meningitis, the second most common opportunistic infection of the CNS associated with AIDS, often presents nonspecifically. Patients may have prolonged fever (often low grade) with or without headache, and altered mental status. Less frequently seen are focal neurological deficits, seizures, meningismus, and photophobia. Extracranial disseminated disease occurs in up to 50% of patients. *(Grant and Armstrong, pp. 457–459; Luft and Remington, pp. 211–222; Noble, p. 942)*

7. **(C)** In toxoplasmic encephalitis, the CSF may be completely normal or may show mild pleocytosis and elevated protein. Although the presence of IgG toxoplasma antibodies in serum does not predict the development of toxoplasmic encephalitis in patients, its absence argues strongly against the presence of disease in a patient with intracerebral lesions. However, more sensitive assays are needed to improve diagnosis. Production of toxoplasma-specific IgG antibodies in the CSF and serum may be useful in diagnosing active CNS infection. The CSF of patients with cryptococcal meningitis may reveal normal glucose and protein with absence of pleocytosis. Latex agglutination detects cryptococcal polysaccharide antigen in serum and CSF, a positive titer indicating active disease. Less commonly, an India ink stain of the CSF may reveal organisms with their typical large capsules. CSF cryptococcal antigen titers are serially followed to determine response to therapy; however, serum titers may remain high and cannot be correlated with clinical improvement. *(Grant and Armstrong, pp. 457–459; Luft and Remington, pp. 211–222; Noble, p. 941)*

8. **(C)** Duration of initial treatment of toxoplasmic encephalitis is approximately 6 weeks, providing there is steady improvement of intracerebral lesions on neuroradiographic imaging. Chronic suppressive therapy is required indefinitely to prevent the recurrence of lesions or the development of new lesions.

Although the combination of pyrimethamine with sulfadiazine or clindamycin is highly active against the proliferative form of *Toxoplasma gondii*, it is not effective against the dormant cyst. Therefore, if therapy is withdrawn, relapse may occur in up to 80% of cases. Pyrimethamine at 25 to 50 mg daily and sulfadiazine at 2 to 4 g daily or clindamycin 300 mg qid, both taken orally with folinic acid, appear to be an adequate suppressive regimen. Recurrences may still present on suppressive treatment, requiring reinitiation of high-dose therapy. Initial management of cryptococcal meningitis usually consists of daily amphotericin B until the patient is stable and becomes afebrile and free of nausea, vomiting and headache. Treatment can then be changed to oral fluconazole 400 mg daily to complete an 8- to 10-week course. Maintenance therapy with fluconazole 200 mg daily should begin immediately to prevent relapse. Adverse effects of fluconazole include skin rash, nausea, vomiting, abdominal pain, diarrhea, and elevated SGOT and SGPT. *(Grant and Armstrong, pp. 459–462; Luft and Remington, pp. 211–222; Noble, p. 941; Saag et al, pp. 83–94)*

9. **(C)** The cumulative incidence of reported AIDS cases in the United States is disproportionately higher in African-Americans and Hispanics. From the reporting period 1981–1987 to 1993–1995, the proportion of cases among whites decreased from 60% to 43%, whereas the proportion among blacks and Hispanics increased from 25% to 38% and from 14% to 18%, respectively. During 1994, rates per 100,000 population for reported AIDS cases were 48 in the Northeast and 13 in the Midwest. The rates were nearly identical in the South (31/100,000) and the West (29/100,000). The proportion of adult AIDS cases in women has increased over time. As of November 1995, the percentage of reported AIDS cases in women had risen to 18%. Close to 90% of HIV infection in children occurs in those born to women who are at risk of HIV infection. Women at increased risk should be counseled, tested for HIV antibody status, and advised of the risk of HIV transmission to fetus should pregnancy arise. From 1993 to 1995, higher proportions of

cases among those ages 13–29 occurred in small (50,000–499,999) metropolitan statistical areas (MSAs) and non-MSAs (rural areas) in the South and Midwest than in the Northeast and West. *(CDCP, First 500,000 AIDS Cases, pp. 849–851; CDCP, HIV/AIDS Surveillance, pp. 1–23)*

10. **(A)** The first step in evaluating the presence of HIV infection is the HIV antibody status using the enzyme-linked immunosorbent assay (ELISA) technique. HIV antibodies may be detected by this screening method 1 to 2 months after the onset of acute illness. If this test is found to be positive, it is confirmed by the more specific Western blot (WB) method of HIV antibody detection. HIV serum p24 antigen may be detected by ELISA in the period prior to antibody seroconversion but is less sensitive than antibody status and may be present in the serum for only a brief time. Persistent p24 antigenemia or the reappearance of antigenemia may be associated with poor clinical outcome. In vitro culture of HIV is used in clinical trials and in research, but is rarely indicated in routine practice. T-lymphocyte subset studies are routinely used only in known HIV-infected patients. Major subsets include CD4+ (T-helper) cells and CD8 (T-suppressor) cells. A decrease in absolute number of CD4 cells generally correlates with a decline in function of the immune system and an increase in risk of opportunistic infection. *(Tindall et al, pp. 329–338)*

11. **(D)** Progressive multifocal leukoencephalopathy (PML) results from destruction of oligodendrocytes by the JC papovavirus, a DNA "slow" virus. Neurological deterioration occurs with diminished mental acuity, visual impairment, cranial nerve and motor dysfunction, and, in terminal stages, altered consciousness. Neuroradiographic imaging reveals hypodense white matter lesions with irregular borders without contrast enhancement or mass effect on CT and multifocal demyelination on MRI. Definitive diagnosis requires brain biopsy. There is no standard treatment available; however, experimental treatments include interferon, vidarabine, cy-

tarabine, and zidovudine (AZT). To date, results have been disappointing. Primary central nervous system (CNS) lymphoma commonly presents with symptoms of confusion and memory loss, as well as hemiparesis, seizures, headache, aphasia, or cranial nerve palsies. Single or multiple lesions that are frequently hypodense and contrast enhancing are seen on CT or MRI scanning of the head. These lesions may be indistinguishable from toxoplasmosis; therefore, brain biopsy may be necessary for confirmation. Treatment for primary CNS lymphoma involves whole-brain irradiation sometimes combined with a short course of steroids; however, survival is not significantly improved. Combination chemotherapy is being studied. HIV-infected patients are at increased risk for all forms of tuberculosis, both pulmonary and extrapulmonary; the latter includes TB meningitis. To date, there are no studies documenting an increased risk of bacterial meningitis in HIV-infected patients. *(Chaisson and Griffin, pp. 79–82)*

12. **(C)** HIV may be transmitted from mother to neonate during intrauterine life as well as during delivery. HIV antibodies cross the placenta; thus, the positive HIV antibody status of the infant may reflect the presence of maternal antibodies. Symptoms of HIV infection, fever, chronic diarrhea, and thrush may appear as early as 5 months of age. There often is a decrease in weight gain and linear growth and an increase in infections such as otitis media and pneumonia. Staphylococcal and gram-negative infections begin to occur. Chronic lymphocytic infiltrative pneumonia (LIP) and chronic parotid enlargement are common in children. LIP appears on chest x-ray as interstitial, usually bilateral, infiltrates. PCP is the most common opportunistic infection in children, but others include *Mycobacterium avium* complex (MAC), toxoplasmosis, viral, cryptococcal, and other fungal infections. Kaposi's sarcoma occurs rarely in children, but lymphomas are seen frequently. Neurological involvement, primarily progressive encephalopathy, has been described in more than half of pediatric AIDS cases. *(Grossman, pp. 533–541)*

13. **(D)** Diarrhea, weight loss, and abdominal cramps are common presenting symptoms in HIV-infected patients. Although AIDS-wasting syndrome (HIV infection without superimposed enteric infection) is frequently seen in AIDS patients, intestinal infection should first be excluded. Initial evaluation should include stool culture for routine bacterial pathogens, including *Salmonella*, *Shigella*, *Campylobacter*, and *Yersinia*. Therapy is directed at each specific organism and should be of 1 to 2 weeks' duration. Stool examination for ova and parasites may reveal *Giardia lamblia* and *Entamoeba histolytica*, and assay for *Clostridium difficile* toxin should be obtained, all of which are associated with acute enteritis. *Cryptosporidium* and *Isospora belli*, two atypical parasitic infections common in patients with AIDS, are easily identified by examining the stool with acid-fast stain. In patients with cryptosporidiosis, symptoms develop insidiously and become more severe with deterioration of the immune system. Symptoms may include voluminous (1 to 25 L daily) diarrhea, weight loss of more than 10% of total body weight, severe abdominal pain, and dehydration. The biliary tract may become involved, causing nausea and vomiting. Nonspecific treatment of cryptosporidiosis is empiric and depends on the use of antidiarrheal agents (opiates, diphenoxylate, and loperamide), nutritional management, and fluids. Hyperimmune bovine colostrum (HBC), a promising treatment under investigation, has been shown to ameliorate symptoms. Other potentially effective treatments include three macrolide antibiotics (azithromycin, clarithromycin, and roxithromycin), paromycin, a nonabsorbable aminoglycoside, and octreotide, a synthetic cyclic octapeptide analog of somatostatin. Isosporiasis is diagnosed less frequently than cryptosporidiosis, but the symptoms are indistinguishable. Other chronic causes of enteritis include *Mycobacterium avium* complex (also demonstrated on acid-fast stain), CMV, and Kaposi's sarcoma. Blood cultures for CMV and MAC would be useful in detecting those infections, and treatment would be aimed at the specific organism.

If the evaluation reveals no specific pathogen, sigmoidoscopy/colonoscopy with biopsy would be an appropriate last step. Barium enema would be least helpful in diagnosing the etiology of diarrhea in HIV-infected patients. *(Bartlett et al, pp. 726–735; Petersen, pp. 903–909; Chaisson and Griffin, pp. 79–82)*

14. **(D)** Didanosine (ddI) and zalcitabine (ddC) are both nucleoside analogs found to be inhibitors of HIV reverse transcriptase, thereby inhibiting HIV replication. Peripheral neuropathy, characterized by distal numbness, tingling, or pain, occurs in 13% to 34% of patients on ddI and 17% to 31% of patients on ddC. Other adverse effects for ddI include elevations in serum uric acid and triglyceride levels, headache, diarrhea, and retinal depigmentation; and for ddC include oral and esophageal ulcers, rash, cardiomyopathy, and congestive heart failure. Both ddI and ddC can be used as alternate antiretroviral therapy in patients who become intolerant of zidovudine or display disease progression (decline in CD4$^+$ cell count or development of constitutional symptoms or opportunistic infection). Clinical studies examining combination therapy (such as AZT combined with ddI or ddC) are encouraging. Because of problems with viral resistance, drug failure, and drug toxicity, emphasis is now being placed on combination drug regimens in HIV therapy. Dosing of ddI is 200 mg (two 100-mg tablets) twice daily in patients weighing >60 kg and 125 mg (one 100-mg and one 25-mg tablet) twice daily in patients weighing <60 kg. Administration should take place on an empty stomach, and two tablets should be taken at each dose so that adequate buffering is provided to prevent gastric acid degradation of ddI. Dosing of ddC is 0.75 mg every 8 hours orally, with a dose reduction to 0.375 mg every 8 hours for mild drug toxicity or dose interruption for severe toxicity. Pancreatitis, ranging from mild abdominal pain and elevated serum amylase concentrations to fatal disease, occurs in 5% to 10% of patients on ddI and <1% of patients taking ddC. *(Hirsch and D'Aquila, pp. 1686–1695; Noble, pp. 394–395; Sommadossi, pp. S7–S15)*

15. **(A)** The most common causative agents of fungal infections in HIV patients are *Candida* species. Oral candidiasis is a marker of an impaired immune system, and candidal infections of the esophagus, trachea, bronchi, or lungs are recognized as indicator diseases for AIDS. Candidal esophagitis seldom occurs in patients with CD4 counts higher than 100 cells/mm^3 and is frequently diagnosed on the basis of its characteristic presentation (odynophagia, dysphagia, a feeling of obstruction, substernal chest pain, or a combination of these). Experienced radiologists may be able to distinguish *Candida* esophagitis from those caused by herpes virus or cytomegalovirus without the need for endoscopy or radiologic interventions. An esophageal contrast study may reveal widely separated plaques on a normal background mucosa, diffuse plaque formation without ulcers, or a grossly irregular esophagus caused by multiple plaques and ulcers. *Candida* esophagitis may also be diagnosed using blind brushings of the esophagus through a nasogastric tube. CMV and herpes virus esophagitides also present with odynophagia, retrosternal chest pain, and dysphagia. Cultures of biopsy specimens for the diagnosis of CMV are not helpful because they are often negative or represent blood contamination. Diagnosis is made, rather, by histopathologic examination of biopsy materials. Only one study has demonstrated Epstein-Barr virus in cells biopsied from esophageal ulcers. Although herpes simplex virus infections are common in AIDS patients and HSV may cause esophagitis, the most common syndrome is perianal or perineal ulceration. *(DeVita et al, pp. 236–237, 269, 272, 368, 379)*

16. **(E)** Zidovudine interferes with HIV replication by competitive inhibition of the viral enzyme reverse transcriptase, but has no effect on previously infected cells. A 1987 study seemed to indicate that AIDS or ARC patients receiving 1,500 mg/day of zidovudine had significantly fewer opportunistic infections, increased CD4 counts, and weight gain than patients receiving a placebo. Following FDA approval of zidovudine for AIDS patients with a prior episode of *P. carinii* pneu-

monia whose CD4 count was below 200/mm^3, it was learned that 500 to 600 mg/day was better tolerated and as efficacious as higher doses. In 1996, accepted dosage is 200 mg every 8 hours, with periodic complete blood count monitoring and evaluation for potential side effects. Early investigators recommended beginning zidovudine in symptomatic and mildly symptomatic patients with CD4 counts between 200 and 500/mm^3. However, preliminary results of the Concorde I study found that rates of disease progression did not differ between treatment and placebo groups after 3 years. Current thinking is that zidovudine prolongs the period during which patients are asymptomatic or have only mild symptoms, but makes little difference in survival. Toxicities associated with zidovudine include myelosuppression, myopathy, headache, insomnia, flu-like illness, fevers, abdominal discomfort, nausea, and a bluish discoloration of the nail beds. Rarely patients experience lactic acidosis and hepatomegaly with steatosis. Pancreatitis and peripheral neuropathy are toxicities of ddI and ddC; hyperuricemia is associated with ddI and urticaria with ddC. *(Hirsch and D'Aguila, pp. 1686–1695; Noble, p. 934)*

17. **(A)** Trends of newly diagnosed HIV infections in the United States in groups at recognized risk have changed over time. Evidence indicates a decrease in the incidence of new infections in men who have sex with men, reflecting reduced high-risk sexual behavior in this population. The risk of new infection in hemophiliacs has decreased dramatically with the development in 1984 of heat treatment of clotting factor concentrates. The incidence of new infection in IV drug users and their heterosexual partners appears to be increasing. Seroprevalence in IV drug users is strongly associated with the number of persons with whom needles are shared and the use of shooting galleries. Effective interventions for behavior change are difficult but essential to persuade IV drug users not to share needles or to clean needles and drug paraphernalia with bleach. The incidence of new HIV infection in people with no known risk factors remains between 3% and 6%; however, 75% are reclassi-

fied into known-risk categories following additional questioning. The incidence among persons reported as infected through heterosexual contact in 1993 increased 23%. *(CDCP, HIV/AIDS Surveillance, pp. 1–23; CDCP, Update: Trends in AIDS diagnosis; Wolfsy, pp. 307–319)*

18. **(A)** The Centers for Disease Control and Prevention (CDCP), in collaboration with the Council of State and Territorial Epidemiologists (CTSE), expanded the AIDS surveillance case definition effective January 1, 1993. The expanded definition included pulmonary tuberculosis (TB), recurrent pneumonia, and invasive cervical cancer, reflecting the importance of these diseases in the HIV epidemic. Pulmonary TB is the most common type of TB in HIV-infected patients. Patients co-infected with HIV and TB have a substantially increased risk of developing active TB than patients without HIV infection. With the exception of conditions included in the 1987 AIDS surveillance case definition, pneumonia is the leading cause of HIV-related morbidity and mortality. Two or more recurrent episodes of pneumonia in a 1-year period are required for AIDS case reporting. Multiple episodes of pneumonia are more strongly associated with immunosuppression than are single episodes. Several studies have found an increased prevalence of cervical dysplasia, a precursor lesion for cervical cancer, among HIV-infected women. This finding usually is associated with greater immunosuppression, and HIV infection may adversely affect the clinical course and treatment of cervical dysplasia and cancer. Invasive cervical cancer is preventable by the proper recognition and treatment of cervical dysplasia. Kaposi's sarcoma and *P. carinii* pneumonia were included in the earlier case definition. Coexisting syphilis is not unusual in AIDS patients and diarrhea is a common symptom, but neither is included in the case definition per se. *(CDCP, 1993 revised classification system, pp. 1–9)*

19. **(D)** Now that *P. carinii* pneumonia has declined in frequency, disseminated *Mycobacterium avium* complex (DMAC) infection seems to be the most common opportunistic complication found in AIDS patients in the United States, oc-

curring in up to 40% of late-stage HIV-infected patients. The patients at greatest risk for DMAC are those with profoundly depressed CD4$^+$ T-lymphocyte counts below (50/mm^3). DMAC frequently produces symptoms of chronic fever, diaphoresis, and weight loss; also associated are diarrhea, anorexia, and chronic abdominal pain with hepatosplenomegaly. It often infects bone marrow, causing anemia and granulocytopenia. Anemia may be profound enough to require chronic transfusions. DMAC may be found in virtually any organ in the body, including the spleen, liver, lymph nodes, lungs, kidneys, adrenals, and gastrointestinal tract. Patients with DMAC should be treated to reduce mycobacterial load and alleviate symptoms; however, it has not been proven that treatment elicits a durable response or extends survival. DMAC is a multiresistant organism, but treatment has improved with the new broad-spectrum long-acting macrolide antibiotics. Clarithromycin at a dose of 500 mg to 1 g twice daily is the preferred first agent with azithromycin as an alternative. Either macrolide in combination with ethambutol, clofazimine, rifampin, refabutin, ciprofloxacin, or amikacin improves symptoms and reduces bacteremia. *(Benson and Ellner, pp. 7–20; Noble, p. 955)*

20. **(A)** One of the major advances in HIV treatment has been the development of prophylactic regimens to prevent *Pneumocystis carinii* pneumonia (PCP), prompting the U.S. Public Health Service task force to issue guidelines on PCP prophylaxis. Secondary prophylaxis should be started after a patient has been treated for a first episode of PCP. Primary prophylaxis should begin when an HIV-infected patient's CD4$^+$ cell count falls below 200 cells/mm^3 or a CD4 cell percentage below 20, or an HIV-infected patient develops oral thrush or unexplained fevers over 100°F for longer than 2 weeks (even if the CD4$^+$ count is above 200 cells/mm^3). To monitor a patient's immune system more closely, CD4$^+$ cell counts should be measured every 3 months. The first-line agent for PCP prophylaxis is trimethoprim-sulfamethoxazole (TMP-SMX). Although optimal dosage is unknown, the dose recommended in the new guidelines is one double-strength tablet (160 mg TMP plus

800 mg SMX) once a day. Smaller doses may be equally effective and less toxic. Approximately 25% of patients are unable to tolerate TMP-SMX secondary to bone marrow suppression or skin and other allergic reactions. For patients experiencing myelosuppression secondary to zidovudine, TMP-SMX may not be an appropriate choice for PCP prophylaxis. The leading candidate for a second-line agent is Dapsone at a dosage of 50 to 100 mg daily, although there have been reports that doses as low as 100 mg twice weekly may also be effective. Side effects include skin rash, nausea, vomiting, abdominal pain, and headache. The combination of Dapsone and pyrimethamine is effective in preventing both PCP and toxoplasmosis. Added folinic acid minimizes marrow toxicity. Aerosolized pentamidine (AP), which in 1989 was the first drug approved by the FDA for PCP prophylaxis, has since been shown to be less effective than TMP-SMX. AP at a dose of 300 mg once monthly is recommended for PCP in patients who are unable to tolerate SMX-TMP. Ciprofloxacin, clarithromycin, and rifampin are not recommended treatments for PCP prophylaxis. *(CDCP, Recomendations for prophylaxis against PCP for adults and adolescents infected with HIV. MMWR. 1992; 41: RR-4, 141; Noble, p. 958; CDCP, 1993 revised classification system for HIV infection and expanded surveillance case definition for AIDS among teenagers and adults. MMWR. 1993; 41: RR 17, 1–19)*

21. **(C)** HIV infection of the nervous system causes significant morbidity and mortality. It can affect not only the central nervous system, but also the peripheral and autonomic systems. Disease can be caused both by primary HIV infection and by opportunistic infection due to the patient's depressed immune state. Many of the drugs used to treat HIV/AIDS are neurotoxic and add to the complex presentation of AIDS patients with neurological symptoms. In any case, the presentation of the AIDS patient with neurological complications differs dramatically from a patient without HIV infection presenting with the same disease. The mechanisms that lead to nervous system damage are varied and, in many cases, poorly understood. *(Noble, p. 940)*

22. **(B)** In 1983, the self-deferral program of volunteer blood donors who thought they may be at risk for HIV infection was begun in an attempt to reduce HIV transmission through blood transfusions. However, it was not until April 1985 that HIV-antibody testing of donated blood was instituted. This dramatically decreased the risk of HIV transmission to blood recipients. Although blood recipients often wish to have blood donated by family members, this does not decrease the risk of HIV transmission, as risk factors for HIV infection in family members are usually not known or not admitted. Sexual transmission is responsible for the majority of AIDS cases; thus, safer sex practices have become essential. Receptive anal intercourse carries the greatest risk of infection to homosexual men and female partners of bisexual men. The use of latex condoms with or without nonoxynol-9 (a spermicide displaying HIV viricidal activity) reduces the risk of HIV transmission. Nonoxynol-9 inhibits or kills HIV in vitro, but has untested effectiveness in actual sexual situations. The presence of genital ulcers increases the risk of HIV transmission, likely because of increased contact with blood at the ulcer site. Therefore, sexually transmitted diseases that present with genital ulcers increase the risk of HIV transmission. *(CDCP, HIV/AIDS Surveillance, pp. 1–23; DeVita et al, p. 570; Jaffe and Lifson, pp. 299–306; Wolfsy, pp. 307–319)*

23. **(A)** The risk of HIV transmission to health care workers has been evaluated and demonstrated to be approximately 0.33% (1 in 300) following a single needlestick exposure to HIV-infected blood. Although the incidence of transmission is low, the magnitude of the risk emphasizes the need for effective infection control procedures. Universal precautions, such as treating all blood and body fluids as though they were infected with HIV, reduce the risk of occupational exposure. Protective measures include handwashing before and after patient contact, proper disposal of sharp objects, no recapping of needles, use of gloves when handling blood or body fluids/tissues, and use of goggles and gowns when splatter of body fluids is anticipated. The use of masks is necessary only with procedures during

which there is aerosolization of body fluids or with contagious airborne diseases. No cases of HIV transmission to health care workers from contact with body fluids other than blood have been documented. Zidovudine has been given prophylactically to people who have been inoculated with HIV-infected blood in an effort to prevent seroconversion. There has been no documentation to date to prove its effectiveness in such circumstances, and there have been anecdotal reports of the failure of zidovudine in preventing infection. The potential for HBV transmission to health care workers after accidental exposure is much greater than HIV transmission. Studies demonstrate that 10% to 30% of health care workers have serologic evidence of past or present HBV exposure. Twelve thousand health care workers become infected with HBV each year, of which 700 to 1,200 become chronic carriers. *(Gerberding and Henderson, pp. 1179–1185; Henderson et al, pp. 740–746)*

24. **(D)** CMV infection in AIDS patients is quite common and can cause several clinical illnesses, most frequently chorioretinitis, gastrointestinal disease, and pneumonia. Culture of CMV from pulmonary secretions or lung tissue is common, but its isolation does not always indicate active disease. Many patients with pulmonary disease and CMV isolation from the lung have concomitant infections, thereby raising doubt as to whether CMV is a true pulmonary pathogen. CMV is considered a possible pathogen when CMV-infected cells are seen histopathologically in tissue specimens. Therapy with ganciclovir or foscarnet should be considered when CMV is felt to be documented as a pulmonary pathogen and the patient's clinical course is deteriorating. HSV infection, common in HIV-infected patients, may cause oral, genital, and anorectal lesions, as well as esophagitis and other organ involvement. The severity of illness depends on the degree of immunosuppression in the patient and site of infection. Prompt administration of therapy (acyclovir or foscarnet for acyclovir-resistant HSV) for active infection reduces morbidity and the risk of serious complications. Topical acyclovir, although reducing virus shedding, does not reduce the

formation of new lesions or risk of dissemination. Recurrent VZV infection manifesting as shingles occurs commonly in immunosuppressed HIV-infected patients. Dissemination of VZV to lung, liver, and central nervous system has been associated with a high mortality rate. This life-threatening disease process warrants hospitalization and treatment with high-dose IV acyclovir or foscarnet for acyclovir-resistant VZV. Varicella pneumonia may present with mild symptoms or with severe hypoxia and respiratory failure. Patients should be treated with intravenous acyclovir. *(Drew, pp. 495–509; Studies of Ocular Complications of AIDS Research Group, in Collaboration with the AIDS Clinical Trials Group, pp. 213–220)*

25. **(A)** Kaposi's sarcoma (KS) is the most frequent AIDS-associated malignancy and is seen primarily in homosexual men. Unlike classic KS, which presents with relatively indolent cutaneous lesions, KS in AIDS patients often is aggressive and can be found as cutaneous lesions, visceral lesions, or both. Cutaneous KS can appear on any body surface but is commonly seen on the face and in the oral cavity. KS may cause pulmonary disease, gastrointestinal disease leading to gastric outlet obstruction, or gastrointestinal bleeding and cause lymphatic obliteration leading to severe lymphedema. Pulmonary KS may be seen on chest x-ray as nodular infiltrates, with or without pleural effusions, and patients often present with shortness of breath, hemoptysis, and dyspnea. Definitive diagnosis of Kaposi's sarcoma is readily made by biopsy. Radiotherapy is an effective palliative treatment for KS lesions; however, progression and dissemination are not altered with treatment and prognosis is not improved. Multiple cytotoxic chemotherapeutic agents have been used to treat visceral KS with varying response rates. Most of these agents, including vincristine, vinblastine, doxorubicin, etoposide, and bleomycin, have been associated with severe toxicities. Alpha-interferon administered parenterally has proven effective against KS, particularly in patients with early disease who do not yet have marked depletion of CD4$^+$ cells. *(Krown, pp. 24–29; Mitsuyasu, pp. 511–523)*

REFERENCES

Bartlett JG, Belitsus PC, Sears CL. AIDS enteropathy. *Clin Infect Dis.* October 1992; 15: 726–735.

Bartlett JF, Feinberg, J. Update on management of opportunistic infections in patients with HIV infection. *Infect Dis Clin Pract.* 1993; 2: 233–246.

Benson CA, Ellner JJ. *Mycobacterium avium* complex infection and AIDS: Advances in theory and practice. *Clin Infect Dis.* July 1993; 17: 7–20.

Bozzette SA, Sattler FR, Chiu J, et al. A controlled trial of early adjunctive treatment with corticosteroids for *Pneumocystis carinii* pneumonia in the acquired immunodeficiency syndrome. *N Eng J Med.* December 1990; 323: 1451–1457.

Centers for Disease Control and Prevention. First 500,000 AIDS cases—United States, 1995. *MMWR.* 1995; 44: 849–853.

Centers for Disease Control and Prevention. *HIV/AIDS Surveillance, Year-End Edition. U.S. Cases Reported through December 1992.* Atlanta, GA: 1993; 1–23.

Centers for Disease Control and Prevention. 1993 revised classification system for HIV infection and expanded surveillance case definition for AIDS among teenagers and adults. *MMWR.* 1993; 41: RR 17, 1–19.

Centers for Disease Control and Prevention. Recommendations for prophylaxis against PCP for adults and adolescents infected with HIV. *MMWR.* 1992; 41: RR–4, 141.

Centers for Disease control and Prevention. Update: Trends in AIDS diagnosis and reporting under the expanded surveillance definition for adolescents and adults—United States, 1993. MMWR. 1994; 43: 826–831.

Chaisson R, Griffin D. Progressive multifocal leukoencephalopathy in AIDS. *JAMA.* 1990; 264: 79–82.

DeVita, Jr., VT, Hellman S, Rosenberg SA. *AIDS: Etiology, Diagnosis, Treatment and Prevention,* 4th ed. Philadelphia: Lippincott–Raven; 1997.

Drew WL. Herpesvirus infections. How to use ganciclovir and acyclovir. *Infect Dis Clin North Am.* 1988; 2(2): 495–501.

Gerberding JL, Henderson DK. Management of occupational exposures to bloodborne pathogens: Hepatitis B virus, hepatitis C virus and HIV. *Clin Infect Dis.* June 1992; 14: 1179–1185.

Grant IH, Armstrong D. Fungal infections in AIDS. Cryptococcus. *Infect Dis Clin North Am.* 1988; 2(2): 457–464.

Grossman M. Children with AIDS. *Infect Dis Clin North Am.* 1988; 2(2): 533–541.

Henderson DK, Fahey BJ, Willy M, et al. Risk for occupational transmission of human immunodeficiency virus type 1 (HIV-1) associated with clinical exposures: A prospective evaluation. *Ann Intern Med.* 1990; 113: 740–746.

Hirsch MS, D'Aguila RT. Therapy for human immunodeficiency virus infection. *N Eng J Med.* 1993; 328: 1686–1695.

Jaffe HW, Lifson AR. Acquisition and transmission of HIV. *Infect Dis Clin North Am.* 1988; 2(2): 299–306.

Krown SE. Evolving therapeutic options for Kaposi's sarcoma. *HIV Adv Res Ther.* October 1992; 2(3): 24–29.

Luft BJ, Remington JS. Toxoplasmic encephalitis in AIDS. *Clin Infect Dis.* August 1992; 18: 211–222.

Mitsuyasu RT. Kaposi's sarcoma. *Infect Dis Clin North Am.* 1988; 2(2): 511–523.

Noble, J. *Textbook of Primary Care Medicine.* St. Louis, MO: Mosby; 1996.

Petersen C. Cryptosporidiosis in patients infected with the human immunodeficiency virus. *Clin Infect Dis.* December 1992; 15: 903–909.

Saag MS, Powderly WG, Cloud GC, et al. Comparison of amphotericin B with fluconazole in the treatment of acute AIDS-associated cryptococcal meningitis. *N Eng J Med.* January 1992; 326: 83–94.

Sommadossi JP. Nucleoside analogs: Similarities and differences. *Clin Infect Dis.* February 1993; 16: S7–S15.

Studies of Ocular Complications of AIDS Research Group, in Collaboration with the AIDS Clinical Trial Group. Mortality in patients with the acquired immunodeficiency syndrome treated with either foscarnet or ganciclovir for cytomegalovirus retinitis. *N Eng J Med.* January 1992; 362: 213–220.

Tindall B, Cooper DA, Donovan B, Pennt R. Primary human immunodeficiency virus infection. Clinical and serologic aspects. *Infect Dis Clin North Am.* 1988; 2(2): 329–341.

Wofsy CB. Prevention of HIV transmission. Infect *Dis Clin North Am.* 1988; 2(2): 307–319.

Internal Medicine: Dermatology
Questions

William H. Fenn, MM, PA-C

DIRECTIONS (Questions 1 through 12): Each of the numbered items or incomplete statements in this section is followed by answers or by completions of the statement. Select the ONE lettered answer or completion that is BEST in each case.

Questions 1 through 12

1. A 6-year-old child with a history of antecedent upper respiratory infection presents with two 1.5- to 2.5-cm round areas of honey-colored crusts on an erythematous base to the area of the right nasal ala. The most likely diagnosis is

   (A) candidiasis
   (B) cellulitis
   (C) erysipelas
   (D) impetigo
   (E) varicella

2. First-line therapy for acute tinea pedis may include

   (A) clotrimazole
   (B) griseofulvin
   (C) nystatin
   (D) salicylic acid
   (E) triamcinolone

3. Which of the following does not exhibit the Koebner phenomenon?

   (A) lichen planus
   (B) pityriasis rosea
   (C) psoriasis

   (D) verruca(e)
   (E) contact dermatitis

4. A 24-year-old Caucasian American female presents with a 1-cm nontender mobile firm nodule on her left shin, present without changes for "several months." The lesion dimples inward when gently squeezed from the sides. The most likely diagnosis is

   (A) benign familial keratoma
   (B) dermatofibroma
   (C) epidermal inclusion cyst
   (D) keratoacanthoma
   (E) lipoma

5. Which of the following topical steroids is appropriate in the treatment of a localized allergic contact dermatitis on the face?

   (A) Temovate (clobetasol propionate) 0.05% cream
   (B) Hytone (hydrocortisone) 2.5% cream
   (C) Cyclocort (amcinonide) 0.1% ointment
   (D) Lidex (fluocinonide) 0.05% cream
   (E) Halog (halcinonide) 0.1% ointment

6. Which of the following is the most appropriate type of testing if the diagnosis of pityriasis rosea is in doubt?

   (A) chest x-ray
   (B) darkfield microscopy
   (C) KOH prep (potassium hydroxide)
   (D) skin biopsy
   (E) serologic testing

7. A 56-year-old male presents with a 0.9-cm pearly umbilicated papule with telangiectasia to the left temple, with a weathered appearance to the facial skin. The most likely diagnosis is

   (A) basal cell carcinoma
   (B) Bowen's disease (carcinoma in situ)
   (C) keratoacanthoma
   (D) nodular melanoma
   (E) squamous cell carcinoma

8. The most likely diagnosis for a severely pruritic, rough, erythematous, scaly lesion on the lateral aspect of the ankle that started from what was thought to be a mosquito bite 3 months before is

   (A) allergic contact dermatitis
   (B) psoriasis
   (C) systemic lupus erythematosus
   (D) lichen simplex chronicus
   (E) pemphigus vulgaris

9. A necrotic skin ulcer is most commonly associated with the bite of a

   (A) gypsy moth
   (B) brown recluse spider
   (C) scabies mite
   (D) black widow spider
   (E) scorpion

10. A 7-year-old patient presents with pruritic erythematous linear eruptions consisting of papules and small vesicles occurring primarily on the distal extremities. The eruption occurred approximately 24 hours after a cub scout field trip, and secondary excoriations are present. The most likely diagnosis is

    (A) atopic dermatitis
    (B) eczematous dermatitis
    (C) Rhus (plant) dermatitis
    (D) toxic epidermal necrolysis
    (E) viral exanthem

11. Acne is exacerbated by all of the following EXCEPT

    (A) cosmetics
    (B) emotional stress
    (C) topical steroids
    (D) mechanical stress
    (E) food

12. A KOH prep (potassium hydroxide) showing a "spaghetti and meatballs" pattern is associated with

    (A) tinea capitis
    (B) tinea corporis
    (C) tinea cruris
    (D) tinea pedis
    (E) tinea versicolor

DIRECTIONS (Questions 13 through 28): Each group of items in this section consists of lettered headings followed by a set of numbered words or phrases. For each numbered word or phrase, select the ONE lettered heading that is most closely associated with it. Each lettered heading may be selected once, more than once, or not at all.

Questions 13 through 16

Select the viral skin problem for each of the cutaneous lesions.

    (A) verruca vulgaris
    (B) herpes zoster
    (C) molluscum contagiosum
    (D) ecthyma contagiosum
    (E) erythema infectiosum

13. Grouped vesicles, unilateral along a dermatome

14. Slapped face appearance

15. 1.5-cm nontender, dome-shaped bulla with central crusting on the hand of a veterinarian

16. Dome-shaped papules with central umbilication

Questions 17 through 20

Match the appropriate diagnostic test with the listed diagnosis.

(A) syphilis

(B) erythrasma

(C) herpes simplex

(D) tinea corporis

(E) scabies

17. KOH prep (potassium hydroxide)

18. Tzanck smear

19. Darkfield microscopy

20. Mineral oil scrape

Questions 21 through 24

For each characteristic exam finding, select the most likely associated disease or disorder.

(A) Auspitz sign

(B) Dennie's lines

(C) Dimple sign

(D) Nikolsky's sign

(E) Wickham's striae

21. Atopic dermatitis

22. Lichen planus

23. Pemphigus vulgaris

24. Psoriasis

Questions 25 through 28

For each of the following chronic disorders, select the appropriate maintenance therapy.

(A) low-medium potency topical cortico-steroids

(B) medium-high potency topical cortico-steroids

(C) systemic steroids

(D) topical retinoids

(E) systemic retinoids

25. Atopic dermatitis

26. Acne vulgaris

27. Psoriasis

28. Eczematous dermatitis

DIRECTIONS (Questions 29 through 36): Each of the numbered items or incomplete statements in this section is followed by answers or by completions of the statement. Select the ONE lettered answer or completion that is BEST in each case.

29. Which of the following is caused by exposure to ultraviolet light (sunlight)?

(A) actinic keratosis

(B) erythroderma

(C) keratosis piliaris

(D) seborrheic dermatitis

(E) seborrheic keratosis

30. A nonpainful macule that appears ecchymotic and is palpably firm most likely represents

(A) capillary hemangiomata

(B) cutaneous sarcoidosis

(C) Kaposi's sarcoma

(D) porphyria cutanea tarda

(E) Stevens–Johnson syndrome

31. Topical preparations containing ketoconazole are useful alone in the definitive treatment of which of the following?

(A) tinea capitis

(B) tinea manuum

(C) onychomycosis

(D) seborrheic dermatitis

(E) eczematous dermatitis

32. A 26-year-old male presents with what appears on exam to be tinea cruris. Examination under ultraviolet light (Wood's lamp) shows coral-red fluorescence. The most likely diagnosis is

(A) chancroid

(B) erythrasma

(C) lymphogranuloma venereum

(D) scabies

(E) tinea incognito

33. Mongolian spots usually

    (A) disappear in childhood
    (B) are a malignancy indicator
    (C) occur on the face
    (D) occur in Caucasian patients
    (E) are an acquired lesion

34. The category of drug most likely to induce erythema nodosum is

    (A) antihistamines
    (B) macrolide antibiotics
    (C) oral contraceptives
    (D) sulfonylureas
    (E) tricyclic antidepressants

35. A 25-year-old female presents with intense pruritus to the elbows for 3 days. Contact history is unrevealing. Past medical history is remarkable for malabsorptive disease. Exam reveals marked excoriation to the posterior elbows with a few intact small vesicles in a group. The most likely diagnosis is

    (A) bullous pemphigoid
    (B) contact dermatitis
    (C) dermatitis herpetiformis
    (D) pemphigus erythematosus
    (E) scabies

36. Which of the following is a treatment of choice for rosacea?

    (A) corticosteroids
    (B) metronidazole
    (C) sun-blocking agents
    (D) tetracycline
    (E) vasoconstrictors

Answers and Explanations

1. **(D)** Impetigo is a superficial skin infection caused by streptococcal or staphylococcal species. It is seen most often in children, especially after viral upper respiratory infections, and often on the face. The hallmark diagnostic appearance is the presence of honey-colored crusting. Candidiasis is a superficial fungal infection that would be highly uncommon on the face and that is characterized by deep red satellite lesion and frequently a whitish scale. Cellulitis is a somewhat deeper bacterial infection that often occurs without scale. Erysipelas is a specific variant of cellulitis characterized by palpable "step-off" margins. Varicella is a viral disorder of childhood that displays widespread lesions in several stages: the classic lesion is the "dewdrop on a rose petal." (*Sauer and Hall, p. 155*)

2. **(A)** Clotrimazole is a topical antifungal agent in the imidazole group, low in cost, extremely low in side effects, and highly effective against dermatophytic organisms. Griseofulvin also has activity against the causative organisms, but has significant systemic side effects and thus should not be considered for initial treatment. Nystatin is an antifungal agent specific for *Candida albicans* and has no activity against the causative species for tinea pedis. Salicylic acid is a mild keratolytic agent with no clinical antifungal activity. Triamcinolone is a corticosteroid with anti-inflammatory properties but no antifungal properties. (*Sauer and Hall, pp. 210–216; Fitzpatrick et al, 1996, pp. 98–100*)

3. **(B)** The Koebner phenomenon is a well-known, but somewhat poorly understood, occurrence whereby the lesion(s) of a disorder will spread isomorphically to nearby areas of the skin, usually in a linear fashion. A frequently postulated mechanism is trauma, particularly in psoriasis and lichen planus, although viral seeding likely is a factor in verrucae. Both trauma and secondary spread of the offending agent via excoriation may play a factor in contact dermatitis. The Koebner phenomenon has not been observed in pityriasis rosea: the linear distribution that frequently occurs is simply a manifestation of the disorder itself. (*Lookingbill and Marks, pp. 138, 184*)

4. **(B)** Dermatofibromas are common small benign tumors, thought most likely to arise from trivial trauma. Thus, in the United States, the most common site is the anterior shin of women, presumably from shaving. They are well-demarcated and display a positive "dimple" sign: the tumor invaginates slightly when compressed from the sides resulting in a characteristic dimpling. No other disorder manifests this sign. Epidermal inclusion cysts are benign keratin-containing lesions that often have a central punctum. Keratoacanthomas are rapidly growing vegetative lesions. Lipomas are benign fatty tumors that are somewhat irregular and relatively less mobile. (*Fitzpatrick et al, 1993, pp. 1201–1203*)

5. **(B)** Hytone (hydrocortisone) 2.5% is the drug of choice among those listed for treatment of any lesion on the face because of its low potency. Topical corticosteroids can be grouped in at least four separate groups, which include low-potency, mid-potency high-potency, and ultra-high-potency categories, based on their strength of activity. The other four drugs listed are either in the high-potency or ultra-high-potency groups and should never be used on thin skin, such as the face, or in areas where they would be occluded, such as the groin or the intertriginous areas of the skin. High-potency steroids are useful primarily on very thick skin or on severely hyperkeratotic lesions, such as psoriasis. High-potency steroids used either on the face or in the intertriginous areas can cause severe atrophy. *(Sauer and Hall, pp. 40–43)*

6. **(E)** The rash of pityriasis rosea is similar to a pattern associated with secondary syphilis. This is especially true if there is no complaint of pruritus. Serologic testing is indicated in such cases to rule out secondary syphilis. Chest x-rays have no value in either diagnosis. Darkfield microscopy is indicated in the diagnosis of primary, not secondary, syphilis. A potassium hydroxide prep may be useful in differentiating atypical pityriasis rosea from dermatophytosis, but does not rule out the overriding concern for secondary syphilis. Skin biopsy would be of limited use in establishing the diagnosis and represents an unnecessary invasive procedure. *(Sauer and Hall, pp. 107–110; Lookingbill and Marks, pp. 149–151)*

7. **(A)** Any ulcerative or umbilicated lesion in a sun-exposed area should raise the possibility of neoplasm, and even more so when the background skin suggests significant exposure. The pearly appearance and associated telangiectasia are consistent with classic basal cell carcinoma. Basal cell carcinomas are more common in males and increase in incidence with age, particularly after 50. Bowen's disease is a form of squamous cell carcinoma that usually appears as a scaly erythematous patch and may be confused with a chronic dermatitis. Keratoacanthomas are benign le-

sions that grow quite rapidly to become vegetative or ulcerative. Nodular melanomas involve various levels of irregular hyperpigmentation. *(Sauer and Hall, pp. 331–333; Lookingbill and Marks, pp. 78–86, 95)*

8. **(D)** Lichen simplex chronicus is a commonly seen chronic area of dermatitis, occurring in response to repeated scratching and/or rubbing. The most distinctive feature is lichenification, and the lesions are usually fairly well circumscribed. The most common sites are back of the neck, lower legs, ankles, wrists, and forearms. It frequently begins in response to some small local irritation, such as an insect bite. A scratch–itch cycle is initiated, which results in thickening of the skin and chronic irritation. Contact dermatitis usually is of a much shorter duration and comes on much more suddenly in the acute erythematous stage. Psoriasis usually has a much more sharply demarcated border, is less pruritic, and occurs in multiple lesions. Systemic lupus erythematosus is usually an ill-defined lesion, mostly affecting the face, arms, shoulders, and upper trunk but can affect the hands. The lesions are more violaceous than those of lichen simplex chronicus. Pemphigus vulgaris is a vesiculobullous disease. *(Sauer and Hall, pp. 107–110)*

9. **(B)** The brown recluse spider, often called the fiddleback spider because of the violin-shaped figure on its thorax, bites when humans accidentally disturb its habitat. The initial bite often is painless with the wound starting as a small erythematous papule over the first 6 to 12 hours, progressing to a blister and/or skin necrosis. The resultant necrotic skin ulcer heals slowly and may require a skin graft. The gypsy moth (*Lymantria dispar*), a caterpillar species, may cause irritation with its histamine-containing hairs. The lesions in this case may appear as grouped vesicles and/or bullae. Papules and vesicles are the most common lesions of scabies, but the burrow is the most characteristic and diagnostic feature. The black widow spider, also called the hourglass spider, has a neurotoxic venom that produces minimal local reactions. Generalized pain may occur within 1

to 8 hours. Characteristically, the crampy abdominal pain may be associated with pain in the flanks or chest and confused with acute appendicitis, renal colic, or acute myocardial infarction. Nausea and vomiting accompany most bites. Scorpions are of primary medical interest in tropical or desert areas, such as the southwestern United States, Mexico, and the Middle East. Their venom induces complex cardiac arrhythmias. (*Fitzpatrick et al, 1993, pp. 2815–2818*)

10. **(C)** Plant dermatitis secondary to exposure to an oleoresin found in the Rhus species such as poison ivy is a common complaint. Most exposures involve the extremities, hence this is the most common site of the lesions. As with all allergic contact dermatitis, the time from contact to onset is usually less than 1 day, resulting in pruritic papules and vesicles. A characteristic of plant dermatitis is the linearity of the eruption, which is attributable to the usual patterns of contact. Atopic and eczematous dermatitis usually do not have such an abrupt onset, involve additional areas, and do not usually display linearity. Toxic epidermal necrolysis is a disorder almost exclusively of adults and presents with dramatic widespread epidermal sloughing and systemic symptomatology. Viral exanthems may occur in many patterns, however onset only on the distal extremities would be uncommon. (*Isselbacher et al, p. 225; Sauer and Hall, pp. 78–79; Fitzpatrick et al, 1996, p. 334*)

11. **(E)** Food does not appear to be an exacerbating factor with acne vulgaris. However, some patients cling to the belief that their flare-ups are associated with certain foods, particularly with the ingestion of chocolate. Although there is no scientific evidence for this, it is better to eliminate those dietary agents in these cases. Some authors fail to make the distinction between scientific principles and patient prejudices. Cosmetics, with their multiple chemical components, have been found to exacerbate acne, although those labeled noncomedogenic probably do not induce *new* lesions. Just as stress can worsen diseases such as hypertension or diabetes, it can exac-

erbate acne as well. Topical corticosteroids and repetitive trauma to the skin, such as rubbing, can exacerbate acne. (*Fitzpatrick et al, 1993, pp. 709–724*)

12. **(E)** A potassium hydroxide prep may be positive for hyphae and spores in any dermatophytosis. In general, however, the specific organism cannot be identified. However, the pattern displayed by pityrosporum orbiculare (previously called malassezia furfur), the etiologic organism in tinea versicolor, does display a characteristic appearance suggestive of "spaghetti and meatballs." Many clinicians have not seen this pattern, however, as the clinical appearance of the disorder is usually characteristic enough to establish the diagnosis without a potassium hydroxide prep. (*Isselbacher et al, p. 277; Fitzpatrick et al, 1993, p. 2464*)

13. **(B)** The most distinctive feature of herpes zoster is the localization of the rash. Its characteristic rash is nearly always unilateral, does not cross the midline, and is limited in most cases to the area of skin supplied by a single sensory dermatome. Lesions rarely occur below the elbows or knees. (*Fitzpatrick et al, 1993, p. 2552*)

14. **(E)** Erythema infectiosum, or "Fifth disease," is a mild, febrile exanthematous disease of viral etiology. There is usually little or no prodrome. Fifth disease begins as a low-grade fever, with or without conjunctivitis, upper respiratory infection, itching, and nausea and vomiting. In many cases, this vague early period is followed by a confluent erythema over the cheeks. This rash is the so-called slapped face appearance. It is typical for signs and symptoms to occur, then abate, only to reappear, especially in times of stress. This may happen for a period of weeks. (*Isselbacher et al, pp. 685–686*)

15. **(D)** Ecthyma contagiosum (Orf) is a contagious viral disorder caused by a poxvirus, which is usually contracted from infected sheep and goats and is seen in shepherds, slaughterhouse workers, shearers, veterinari-

ans, and laboratory workers. The lesions are usually 1 to 2 cm in size and generally asymptomatic. The diagnosis is usually based on the clinical appearance of the lesion, the location of the lesion, and a history of exposure to an infected animal. *(Fitzpatrick et al, 1993, pp. 2603–2606)*

16. **(C)** Molluscum contagiosum is a benign viral disease of the skin caused by a poxvirus. It affects children much more often than adults. It may be transmitted by sexual contact, although that is only one route of spread. The lesions are individual, discrete, smooth, pearly to flesh-colored, dome-shaped papules. Often these lesions have a central umbilication and a mildly erythematous base. *(Sauer and Hall, p. 199)*

17. **(D)** Tinea corporis is a superficial fungal infection of the stratum corneum caused by fungi in the trichophyton, microsporum, or, less commonly, epidermophyton families. The fungus is readily identified in 10% KOH by visualizing the hyphae. Wood's lamp examination is not useful. *(Fitzpatrick et al, 1993, p. 2495)*

18. **(C)** Herpes simplex (HSV) infections may be rapidly diagnosed by obtaining cells from the base of the lesion and making a smear on a glass slide. This slide is then stained with Wright's stain or Giemsa's stain and examined for multinucleated giant cells. This is a Tzanck smear, which is positive in at least 75% of early herpetic (not just simplex) infections. *(Fitzpatrick et al, 1996, pp. 71, 73, 308)*

19. **(A)** Syphilis is a communicable disease caused by *Treponema pallidum*. The diagnosis of primary syphilis may be made by detecting the organism in early lesions. Serum from moist lesions or scrapings of the base of dry lesions when viewed with a darkfield microscope may reveal characteristic movements of *T. pallidum*. These include corkscrew rotation, a gentle bending like a bamboo pole, and a spiral spring shortening and lengthening. *(Fitzpatrick et al, 1993, p. 52)*

20. **(E)** The mineral oil technique of Muller and colleagues is excellent for isolating the mite that causes scabies. In this technique, a drop of sterile mineral oil is placed on a sterile scalpel blade. The oil is then applied to the surface of a burrow or papule. The burrow or papule is then scraped vigorously to remove the entire top of the papule. Tiny flecks of blood will appear in the oil, and when viewed under the microscope should reveal mites, ova, and/or feces. *(Fitzpatrick et al, 1993, p. 51)*

21. **(B)** The presence of Dennie–Morgan lines (often truncated to Dennie's lines) or prominent infraorbital folds is associated with allergic or atopic disease. They are characteristic, but their absence does not exclude the diagnosis. *(Lookingbill and Marks, p. 128)*

22. **(E)** Close examination of the surface of lesions in lichen planus will reveal fine, reticulate white lines. These are Wickham's striae, a useful finding in differentiating the diagnosis from other disorders. *(Lookingbill and Marks, p. 184)*

23. **(D)** In bullous disease, a useful exam technique is to apply gentle lateral pressure to an intact bulla. Extension of the bulla, sometimes accompanied by a palpable "unzipping" sensation, is a positive Nikolsky's sign seen only in pemphigus vulgaris. *(Isselbacher et al, p. 285; Fitzpatrick et al, 1993, pp. 50–51; Lookingbill and Marks, p. 172)*

24. **(A)** Auspitz's sign occurs when the gentle removal of scale associated with an eruption results in punctate bleeding points underneath. This is classically associated with psoriasis, although some authors believe it is not that specific. *(Fitzpatrick et al, 1993, pp. 33, 51, 773)*

25. **(A)** Atopic dermatitis may require several considerations for maintenance therapy, including hydration, emollients, and antipruritics. In severe cases, short bursts of oral steroids or higher-potency topical steroids may be necessary. However, these are con-

traindicated for maintenance therapy, and the use of steroids of potency above the low-medium range may induce tachyphylaxis. *(Isselbacher et al, p. 274)*

26. **(D)** Acne is a chronic disorder that generally does require prolonged therapy. Both topical and systemic steroids are well known to aggravate acne. Systemic retinoids (isotretinoin, Accutane) may be very useful in select cases of severe acne, but are prescribed within very strict time frames, and not on a maintenance basis. Topical retinoids (tretinoin, Retin-A) are very useful agents for maintenance control until such time as the disorder spontaneously remits. *(Lookingbill and Marks, pp. 189–194)*

27. **(B)** The hyperkeratotic plaques of psoriasis make low-strength steroids generally ineffective and require the use of higher potency topical steroids. The principle of using the lowest potency to achieve the desired effect still applies, but medium to high potencies will be required. It is important that the clinician recognize this, as overcautious use of a low-potency steroid, which will not be effective in this disorder, will often result in a patient who feels you do not take his or her problem seriously. Occasional use of systemic steroids may be required for severe exacerbations, but only for a short burst, not for maintenance. Promising research in retinoids may produce preparations that are beneficial for long-term use, but at present, available retinoids are useful only for select patients for short-term administration. *(Fitzpatrick et al, 1993, pp. 40–51; Lookingbill and Marks, pp. 138–142)*

28. **(A)** The explanation for Question 24 also applies to eczematous dermatitis. Indeed, atopic and eczematous disorders share many similarities. There continues to be taxonomic debate on whether these are related disorders, totally different disorders, or if one is simply a variation of the other. *(Fitzpatrick et al, 1993, pp. 16–27; Lookingbill and Marks, pp. 120–130)*

29. **(A)** Actinic keratoses are the direct result of excessive cumulative exposure to the ultravi-olet band of sunlight and are regarded as premalignant lesions with a higher incidence of degeneration to squamous cell carcinoma. Their detection and prompt management are a key to preventing progressive neoplasia. Erythroderma is a dramatic exfoliative disorder that may arise from a preexisting condition and/or drug reaction. Although the diffuse erythema may casually resemble a mild sunburn, the appearance is misleading. Keratosis piliaris is a common follicular disorder with no association to sun exposure. Seborrheic dermatitis is a complex disorder associated with *Pityrosporum orbiculare.* Although it is not clear that the organism is causative, and other mechanisms such as reaction to seasonal changes in body oils have been postulated, it is clearly not caused by sun exposure. Seborrheic keratoses, despite the similarity in nomenclature, are unrelated benign epidermal tumors that may be inherited as an autosomal dominant trait. *(Fitzpatrick et al, 1993, pp. 551, 804–807, 855–858, 2956)*

30. **(C)** Kaposi's sarcoma is a vascular neoplasm with increased incidence in HIV-positive persons. It frequently appears initially similar to a bruise, but is almost always palpably firm. Capillary hemangiomata also are vascular, but, as there is no extravascular blood, there is no ecchymotic appearance. Porphyria cutanea tarda consists largely of bullae, but there may well be painful ecchymotic areas in easily traumatized skin. There will be no firmness to palpation however. Sarcoid is a complex disorder that may present with a number of lesion types; ecchymoses are not generally associated. Stevens–Johnson syndrome is the severe form of erythema multiforme, which, as the name suggests, may have lesions of many forms. Ecchymoses are not classically seen, but when they are there would not likely be any degree of palpable firmness. *(Fitzpatrick et al, 1993, pp. 432–437, 544–546, 432–437; Lookingbill and Marks, pp. 243–245)*

31. **(D)** Tinea capitis and onychomycosis are dermatophytic infections involving the keratin extensions of the epidermis, the scalp

hairs and nails, respectively. Topical medications of any type are ineffective in penetrating these structures. Similarly tinea manuum, a dermatophytic infection of the palms of the hands, does not respond to topical agents alone, perhaps because of the highly keratotic epidermis. Seborrheic dermatitis is a disorder primarily of the facial and scalp skin that is associated with a superficial overgrowth of *Pityrosporum orbiculare*, which responds to topical ketoconazole. Eczematous dermatitis is an inflammatory disorder without a fungal component. *(Fitzpatrick et al, 1996, pp. 102–112; Lookingbill and Marks, pp. 120–123, 130–131, 281–283)*

32. **(B)** Erythrasma is a superficial bacterial infection caused by *Corynebacterium minutissimum*. When seen in the inguinal area, as is common, it is easily mistaken for tinea cruris. However, examination under a Wood's lamp will show a clear "coral-red" appearance due to the production of porphyrin by the causative organism. This is a diagnostic indicator that is not seen in other disorders. *(Sauer and Hall, pp. 163–164)*

33. **(A)** Mongolian spots are congenital and usually disappear, depending on the size, within a few years. Mongolian spots may persist into adulthood, with a 3% to 4% incidence in the Japanese. Mongolian spots are almost always located in the lumbosacral area and on the buttocks. When seen on the face, they may be confused with a nevus of Ota. One point of difference in the pigmentation of the mongolian spot is a blue-black macule of varying sizes, whereas the nevus of Ota has a characteristic mottling with blue and brown spots. The nevus of Ota is not congenital and may persist through life. Laser therapy offers hope to decrease the color intensity with both. Mongolian spots are observed in more than 90% of the Asiatic and American Indian races, less frequently in blacks, and in less than 10% of whites. *(Fitzpatrick et al, 1993, pp. 978–979)*

34. **(C)** Erythema nodosum is an inflammatory pattern of panniculus involving the lower ex-

tremities. It is caused by diverse mechanisms, one of which is a drug reaction. Although an individual drug reaction is impossible to predict, clearly oral contraceptives have the highest incidence of association with this disorder. *(Isselbacher et al, p. 283; Sauer and Hall, pp. 118–119, Fitzpatrick et al, 1996, pp. 478–479)*

35. **(C)** Dermatitis herpetiformis (DH) is an intensely pruritic vesicular disorder whose lesions show a predilection for the extensor surfaces of the elbows and knees as well as the buttock and sacral area. It is twice as common in females as in males, and about 20% of patients have a concomitant gluten-sensitive enteropathy (nontropical sprue). The lesions occur in groups and are often obscured by marked excoriation. Pemphigoid and pemphigus are bullous disorders that manifest with more widespread and larger bullae of little pruritus in an older age group. Scabies also is highly pruritic, but the lesions tend to be either serpiginous or diffuse. Contact dermatitis is a reasonable consideration, but the pattern would be unusual without a positive contact history (unreliable as it may be), and the presence of malabsorptive disease clearly makes DH much more likely. *(Isselbacher et al, pp. 286–288; Sauer and Hall, pp. 248–249)*

36. **(D)** Rosacea is a chronic acneform inflammation of the face whose etiology is unclear. Tetracycline (or erythromycin) still is the treatment of choice for this disorder, which usually manifests several recurrences before resolving spontaneously. Topical metronidazole is an alternative for those patients who do not respond to or cannot tolerate tetracycline. Some feel sun exposure aggravates the condition, but sun screens are not a direct treatment per se. The disorder usually involves telangiectasia, but vasoconstrictors are of no value. Rosacea may be accompanied by seborrheic dermatitis, which can be treated with 1% hydrocortisone. This, however, does not improve the rosacea, and indeed strong corticosteroids are well known to aggravate the disease. *(Fitzpatrick et al, 1993, pp. 732–734)*

REFERENCES

Fitzpatrick TB, Eisen AZ, Wolff K, Freedburg IM, Austen KF. *Dermatology in General Medicine*, 4th ed. New York: McGraw-Hill; 1993.

Fitzpatrick TB, Johnson RA, Polano MK, Suurmond D, Wolff K. *Color Atlas and Synopsis of Clinical Dermatology*, 3rd ed. New York: McGraw-Hill; 1996.

Isselbacher KJ, Braunwald E, Fauci AS, Kasper DL, Martin JB, Wilson JD. *Harrison's Principles of Internal Medicine*, 13th ed. New York: McGraw-Hill; 1994.

Lookingbill DP, Marks JG. *Principles of Dermatology*, 2nd ed. Philadelphia: Saunders; 1993.

Sauer GC, Hall JC. *Manual of Skin Diseases*, 7th ed. pp 190–191. Philadelphia: Lippincott–Raven Publishers; 1996.

Internal Medicine: Renal
Questions

Brenda L. Jasper, PA-C

DIRECTIONS (Questions 1 through 7): Each of the numbered items or incomplete statements in this section is followed by answers or by completions of the statement. Select the ONE lettered answer or completion that is BEST in each case.

Questions 1 through 7

1. Of the following signs and symptoms listed, which is LEAST likely to be associated with acute pyelonephritis?

   (A) nausea and vomiting
   (B) leukocytosis
   (C) costovertebral angle (CVA) tenderness or pain on deep abdominal palpation
   (D) frequency and urgency
   (E) fever and chills

2. The filtrate that enters the proximal tubule immediately after the glomerulus should contain most all substances present in the plasma EXCEPT

   (A) sodium
   (B) potassium
   (C) protein
   (D) creatinine
   (E) water

3. Mr. Smith is seen in the office for a routine exam. One year ago his creatinine was normal at a level of 1.0 mg/dL. Labs today reveal an elevated creatinine of 2.0 mg/dL. Which of the following BEST describes the reaction of his glomerular filtration rate (GFR)?

   (A) an inconsequential finding
   (B) decrease in GFR from 120 to 60 mL/min
   (C) increase in GFR from 60 to 120 mL/min
   (D) decrease in GFR from 60 to 30 mL/min
   (E) increase in GFR from 30 to 60 mL/min

4. In which of the following renal diseases see eosinophils appear in the urine?

   (A) acute tubular necrosis
   (B) diabetic nephropathy
   (C) hypertensive nephrosclerosis
   (D) interstitial nephritis
   (E) lupus nephritis

5. White blood cell casts are most often seen with

   (A) urethral syndrome
   (B) acute pyelonephritis
   (C) cystitis
   (D) drug-induced tubulointerstitial nephritis
   (E) renal tuberculosis

6. You are asked to see a diabetic patient with retinopathy and hypertension. On examination, the patient's blood pressure is 180/90. Urinalysis shows 300 mg/dL protein, blood urea nitrogen (BUN) 22 mg/dL, creatinine 1.5 mg/dL. Which of the following antihypertensives would be best in this setting?

(A) calcium-channel blocker
(B) nitrates
(C) alpha-blocker
(D) diuretic
(E) angiotensin-converting enzyme inhibitor

7. In the absence of infection, approximately 90% of renal calculi are composed of

(A) calcium compounds
(B) uric acid compounds
(C) cystine compounds
(D) magnesium compounds
(E) ammonium compounds

DIRECTIONS (Questions 8 through 12): Each group of items in this section consists of lettered headings followed by a set of numbered words or phrases. For each numbered word or phrase, select the ONE lettered heading that is most closely associated with it. Each lettered heading may be selected once, more than once, or not at all.

Questions 8 through 12

Of the causes of hematuria and proteinuria listed as (A)–(E) below, select a single BEST response to the following statements.

(A) nephrotic syndrome
(B) multiple myeloma
(C) Berger's disease (IgA nephropathy)
(D) Goodpasture's syndrome
(E) systemic lupus erythematosus

8. These patients present with massive proteinuria but few formed elements (cells, casts, etc.) in their urine.

9. This disorder, caused by circulating immune complexes, presents in early adulthood and waxes and wanes between gross and microscopic hematuria. The disease progresses over a long time and is associated with slowly progressive renal impairment.

10. Patients with this complaint develop hemoptysis in association with rapid-onset renal insufficiency.

11. Illness often associated with rash, renal insufficiency, and arthritis.

12. Light chain immunoglobulins are seen in the urine of patients with this disease.

DIRECTIONS (Questions 13 through 15): Each of the numbered items or incomplete statements in this section is followed by answers or by completions of the statement. Select the ONE lettered answer or completion that is BEST in each case.

Questions 13 through 15

13. A 72-year-old black male presents after several days of voiding difficulty complaining of complete loss of urine production, although he has the desire to void. He denies fever, chills, or recent illness. He admits to a 22-year history of diabetes mellitus and a 2-pack-per-day smoking habit. The most likely cause of his oliguria/anuria is

(A) prerenal anuria due to congestive heart failure (CHF)
(B) postrenal anuria due to renal calculi
(C) intrinsic renal disease due to bilateral renal cortical necrosis
(D) diabetic nephropathy
(E) postrenal anuria due to bladder outlet obstruction

14. All of the following are examples of a prerenal state EXCEPT

(A) interstitial nephritis
(B) renal hypoperfusion
(C) gastrointestinal hemorrhage
(D) excessive diuresis
(E) dehydration

15. A 32-year-old bank executive presents with a 24-hour history of fever, chills, perineal pain and frequency, urgency, and nocturia. He denies being at risk for sexually transmitted disease and has had no urethral discharge. On physical examination, he is noted to have an acutely inflamed prostrate. The treatment of choice for his diagnosis is

(A) amoxicillin 500 mg qid for 30 days
(B) ciprofloxacin 500 mg bid for 30 days
(C) trimethoprim-sulfamethoxazole (160/800 mg) bid for 10 days
(D) amoxicillin 500 mg qid for 10 days
(E) doxycycline 100 mg bid for 10 days

DIRECTIONS (Questions 16 through 20): Each group of items in this section consists of lettered headings followed by a set of numbered words or phrases. For each numbered word or phrase, select the ONE lettered heading that is most closely associated with it. Each lettered heading may be selected once, more than once, or not at all.

Questions 16 through 20

Match the list of disorders of the scrotum and its contents below to the single BEST response in the statements.

(A) cryptorchism
(B) testicular tumors
(C) testicular torsion
(D) acute epididymitis
(E) hydrocele

16. A life-threatening disorder in young men whose only sign may be a painless mass

17. An effusion of fluid in the potential space in the tunica vaginalis

18. Increases chance of testicular malignancy

19. Is an indication for emergent surgical consultation in attempt to save testicle

20. May be associated with urinary tract infection (UTI) or urethritis, especially chlamydia

DIRECTIONS (Questions 21 through 43): Each of the numbered items or incomplete statements in this section is followed by answers or by completions of the statement. Select the ONE lettered answer or completion that is BEST in each case.

Questions 21 through 43

21. Which of the following statements does NOT describe the effects of Angiotensin II?

(A) potent vasoconstrictor
(B) increased aldosterone secretion
(C) increased renal sodium retention
(D) produced in response to low renin levels
(E) increased systemic vascular resistance

22. All of the following diuretics are considered potassium sparing EXCEPT

(A) triamterene
(B) amiloride
(C) hydrochlorothiazide
(D) spironolactone
(E) A and C

23. The leading cause of chronic renal failure is

(A) glomerulonephritis
(B) diabetes mellitus
(C) hypertension
(D) polycystic kidney disease
(E) systemic lupus erythematosus

24. Calculate the anion gap in a patient with the following labs: blood urea nitrogen (BUN) 10 mg/dL, creatinine 1.0 mg/dL, sodium 145 meq/L, potassium 3.0 meq/L, chloride 105 meq/L, bicarbonate 15 meq/L

(A) 35
(B) 25
(C) 32
(D) 43
(E) 27

25. A 41-year-old woman presents for evaluation of renal stones. She is found to have hypercalciuria, hypercalcemia, and hypophosphatemia. What underlying disease would you suspect?

    (A) renal tubular acidosis
    (B) gout
    (C) idiopathic hypercalciuria
    (D) hyperparathyroidism
    (E) sarcoidosis

26. A reduction in what hormone produced by the kidney contributes to anemia in renal failure?

    (A) antidiuretic hormone
    (B) 1,25-dihydroxyvitamin D
    (C) aldosterone
    (D) erythropoietin
    (E) parathyroid hormone

27. The anemia of chronic renal failure is typically

    (A) hypochromic microcytic
    (B) normochromic microcytic
    (C) normochromic normocytic
    (D) normochromic macrocytic
    (E) hypochromic macrocytic

28. Which of the following is NOT a common fluid or electrolyte abnormality seen in chronic renal failure?

    (A) hypomagnesemia
    (B) metabolic acidosis
    (C) hyperkalemia
    (D) hyperphosphatemia
    (E) hypocalcemia

29. Which of the following casts are not indicative of renal disease?

    (A) waxy
    (B) hyaline
    (C) red cell
    (D) white cell
    (E) fatty

30. Findings that may indicate the chronicity of renal failure include all of the following EXCEPT

    (A) azotemia for at least 3 to 6 months
    (B) bilaterally small kidneys by sonogram
    (C) hematuria
    (D) broad casts in urinary sediment
    (E) anemia

31. All of the following are considered nephrotoxins EXCEPT

    (A) radiocontrast agents
    (B) cyclosporine
    (C) aminoglycosides
    (D) cisplatin
    (E) clindamycin

32. A urine output of <400 mL/min is defined as

    (A) anuria
    (B) polyuria
    (C) oliguria
    (D) nocturia
    (E) azotemia

33. All of the following statements are true concerning radiocontrast-induced renal failure EXCEPT

    (A) diabetic patient with a creatinine of 3.0 mg/dL is at higher risk
    (B) creatinine rises after the contrast is given and peaks at 3 to 7 days
    (C) renal function usually returns to baseline
    (D) hydration in high-risk patients is not beneficial
    (E) patients with creatinine less than 1.5 mg/dL are at low risk

34. Which of the following classes of drugs have been used to treat benign prostatic hypertrophy?

    (A) beta-blockers
    (B) alpha-adrenergic blockers
    (C) calcium-channel blockers

(D) diuretics

(E) sympatholytics

35. Which of the following is the LEAST important consideration in adjusting medication doses for a patient with renal insufficiency?

(A) serum electrolytes

(B) serum creatinine

(C) age

(D) weight

(E) sex

36. The most common electrolyte abnormality seen in a hospitalized population is

(A) hypokalemia

(B) hyperkalemia

(C) hyponatremia

(D) hypernatremia

(E) hyperchloridemia

37. The most common cause of respiratory alkalosis is

(A) pneumonia

(B) pulmonary embolism

(C) pulmonary edema

(D) hyperventilation syndrome

(E) salicylate overdose

38. What disease is responsible for the most frequent form of nephrotic syndrome in children?

(A) minimal change disease

(B) membranous nephropathy

(C) IgA nephropathy

(D) poststreptococcal glomerulonephritis

(E) Henoch–Schönlein purpura

39. Red blood cell casts are indicative of

(A) pyelonephritis

(B) multiple myeloma

(C) glomerulonephritis

(D) renal calculi

(E) bladder tumor

40. The most important complication of peritoneal dialysis is peritonitis. The organism responsible for most cases of peritonitis in this setting is

(A) *Candida*

(B) *Escherichia coli*

(C) *Streptococcus*

(D) *Pseudomonas*

(E) *Staphylococcus*

41. A patient with chronic renal failure has the following labs: calcium 9.4 mg/dL (normal 8.5–10.5 mg/dL), phosphorous 10.6 mg/dL (normal 2.5–4.5 mg/dL). Which of the following would be the most appropriate treatment?

(A) potassium phosphate

(B) calcium carbonate

(C) cation-exchange resin

(D) aluminum hydroxide

(E) vitamin D

42. Medullary sponge kidney is diagnosed by

(A) clinical features

(B) urinalysis

(C) sonogram

(D) intravenous pyelogram

(E) angiogram

43. In which of the following cases would renal biopsy be most recommended?

(A) patient with single functioning kidney and creatinine levels of 2.0 mg/dL

(B) patient with 30-year history of diabetes, retinopathy, and proteinuria

(C) 6-year-old child with sudden-onset edema and 10 g/day proteinuria

(D) patient with bilaterally small kidneys, uncontrolled hypertension, and creatinine levels of 5.0 mg/dL

(E) patient with recently diagnosed systemic lupus erythematosus, proteinuria, and creatinine levels of 1.7 mg/dL

DIRECTIONS (Questions 44 through 48): Each group of items in this section consists of lettered headings followed by a set of numbered words or phrases. For each numbered word or phrase, select the ONE lettered heading that is most closely associated with it. Each lettered heading may be selected once, more than once, or not at all.

Questions 44 through 48

Of the acid–base disorders listed as (A)–(E), select a single BEST response to the following statements

 (A) metabolic acidosis
 (B) respiratory acidosis
 (C) metabolic alkalosis
 (D) respiratory alkalosis
 (E) normal

44. Low arterial pH, increased pCO_2, increased bicarbonate

45. Elevated arterial pH, decreased pCO_2, decreased bicarbonate

46. Seen in chronic renal insufficiency

47. Result of excessive diuretic therapy

48. Calculation of the anion gap helpful in determining cause of this acid–base disorder

DIRECTIONS (Questions 49 through 67): Each of the numbered items or incomplete statements in this section is followed by answers or by completions of the statement. Select the ONE lettered answer or completion that is BEST in each case.

Questions 49 through 67

49. Mr. Smith is hospitalized for a swollen left leg and a gram-negative urinary tract infection. On admission, a venogram was negative for deep venous thrombosis. A Foley catheter was inserted with a residual urine volume of 30 cc followed by normal urine volumes. The patient was started on intravenous gentamicin and responded well. Admission labs were: blood urea nitrogen (BUN) 30 mg/dL and creatinine 1.0 mg/dL. Labs remained stable until the eighth hospi-

tal day, at which time his BUN became 40 mg/dL and creatinine 2.6 mg/dL. What is the most likely cause of his renal failure?

 (A) obstructive uropathy
 (B) cholesterol emboli
 (C) aminoglycoside nephrotoxicity
 (D) radiocontrast nephrotoxicity
 (E) volume depletion

50. A patient presents with abrupt onset of edema, azotemia, proteinuria, and cola-colored urine. The most likely diagnosis is

 (A) nephrotic syndrome
 (B) minimal change disease
 (C) acute glomerulonephritis
 (D) obstructive uropathy
 (E) renal calculi

51. A 40-year-old female develops nausea, headache, and seizures 2 days status post hysterectomy. Review of the record indicates patient has received hypotonic fluids intravenously since her surgery. Labs were obtained and show a serum sodium of 110 meq/L. Appropriate initial treatment would be

 (A) fluid restriction
 (B) demeclocycline 300 mg orally twice daily
 (C) hypotonic saline
 (D) isotonic saline
 (E) hypertonic saline

52. An 8-year-old child presents with onset of periorbital and leg edema following a recent viral upper respiratory tract illness. Urinalysis shows microscopic hematuria without red blood cell casts and heavy proteinuria. Which of the following is the most likely diagnosis?

 (A) poststreptococcal glomerulonephritis
 (B) Henoch–Schönlein purpura
 (C) hereditary nephritis
 (D) minimal change disease
 (E) acute leukemia

53. Mrs. Jones completed a course of intravenous methicillin for a staphylococcal infection. She was discharged home and did well for approximately 10 days. She then developed recurrence of fever and a mild rash. She is noted to have an elevated creatinine and eosinophils on her peripheral blood smear. Urinalysis reveals hematuria, pyuria, white blood cell casts, and eosinophiluria. Your diagnosis is

    (A) urinary tract infection
    (B) acute pyelonephritis
    (C) interstitial nephritis
    (D) bladder tumor
    (E) acute poststreptococcal glomerulonephritis

54. Nephrotic syndrome is characterized by all of the following EXCEPT

    (A) proteinuria
    (B) hypoalbuminemia
    (C) edema
    (D) hematuria
    (E) hyperlipidemia

55. A Tenckhoff catheter is used in

    (A) renal angiography
    (B) obstructive uropathy
    (C) hemodialysis
    (D) peritoneal dialysis
    (E) lithotripsy

56. All of the following renal stones are radiopaque EXCEPT

    (A) calcium oxalate
    (B) uric acid
    (C) cystine
    (D) struvite
    (E) calcium phosphate

57. Renal vein thrombosis is most commonly associated with which form of nephrotic syndrome?

    (A) membranous nephropathy
    (B) diabetic nephropathy
    (C) analgesic nephropathy
    (D) reflux nephropathy
    (E) IgA nephropathy

58. Which of the following signs or symptoms is/are seen in uremia?

    (A) fatigue
    (B) nausea
    (C) pericardial friction rub
    (D) asterixis
    (E) all of the above

59. Acute renal failure from urinary tract obstruction can be seen in all of the following EXCEPT

    (A) unilateral ureteral obstruction in a patient with one functioning kidney
    (B) prostatic hypertrophy
    (C) bilateral ureteral obstruction
    (D) calculus in the renal pelvis
    (E) bladder neck tumor

60. Peaked T waves and widening of the QRS complex on an electrocardiograph are indicative of

    (A) hypernatremia
    (B) hypercalcemia
    (C) hyperkalemia
    (D) hypokalemia
    (E) acute myocardial infarction

61. All of the following are considered emergent treatment for hyperkalemia EXCEPT

    (A) peritoneal dialysis
    (B) intravenous regular insulin plus an ampule of D_{50}
    (C) intravenous calcium gluconate
    (D) intravenous sodium bicarbonate
    (E) nebulized albuterol

62. The most serious consequence of rapid correction of hyponatremia is

    (A) hypokalemia
    (B) central pontine myelinolysis
    (C) muscle cramps
    (D) hypernatremia
    (E) fluid overload

63. In treatment of chronic hyponatremia, plasma sodium should be raised by no more than

    (A) 0.1 to 0.5 meq/L/hr
    (B) 0.5 to 1 meq/L/hr
    (C) 2 to 3 meq/L/hr
    (D) 5 meq/L/hr
    (E) 10 meq/L/hr

64. Which of the following factors is/are associated with an adverse prognosis in hypertension?

    (A) black males
    (B) diabetes mellitus
    (C) cardiomegaly
    (D) A and B
    (E) all of the above

65. Which of the following statements is NOT true regarding single-dose antibiotic therapy in the setting of acute *uncomplicated* cystitis?

    (A) safe and efficacious for women
    (B) results in fewer side effects
    (C) most fluoroquinolone antibiotics are effective
    (D) trimethoprim-sulfamethoxazole is effective
    (E) can be used to treat male patients with urinary tract infections

66. Hypertonic saline is indicated in the treatment of

    (A) serum sodium of 130 meq/L
    (B) asymptomatic serum sodium of 125 meq/L
    (C) symptomatic serum sodium of 115 meq/L
    (D) all of the above
    (E) none of the above

67. What amount of proteinuria is diagnostic of nephrotic syndrome?

    (A) 100 mg/dL on urine dipstick
    (B) 350 mg/day
    (C) 1 g/day
    (D) 2.5 g/day
    (E) >3.5 g/day

Answers and Explanations

1. **(D)** Acute pyelonephritis is associated with nausea and vomiting, fever, chills, leukocytosis, costovertebral angle tenderness, or pain on deep abdominal palpation. The patient may or may not have symptoms of cystitis (such as, frequency, urgency, nocturia), and can be suffering from headache or malaise. *(Stamm, pp. 550–551)*

2. **(C)** The glomerulus forms an essentially protein-free filtrate composed of all substances present in plasma at virtually the same concentration as in plasma. There is essentially no protein due to the glomerular membranes restricting movement of high-molecular-weight substance, the exception being some low-molecular-weight substance bound to proteins, such as fatty acids. In diseased kidneys, the glomerular membranes become increasingly permeable to protein and/or the tubules may lose their ability to remove protein. Traditionally, diseases of the kidney have been divided into four pathologic groups—glomerular, tubular, interstitial, and vascular. *(Walker and Mitch, pp. 737–738)*

3. **(B)** Normal GFR in men is approximately 125 mL/min. In a patient with normal renal function, doubling of the serum creatinine represents a loss of approximately 50% of GFR. Using this information, you can make a rough estimation of the loss of GFR with changes in the serum creatinine. For example, assume normal creatinine levels of 1.0 mg/dL and normal GFR of 120 mL/min. A doubling of the serum creatinine from 1

mg/dL to 2 mg/dL represents an approximate reduction in the GFR from 120 mL/min to 60 mL/min (50% of the GFR has been lost). Each additional doubling of the creatinine decreases the *remaining* GFR by approximately one half. When renal function is severely impaired, large increases in the creatinine (ie, as, 8.0 to 16.0 mg/dL) will represent only small decreases in the GFR (approximately 15 to 7 mL/min). This example emphasizes the important impact the initial increase in the serum creatinine has on the GFR. Increased or decreased creatinine production (increased muscle breakdown or decreased muscle mass) also are important factors to be considered when estimating the GFR from the serum creatinine. *(Rose, Chapter 1, p. 6)*

4. **(D)** Interstitial nephritis is most often associated with a hypersensitivity reaction to a drug, although infection may also be a cause. Interstitial edema, interstitial infiltrates, and tubular damage are seen on microscopic exam. Presenting findings can include fever, rash, eosinophilia, pyuria, white blood cell casts, hematuria, and occasional eosinophiluria. In drug-induced interstitial nephritis, there usually is a latent period of several days between administration of the offending agent (usually antibiotic) and onset of symptoms. Some of the antibiotics more commonly associated with interstitial nephritis are penicillins (especially methicillin) and cephalosporins. Other drugs, including nonsteroidal anti-inflammatory drugs, also have

been associated with acute interstitial nephritis. *(Rose, Chapter 8, pp. 389–391)*

5. **(B)** Acute pyelonephritis often presents with fever, chills, flank pain, and dysuria. Urinalysis will reveal pyuria and often white blood cell casts. Cystitis and urethral infections do not affect the kidney and should not have casts. Renal tuberculosis should be considered when there is hematuria and "sterile" pyuria. Drug-induced tubulointerstitial nephritis will produce hematuria, pyuria, proteinuria and, at times, eosinophiluria. *(Walker, pp. 732–733)*

6. **(E)** Angiotensin-converting enzyme (ACE) inhibitors are the drug of choice in this setting. Hypertension has a negative effect on the vascular system, including the intrarenal vessels, resulting in nephrosclerosis. Control of systemic blood pressure can reduce renal vascular damage. In diabetic patients, ACE inhibitors are especially beneficial because of the added effect of reducing intraglomerular pressure and decreasing proteinuria. *(Rose and Brenner, p. 130)*

7. **(A)** Calcium compounds are responsible for approximately 90% of all noninfected, non-struvite stones. The most common compounds are calcium oxalate and calcium phosphate. *(Walker, 1988b, p. 775)*

8. **(A)**; 9. **(C)**; 10. **(D)** *(Walker and Solez)*

11. **(E)** *(Hellmann, p. 775)*

12. **(B)** *(Morrison, p. 83)*

13. **(E)** The complete absence of urine formation is relatively rare, even patients with very poor renal function usually void effectively. Anuria suggests a problem of outlet obstruction. One should consider two possibilities: obstruction above the bladder (rare unless there is a solitary kidney or periureteral metastasis) or bladder outlet obstruction. Bladder outlet obstruction is rare in females but is common in males, especially those who are prone to develop prostate hypertro-

phy, have a history of urethritis (especially gonorrhea), or have had previous instrumentation. Diagnosis and initial treatment can be made by insertion of a bladder catheter. *(Walker, 1988a, p. 757)*

14. **(A)** The major causes of acute renal failure can be divided into three categories: prerenal failure, intrinsic renal failure, and postrenal failure. Prerenal azotemia is a disorder of decreased renal perfusion. It is not generally associated with intrinsic renal disease. Some of the causes include intravascular volume depletion from gastrointestinal losses such as vomiting and diarrhea, burns, dehydration, fluid loss from the kidney as with diuretics, and hemorrhage. Renal hypoperfusion in states of diminished cardiac output also is a prerenal cause of renal failure. Interstitial nephritis is a form of intrinsic renal disease in which the renal parenchyma is affected. Other causes of intrinsic renal disease include bilateral renal artery obstruction, glomerulonephritis, and acute tubular necrosis (ischemic or nephrotoxic). Postrenal failure is caused by obstruction of the urinary tract most commonly associated with enlargement of the prostate or tumors. *(Brady and Brenner, p. 1266)*

15. **(B)** Acute bacterial prostatitis is characterized by irritative bladder symptoms, fever, chills, and perineal discomfort. Pathogens in this disease are usually those associated with urinary tract infection, the gram-negative organisms. Patients usually respond dramatically to antibiotic therapy. Therapy should be continued for at least 30 days to prevent chronic prostatitis. Of the choices listed, ciprofloxacin 500 mg bid for 30 days is correct, because of its superior coverage of gram-negative organisms and the duration of therapy. *(Meares, p. 230)*

16. **(B)** *(Presti and Herr, p. 437)*; **17. (E)** *(McAninch, p. 686)*; **18. (A)** *(McAninch, p. 684)*; **19. (C)** *(McAninch, p. 687)*; **20. (D)** *(Meares, p. 687)*

21. **(D)** Angiotensin II is a hormone with a strong effect on blood pressure. When there

is a decrease in renal perfusion, renin is released. Through a process, renin helps to form angiotensin I, which is then converted to angiotensin II. The conversion of angiotensin I to angiotensin II is helped by an enzyme known as angiotensin-converting enzyme. Angiotensin II is a potent vasoconstrictor that increases systemic vascular resistance to help return the blood pressure to normal. Angiotensin II also has an effect on the kidneys to increase sodium and water retention and stimulate aldosterone secretion. These effects also help to elevate the blood pressure. (*Rose, Chapter 10, pp. 475–476*)

22. **(C)** Triamterene, amiloride, and spironolactone are considered potassium-sparing diuretics. Triamterene and amiloride act to reduce potassium secretion in the distal tubule. Spironolactone acts to inhibit aldosterone. The thiazide diuretics, including hydrochlorothiazide, block sodium reabsorption in the terminal portion of the loop of Henle and the proximal portion of the distal convoluted tubule. This leads to loss of both sodium and potassium in the urine. (*Levinsky, p. 252*)

23. **(B)** In the United States, diabetic nephropathy is the major cause of end-stage renal disease and is the etiology of renal failure in approximately 30% of patients on dialysis. Hypertension and glomerulonephritis are other common causes of chronic renal failure. In addition, inherited polycystic kidney disease and many other systemic diseases can cause renal failure. (*Brenner and Lazarus, pp. 1274–1275; Goldfarb, p. 112*)

24. **(B)** The anion gap can be calculated by subtracting the sum of the measured anions (chloride and bicarbonate) from the major measured cation (sodium). A normal anion gap is between 8 and 16 meq/liter. Increased anion gap acidosis can be seen in ketoacidosis, lactic acidosis, renal failure, and salicylate overdose. A normal anion gap is associated with renal tubular acidosis and gastrointestinal bicarbonate loss. (*Papadakis, p. 818*)

25. **(D)** Primary hyperparathyroidism should be considered in all patients with unexplained hypercalcemia. Renal calculi form as a result of excessive excretion of calcium and phosphate by the kidney. Diagnosis is confirmed by elevated levels of parathyroid hormone. In both idiopathic hypercalciuria and renal tubular acidosis, the serum calcium is normal. (*Coe, 1990, p. 97; Fitzgerald, pp. 1038–1039*)

26. **(D)** Erythropoietin is a hormone produced by cells in the kidney and acts to stimulate maturation of red blood cells in the bone marrow. In patients with chronic renal failure, decreased production of erythropoietin is the main cause of anemia. Recombinant human erythropoietin is now available and is given either subcutaneously or intravenously to increase hematocrit levels. Iron stores must be adequate for erythropoietin to be effective. (*Brenner and Lazarus, p. 1279; Goldberg and Bunn, p. 1716*)

27. **(C)** The anemia of chronic renal failure is typically normochromic, normocytic. Other types of anemia should be investigated and treated appropriately (ie, iron, folate, or vitamin B12 deficiency). In chronic renal failure, decreased erythropoietin production is the main cause of anemia. (*Brenner and Lazarus, p. 1279*)

28. **(A)** Serum magnesium levels can be slightly elevated in patients with chronic renal failure because of decreased excretion of magnesium. For this reason, it is necessary to avoid those medications high in magnesium, such as magnesium-containing laxatives or antacids. (*Brenner and Lazarus, p. 1277; Ahmed and Kopple, p. 291*)

29. **(B)** Casts are cylindrical shaped structures formed from Tamm–Horsfall mucoprotein secreted by cells in the loop of Henle. There are several different types of urinary casts, each with a clinical significance. Hyaline casts contain only mucoprotein and can be seen in normal urine. They also can be seen in the setting of volume depletion or following diuretics. Red cell casts are suggestive of glomerulonephritis or vasculitis. White cell casts are typically seen in tubulointerstitial disease (pyelonephritis) and some glomeru-

lar diseases. Fatty casts are seen in glomerular diseases with nephrotic-range proteinuria. Waxy and broad casts are seen in chronic renal failure. *(Rose, Chapter 1, pp. 23–28)*

30. **(C)** Chronic renal failure implies progressive destruction of nephrons over time, usually months to years. Bilaterally small kidneys, cortical thinning, renal osteodystrophy, symptoms of uremia, anemia, hyperphosphatemia, hypocalcemia, and broad casts in the urine all may indicate chronicity of disease. Proteinuria and hematuria are frequently present but are nonspecific in regard to the chronicity of renal disease. *(Coe and Brenner, pp. 1252–1253)*

31. **(E)** Radiocontrast agents and cyclosporine are nephrotoxic because of their intrarenal vasoconstriction effects. Radiocontrast agents also may cause tubular necrosis. Aminoglycoside toxicity is related to accumulation of the drug in the renal cortex. Cisplatin is a direct tubular toxin. Clindamycin is excreted through the liver and is not nephrotoxic. No dose adjustment is required in renal failure, although, with prolonged use renal function should be monitored. *(Brady and Brenner, p. 1268; Rose, Chapter 3, pp. 88–91; Bennett, p. 580)*

32. **(C)** Oliguria is defined as a decrease in urine output of less than 400 to 500 mL/day. Anuria represents a urine output of less than 50 mL/day. Polyuria is an increase in the total volume of urine, usually more than 2,500 to 3,000 mL/day. Nocturia refers to an increased number of voiding episodes at night. Azotemia refers to elevated serum concentrations of blood urea nitrogen and creatinine. *(Coe, 1994, pp. 236–239)*

33. **(D)** Radiocontrast-induced renal failure occurs more in patients with underlying renal insufficiency and diabetes, especially in those with previously elevated serum creatinine. The risk is low in patients with a creatinine less than 1.5 mg/dL, but risk increases as renal function worsens or other factors are present (diabetes, multiple contrast studies). In most cases, there will be a rise in the creatinine after the contrast study that peaks between 3 to 7 days. The creatinine will usually return to its previous level, but irreversible renal failure can rarely occur. The risk of contrast-induced renal failure can be lessened or prevented by either cautious use or avoidance of contrast material in high-risk patients. If needed, high-risk patients should be adequately hydrated throughout and for several hours after the study to lessen the risk of renal damage. *(Rose, Chapter 3, p. 91)*

34. **(B)** Alpha-adrenergic blockers can be used in the treatment of benign prostatic hypertrophy. Both the prostate and bladder tissues contain alpha-adrenoceptors. Alpha-adrenergic blockers work to block these receptors, causing relaxation of the smooth muscle in the bladder neck and prostate. The result is a decrease in the symptoms of benign prostatic hypertrophy. *(Presti et al, pp. 875-876)*

35. **(A)** Because many drugs are excreted in the urine, knowledge of the renal function is important when dosing medication, especially in patients with renal insufficiency. Drug toxicity or adverse side effects may occur if the drug is dosed improperly. Estimation of the creatinine clearance can help in making the proper drug adjustment for the degree of renal insufficiency. The Cockcroft–Gault equation can be used to calculate creatinine clearance. The formula is:

$$\text{creatinine clearance (mL/min)} = \frac{(140 - \text{age}) \times \text{lean body weight (kg)}}{\text{serum creatinine} \times 72}$$

In female patients, the result is multiplied by .85 because of smaller muscle mass. Appropriate antibiotic adjustments can be made based on the calculated creatinine clearance. *(Bennett, pp. 575–577)*

36. **(C)** Hyponatremia occurs in about 2% of hospitalized patients. It is defined by a serum sodium concentration of less than 130 meq/L and is the most common electrolyte abnormality found in this population. *(Papadakis, p. 801)*

37. **(D)** Hyperventilation syndrome is the most common cause of respiratory alkalosis. Laboratory findings include elevated arterial blood pH and a low pCO_2. *(Papadakis, pp. 816–818)*

38. **(A)** Minimal change (or Nil) disease is a form of idiopathic nephrotic syndrome and is the most common form of nephrotic syndrome in children. It accounts for more than 70% to 80% of cases in children under the age of 16. Minimal change disease also can be seen in adults. In patients over the age of 16, minimal change disease accounts for 15% to 20% of idiopathic nephrotic syndrome cases. *(Glassock and Brenner, pp. 1300–1301)*

39. **(C)** Casts are composed of Tamm–Horsfall mucoprotein secreted in the distal tubules and collecting ducts. Red blood casts suggest glomerular bleeding and are almost always indicative of glomerulonephritis or vasculitis. White blood casts are seen in pyelonephritis. *(Presti et al, p. 858)*

40. **(E)** *Staphylococcus* is the organism responsible for most cases of peritonitis in patients on peritoneal dialysis. Improper technique by the patient in making catheter connections during dialysis exchanges is the entry source in most cases. Abdominal pain, fever, and cloudy dialysis fluid are the presenting symptoms. The enteric bacteria are the second most common organisms seen in peritonitis. Fungal peritonitis is serious and usually requires removal of the peritoneal catheter. *(Miller et al, pp. 176–177)*

41. **(B)** Hyperphosphatemia is commonly seen in patients with chronic renal failure. Dialysis will remove a small amount of phosphorous, but it is necessary to treat the hyperphosphatemia with a phosphate-binding medication to prevent phosphate absorption from the gastrointestinal tract. Calcium carbonate and calcium acetate are the preferred phosphate binders. Products containing magnesium or aluminum are generally avoided because of the potential for accumulation and toxicity in patients with chronic renal failure. *(Papadakis, p. 813)*

42. **(D)** Medullary sponge kidney is an abnormality in which there is cyst formation in the medullary collecting ducts. It is usually asymptomatic and does not impair renal function but can be complicated by renal calculi, urinary tract infections, and hematuria. Medullary sponge kidney is diagnosed by intravenous pyelography. The dilated collecting ducts are identified by their characteristic appearance. *(Avner, pp. 180–181)*

43. **(E)** Renal biopsy is contraindicated in patients with a single functioning kidney, severe hypertension, or an uncorrected bleeding disorder. In certain illnesses such as poststreptococcal glomerulonephritis and diabetes, history and clinical findings often permit diagnosis without obtaining a renal biopsy. In other illnesses such as systemic lupus erythematosus, a renal biopsy is important to identify the type of glomerular disease as treatment is based on the histiological changes. Minimal change disease accounts for most cases of nephrotic syndrome in children and often responds to a course of corticosteroids. For this reason, renal biopsy is reserved for those children who fail to respond to therapy. Renal insufficiency with bilaterally small kidneys is indicative of chronic renal disease. Atrophied and scarred kidneys are not usually biopsied as a reversible disease process is unlikely to be found. In cases of isolated proteinuria and hematuria, other testing such as renal sonogram or labs in addition to the clinical presentation need thorough review before deciding to perform a kidney biopsy. *(Rose and Jacobs, pp. 179–180)*

44. **(B)** Respiratory acidosis is the result of inadequate respiratory ventilation that leads to hypercapnia. Laboratory findings include low arterial pH, elevated pCO_2, and increased serum bicarbonate levels. Causes may include depression of the respiratory center by drugs (sedatives, narcotics), disease (brain tumors, sleep apnea, neuromuscular diseases), and chronic obstructive lung disease. *(Papadakis, pp. 816–817)*

45. **(D)** Respiratory alkalosis is the result of hyperventilation that causes hypocapnia. Labo-

ratory findings include elevated arterial pH, low pCO_2, and decreased bicarbonate levels. Hyperventilation syndrome is the most common cause, but other causes may include high altitude, salicylate overdose, pneumonia, and excessive mechanical ventilation. *(Papadakis, pp. 817–818)*

46. **(A)** The main mechanism of metabolic acidosis in chronic renal failure is the decreased ability of the kidney to excrete acids. A high anion gap is seen because of retention of sulfate and phosphate acid anions. *(Papadakis, pp. 818–820)*

47. **(C)** Metabolic alkalosis is the result of an elevated arterial pH with an increased bicarbonate level. The volume status of the patient and urine chloride levels are helpful in differentiating the causes of metabolic alkalosis. Diuretics act to decrease extracellular volume by causing a loss of sodium chloride and water in the urine. The plasma bicarbonate level will increase because of the contraction of the extracellular fluid. *(Papadakis, pp. 823–824)*

48. **(A)** The anion gap is useful in identifying the causes of metabolic acidosis. It is a measurement of the undetermined anions. The anion gap can be calculated by subtracting the sum of the measured anions (chloride and bicarbonate) from the major measured cation (sodium). A normal anion gap is between 8 and 16 meq/L. Increased anion gap acidosis can be seen in ketoacidosis, lactic acidosis, renal failure, and salicylate overdose. A normal anion gap is associated with renal tubular acidosis and gastrointestinal bicarbonate loss. *(Papadakis, pp. 818–820)*

49. **(C)** There is no indication of volume depletion in this patient or of obstructive uropathy with normal urine volume, no significant urine retention, and normal creatinine on admission. Radiocontrast nephrotoxicity is not likely in this setting considering the time course of the renal failure. Renal failure from contrast agents is associated with an elevation in the serum creatinine following the procedure, peaking of the serum creatinine at

3 to 7 days, then improvement to baseline. Also, contrast-induced renal failure is not usually seen in patients with baseline creatinine levels lower than 1.5 mg/dL. Aminoglycoside nephrotoxicity is the result of an accumulation of the drug in the renal cortex. Therefore, a rise in the serum creatinine is usually not seen until 7 to 10 days after the start of therapy. *(Rose, Chapter 3, p. 65, 91)*

50. **(C)** Acute glomerulonephritis is associated with sudden onset of hematuria, proteinuria, and azotemia. Sodium and water retention are present, causing hypertension and edema. Periorbital edema is common, but edema can be present elsewhere. A reduction in the glomerular filtration rate is due to inflammatory lesions. Prognosis depends on the specific cause of the glomerulonephritis. *(Glassock and Brenner, pp. 1295–1296)*

51. **(E)** A severe hyponatremia can develop within 2 days or less following elective surgery, usually associated with the administration of excessive hypotonic fluids. Premenopausal women are especially at risk. In the presence of central nervous system symptoms, hypertonic saline is the treatment of choice. Over-rapid correction of the serum sodium can result in central pontine myelinolysis. The serum sodium concentration should not be increased by more than 0.5 to 1.0 meq/L/hr with a goal not to exceed serum sodium level of 130 meq/L within the first 48 hours. *(Papadakis, pp. 803–804)*

52. **(D)** Minimal change disease is a form of nephrotic syndrome and accounts for most cases of nephrotic syndrome in children. Presentation typically includes edema, proteinuria, and variable hematuria, but no cellular or granular casts. Minimal change disease often is idiopathic, but some cases have been associated with recent upper respiratory illness and allergic tendencies (milk and pollen). *(Rose and Jacobs, pp. 190–191)*

53. **(C)** Methicillin has been found to have a strong association to interstitial nephritis. Interstitial nephritis is most often associated

with a hypersensitivity reaction to a drug, although infection also can be a cause. Interstitial edema, interstitial infiltrates, and tubular damage are seen on microscopic exam. Presenting findings can include fever, rash, eosinophilia, pyuria, white blood cell casts, hematuria, and occasional eosinophiluria. In drug-induced interstitial nephritis, there is usually a latent period of several days between administration of the offending agent (usually antibiotic) and onset of symptoms. Some of the antibiotics more commonly associated with interstitial nephritis are penicillins (especially methicillin) and cephalosporins. Poststreptococcal glomerulonephritis can be differentiated from interstitial nephritis in that low serum complement levels and red blood cell casts are seen in the former. Furthermore, eliminating the offending drug will improve renal function in cases of interstitial nephritis although this may take months. *(Rose, Chapter 8, pp. 389–392)*

54. **(D)** Normal urinary protein excretion is generally less than 150 mg/day. Protein excretion of more than 3.5 g/day is termed nephrotic range proteinuria and is indicative of glomerular disease. Nephrotic syndrome can be seen in a number of renal diseases. Findings include levels of proteinuria higher than 3.5 g/day, hypoalbuminemia, edema, hyperlipidemia, and a hypercoagulable state. *(Rose, Chapter 5, p. 159)*

55. **(D)** A Tenckhoff catheter is a permanent peritoneal catheter used for peritoneal dialysis. This type of dialysis uses the peritoneal membrane to aid in the removal of solutes and fluids by infusing a dialysate solution into the peritoneal cavity through the catheter and allowing the solution to remain in the peritoneal space for several hours before a new exchange is made. *(Carpenter and Lazarus, p. 1285)*

56. **(B)** Uric acid stones are radiolucent. They are more common in men and are typically seen in acidic urine. Treatment focuses on increasing the urine pH with alkali agents and decreasing overexcretion of uric acid with allopurinol. *(Coe and Favus, pp. 1329–1332)*

57. **(A)** Renal vein thrombosis can be seen in any form of nephrotic syndrome but is most commonly seen in membranous nephropathy. Renal vein thrombosis may be unilateral or bilateral. It is associated with hypercoagulable states, such as nephrotic syndrome, pregnancy, and oral contraceptive use. Symptoms of acute renal vein thrombosis can include fever, flank pain, hematuria, and acute worsening of renal function. In cases of membranous nephropathy, incidence rates as high as 10% to 50% have been reported. Membranoproliferative glomerulonephritis and amyloidosis also are associated with a higher risk of renal vein thrombosis. *(Glassock and Brenner, p. 1300; Badr and Brenner, pp. 1319–1320)*

58. **(E)** There are many signs and symptoms associated with uremia. Several of the most common include: fatigue, nausea, vomiting, anorexia, pallor, pruritis, sleep disorders, lethargy, and anemia. Asterixis, also called flapping tremor, is seen in uremic and other metabolic encephalopathies. Pericarditis can occur as a consequence of uremia and is associated with a pericardial friction rub, pericardial effusion, and chest pain. The presence of pericarditis is an absolute indication to start dialysis. *(Brenner and Lazarus, p. 1277; Miller et al, pp. 165–166)*

59. **(D)** One functioning kidney is capable of clearing waste products. Therefore, for urinary tract obstruction to cause acute renal failure, one of the following must be present: both ureters must be obstructed, unilateral ureteral obstruction in the setting of one functioning kidney, or obstruction between the external urethral meatus and bladder neck (prostatic disease, tumor). *(Brady and Brenner, p. 1269)*

60. **(C)** Electrocardiographic changes of hyperkalemia include peaked T waves, flattening of the P wave, prolongation of the PR interval, widening of the QRS complex, and biphasic QRS-T complexes. In addition, bradycardia may be present. If untreated, ventricular fibrillation or cardiac arrest may result. *(Papadakis, p. 808)*

61. (A) Intravenous calcium acts to antagonize cardiac conduction abnormalities. Intravenous bicarbonate, insulin, and nebulized albuterol act to shift potassium into cells. Peritoneal dialysis involves infusion of a dialysis solution into the peritoneal cavity at regular intervals. The serum potassium is lowered by diffusive removal of potassium and also by transcellular shift of potassium into cells due to the glucose load of the dialysate solution. This is a continuous process that results in a slow decrease in the serum potassium. *(Papadakis, pp. 808–809)*

62. (B) Rapid correction of hyponatremia can result in severe brain damage, including central pontine myelinolysis. For this reason, the serum sodium concentration should be raised by 0.5 to 1 meq/L/hr or by no more than 12 meq/L over the first 24 hours. *(Levinsky, p. 247)*

63. (B) In chronic hyponatremia, the plasma sodium should not be raised by more than 0.5 to 1 meq/L/hr or by more than 12 meq/L over the first 24 hours. Neurological damage, including central pontine myelinolysis, can result from overly rapid correction of hyponatremia. *(Levinsky, p. 247)*

64. (E) Many factors are associated with an adverse prognosis in hypertension. In addition to those listed, other factors include: age, smoking, alcohol use, cholesterol level, obesity, and evidence of end-organ damage (cardiac, eye ground changes, renal or nervous system involvement). *(Williams, p. 1119)*

65. (E) Single-dose antibiotics offer the advantage of less expense, better compliance, and fewer side effects. However, in men, urinary tract infection should be considered a complicated infection and urologic evaluation should be performed to evaluate any urologic pathology or prostatic involvement. Single-dose antibiotic choices may include trimethoprim-sulfamethoxazole, trimethoprim, sulfa, and most fluoroquinolones. Single-dose amoxicillin also can be used but may result in a lower cure rate, especially in

those patients with strains of bacteria resistant to this drug. *(Stamm, p. 552)*

66. (C) Hypertonic saline is used to treat those patients with severe, symptomatic hyponatremia. These symptoms are related to the central nervous system and can include altered sensorium, lethargy, seizures, and coma. Proper calculation must be made so as not to raise the serum sodium by more than 0.5 to 1 meq/L/hr or by more than 12 meq/L over the first 24 hours. Neurological damage, including central pontine myelinolysis, can result from overly rapid correction of hyponatremia. *(Levinsky, p. 247)*

67. (E) Nephrotic syndrome is present when proteinuria is more than 3.5 g/day. *(Coe and Brenner, p. 1253)*

REFERENCES

Ahmed K, Kopple JD. Nutritional management of renal disease. In Greenberg A (ed), *Primer on Kidney Diseases.* San Diego: Academic Press; 1994.

Avner ED. Medullary cystic disease and medullary sponge kidney. In Greenberg A (ed), *Primer on Kidney Diseases.* San Diego: Academic Press; 1994.

Badr KF, Brenner BM. Vascular injury to the kidney. In Isselbacher KJ et al (eds), *Harrison's Principles of Internal Medicine,* 13th ed. New York: McGraw-Hill; 1994.

Bennett WM. Use of drugs in the patient with renal insufficiency. In Rose BD, *Pathophysiology of Renal Disease,* 2nd ed. New York: McGraw-Hill; 1987.

Brady HR, Brenner BM. Acute renal failure. In Isselbacher KJ et al (eds), *Harrison's Principles of Internal Medicine,* 13th ed. New York: McGraw-Hill; 1994.

Brenner BM, Lazarus JM. Chronic renal failure. In Isselbacher KJ et al (eds), *Harrison's Principles of Internal Medicine,* 13th ed. New York: McGraw-Hill; 1994.

Carpenter CB, Lazarus JM. Dialysis and transplantation in the treatment of renal failure. In Isselbacher KJ et al (eds), *Harrison's Principles of Internal Medicine,* 13th ed. New York: McGraw-Hill; 1994.

Coe FL. Alterations in urine function. In Isselbacher KJ et al (eds), *Harrison's Principles of Internal Medicine*, 13th ed. New York: McGraw-Hill; 1994.

Coe FL. The patient with renal stones. In Schrier RW (ed), *Manual of Nephrology: Diagnosis and Therapy*, 3rd ed. Boston: Little, Brown; 1990.

Coe FL, Brenner BM. Approach to the patient with diseases of the kidney and urinary tract. In Isselbacher KJ et al (eds), *Harrison's Principles of Internal Medicine*, 13th ed. New York: McGraw-Hill; 1994.

Coe FL, Favus MJ. Nephrolithiasis. In Isselbacher KJ et al (eds), *Harrison's Principles of Internal Medicine*, 13th ed. New York: McGraw-Hill; 1994.

Fitzgerald PA. Endocrinology. In Tierney LM Jr et al (eds), *Current Medical Diagnosis and Treatment*, 36th ed. Stamford, CT: Appleton & Lange; 1997.

Glassock RJ, Brenner BM. The major glomerulopathies. In Isselbacher KJ et al (eds), *Harrison's Principles of Internal Medicine*, 13th ed. New York: McGraw-Hill; 1994.

Goldberg MA, Bunn HF. Molecular and cellular hematopoiesis. In Isselbacher KJ et al (eds), *Harrison's Principles of Internal Medicine*, 13th ed. New York: McGraw-Hill; 1994.

Goldfarb S. Diabetic nephropathy. In Greenberg A (ed), *Primer on Kidney Diseases*. San Diego: Academic Press; 1994.

Hellmann DB. Arthritis and musculoskeletal disorders. In Tierney LM Jr et al (eds), *Current Medical Diagnosis and Treatment*, 36th ed. Stamford, CT: Appleton & Lange; 1997.

Levinsky NG. Fluids and electrolytes. In Isselbacher KJ et al (eds), *Harrison's Principles of Internal Medicine*, 13th ed. New York: McGraw-Hill; 1994.

McAnich JW. Disorders of the testis, scrotum, and spermatic cord. In Tanagho EA, McAninch JW (eds), *Smith's General Urology*, 14th ed. Norwalk, CT: Appleton & Lange; 1995.

Meares EM. Nonspecific infections of the genitourinary tract. In Tanagho EA, McAnich JW (eds), *Smith's General Urology*, 14th ed. Norwalk, CT: Appleton & Lange; 1995.

Miller RB, Sigala JF, Upham AT. The patient with chronic azotemia, with emphasis on chronic renal failure. In Schrier, RW (ed), *Manual of Nephrology: Diagnosis and Therapy*, 3rd ed. Boston: Little, Brown; 1990.

Morrison G. Kidney. In Tierney LM Jr et al (eds), *Current Medical Diagnosis and Treatment*, 36th ed. Stamford, CT: Appleton & Lange; 1997.

Papadakis MA. Fluid and electrolyte disorders. In Tierney LM Jr et al (eds), *Current Medical Diagnosis and Treatment*, 36th ed. Stamford, CT: Appleton & Lange; 1997.

Presti JC Jr, Herr HW. Genital tumors. In Tanagho EA, McAnich JW (eds), *Smith's General Urology*, 14th ed. Norwalk, CT: Appleton & Lange; 1995.

Presti JC Jr, Stoller ML, Carroll PR. Urology. In Tierney LM Jr et al (eds), *Current Medical Diagnosis and Treatment*, 36th ed. Stamford, CT: Appleton & Lange; 1997.

Rose BD. Acute renal failure—Prerenal disease versus acute tubular necrosis. Chapter 3 in Rose BD, *Pathophysiology of Renal Disease*, 2nd ed. New York: McGraw-Hill; 1987.

Rose BD. Clinical assessment of renal function. Chapter 1 in Rose BD, *Pathophysiology of Renal Disease*, 2nd ed. New York: McGraw-Hill; 1987.

Rose BD. Pathogenesis, clinical manifestations, and diagnosis of glomerular disease. Chapter 5 in Rose BD, *Pathophysiology of Renal Disease*, 2nd ed. New York: McGraw-Hill; 1987.

Rose BD. Pathogenesis of essential hypertension. Chapter 10 in Rose BD, *Pathophysiology of Renal Disease*, 2nd ed. New York: McGraw-Hill; 1987.

Rose BD. Tubulointerstitial diseases. Chapter 8 in Rose BD, *Pathophysiology of Renal Disease*, 2nd ed. New York: McGraw-Hill; 1987.

Rose BD, Brenner BM. Mechanisms of progression of renal disease. Chapter 4 in Rose BD, *Pathophysiology of Renal Disease*, 2nd ed. New York: McGraw-Hill; 1987.

Rose BD, Jacobs JB. Nephrotic syndrome and glomerulonephritis. Chapter 6 in Rose BD, *Pathophysiology of Renal Disease*, 2nd ed. New York: McGraw-Hill; 1987.

Stamm WE. Urinary tract infections and pyelonephritis. In Isselbacher KJ et al (eds), *Harrison's Principles of Internal Medicine*, 13th ed. New York: McGraw-Hill; 1994.

Walker WG. Oliguria and acute renal failure. In Harvey AM et al (eds), *The Principles and Practice of Medicine*, 22nd ed. Norwalk, CT: Appleton & Lange; 1988a.

Walker WG. Renal calculi. In Harvey AM et al (eds) *The Principles and Practice of Medicine,* 22nd ed. Norwalk, CT: Appleton & Lange; 1988b.

Walker WG, Mitch WE. Pathophysiology of uremia and clinical evaluation of renal function. In Harvey AM et al (eds), *The Principles and Practice of Medicine,* 22nd ed. Norwalk, CT: Appleton & Lange; 1988.

Walker WG, Solez K. The proteinurias and hematurias. In Harvey AM et al (eds) *The Principles and Practice of Medicine,* 22nd ed. Norwalk, CT: Appleton & Lange; 1988.

Williams GH. Hypertensive vascular disease. In Isselbacher KJ et al (eds), *Harrison's Principles of Internal Medicine,* 13th ed. New York: McGraw-Hill; 1994.

Internal Medicine: Pulmonary
Questions

Joseph H. Thornton, MPH, PA-C

DIRECTIONS (Questions 1 through 40): Each of the numbered items or incomplete statements in this section is followed by answers or by completions of the statement. Select the ONE lettered answer or completion that is BEST in each case.

Questions 1 through 40

1. The most common cause of hemoptysis is

   (A) tuberculosis
   (B) trauma
   (C) bronchogenic carcinoma
   (D) bronchitis
   (E) pulmonary embolism

2. By which of the following routes may bacteria be introduced into the lungs?

   (A) aspiration
   (B) inhalation
   (C) direct extension
   (D) bacteremia
   (E) all of the above

3. Which of the following is characteristic of pleuritic chest pain?

   (A) It has no relationship to respirations.
   (B) It is frequently associated with redness, swelling, and enlargement of the costal ridges.
   (C) It tends to be distributed along the intercostal nerve zones.
   (D) It is most often bilateral.
   (E) It is usually described as a squeezing pain.

4. A 50-year-old male presents with a history of persistent cough, hemoptysis, and weight loss. He states he has had several lung infections over the past 3 to 4 months. The patient is a 30-pack-per-year smoker and also complains of right shoulder and chest pain. The patient is afebrile, pale, and dyspneic with exertion. The chest x-ray suggests mediastinal widening and perihilar adenopathy. Which of the following diagnoses is most consistent with the given history?

   (A) bronchiectasis
   (B) chronic obstructive pulmonary disease
   (C) chronic bronchitis
   (D) asthma
   (E) bronchogenic carcinoma

5. Which of the following is the most common cause for chronic obstructive pulmonary disease (COPD)?

   (A) air pollution
   (B) recurrent infection
   (C) smoking
   (D) asthma
   (E) trauma

6. Indications for pulmonary function testing include

   (A) evaluation of the type and degree of pulmonary dysfunction
   (B) preoperative evaluation
   (C) follow-up of response to therapy
   (D) surveillance in occupational settings
   (E) all of the above

7. Which of the following tests is the LEAST helpful in the diagnosis of bronchogenic carcinoma?

   (A) sputum cytology
   (B) bronchoscopy and biopsy
   (C) ventilation-perfusion scan
   (D) pulmonary function tests
   (E) CAT scan

8. Which of the following statements regarding asthma is true?

   (A) It is always the result of an infectious process.
   (B) It is characterized by irreversible bronchospasm.
   (C) It is a condition that always begins in childhood.
   (D) The classic clinical triad is cough, wheezing, and dyspnea.
   (E) Women are affected twice as often as men.

9. An intermediate-strength PPD test

   (A) indicates active infection
   (B) is considered positive if 10 mm or more of erythema is present
   (C) is performed intramuscularly
   (D) may be falsely positive if patient is anergic
   (E) should be checked 48 to 72 hours after administration

10. Which of the following is/are true concerning the treatment of tuberculosis (TB) in patients who are not infected with human immunodeficiency virus (HIV)?

    (A) Single-drug regimens are notoriously ineffective.
    (B) Noncompliance is the major cause of treatment failure and drug resistance.
    (C) Initial pharmacological therapy involves a multi-drug regimen.
    (D) Treatment of extrapulmonary TB is the same as for pulmonary TB.
    (E) All of the above are true.

11. A 2-year-old patient is brought to the emergency department by his mother with sudden onset of choking, gagging, coughing, and wheezing. The patient was last seen playing on the floor with several small toys. Vital signs are respiration 28, pulse 120, and temperature 98.6°F. Exam reveals decreased breath sounds over the right lower lobe with inspiratory rhonchi and a localized expiratory wheeze. Chest x-ray shows normal inspiratory views, but expiratory views show localized hyperinflation wih mediastinal shift to the left. The most likely diagnosis is

    (A) viral croup
    (B) subglottic tumor
    (C) foreign-body aspiration
    (D) epiglottitis
    (E) asthmatic bronchitis

12. For the patient in Question 11 the correct way to progress in the treatment of this case would be

    (A) chest physiotherapy
    (B) cool-mist therapy with racemic epinephrine
    (C) bronchoscopy as soon as possible
    (D) intubation as soon as possible
    (E) antibiotics with antitussives

13. All of the following are characteristic physical findings in a patient with pneumothorax EXCEPT

    (A) trachea may deviate to the opposite side
    (B) hyperresonant percussion note over affected area

(C) prominent wheezes throughout both lung fields

(D) decreased to absent breath sounds over affected area

(E) decreased to absent tactile fremitus over affected area

14. A spontaneous pneumothorax is most likely in

(A) a male patient 2 to 10 years of age

(B) a female patient 2 to 10 years of age

(C) a male patient 15 to 35 years of age

(D) a female patient 15 to 35 years of age

(E) a patient 40 to 50 years of age

15. Deep regular respirations with periods of apnea BEST describe

(A) Cheyne–Stokes respiration

(B) Biot's breathing

(C) Kussmaul's respiration

(D) stridulous breathing

(E) apnea

16. All of the following physical findings are consistent with a consolidated pneumonia EXCEPT

(A) rales

(B) increased vocal fremitus

(C) dullness with percussion

(D) decreased whispered pectoriloquy

(E) presence of egophony

17. A 19-year-old female is involved in an automobile accident; she is hospitalized with a fractured femur. Her past medical history is unremarkable, except for the fact that she has been taking birth control pills for the past 2 years. The patient suddenly develops dyspnea, cough, and anxiety, with retrosternal chest pain. Vital signs are pulse 120, respiration 32, blood pressure 120/80, and temperature 100.1°F. Chest x-ray shows mild bilateral atelectasis, and the ECG is normal. The most likely diagnosis is

(A) pneumonia

(B) myocardial infarction

(C) pulmonary embolism

(D) costochondritis with hyperventilation

(E) unrecognized pneumothorax

18. The most sensitive test to confirm your diagnosis for the patient in Question 17 would be

(A) CT scan of the chest

(B) serial ECGs

(C) arterial blood gases

(D) ventilation-perfusion scan

(E) serum cardiac enzymes

19. Which of the following tests are best used to differentiate between restrictive and obstructive pulmonary disease?

(A) arterial blood gases

(B) ventilation-perfusion scanning

(C) forced expiratory volume in 1 second divided by the force vital capacity (FEV_1/FVC)

(D) chest x-ray

(E) pulse oximetry

20. The drug of choice in the treatment of pneumococcal pneumonia is

(A) dicloxacillin

(B) gentamycin

(C) penicillin

(D) ticarcillin

(E) vancomycin

21. The major cell types of bronchogenic carcinoma include all of the following EXCEPT

(A) adenocarcinoma

(B) large cell carcinoma

(C) infiltrating ductal carcinoma

(D) small cell carcinoma

(E) squamous cell carcinoma

22. Which of the following is NOT a clinical finding associated with adult respiratory distress syndrome (ARDS)?

    (A) tachypnea
    (B) air bronchogram
    (C) cardiomegaly
    (D) multiple organ failure
    (E) diffuse patchy infiltrate

23. Which of the following factors may precipitate an asthma attack?

    (A) anxiety
    (B) air pollution
    (C) exercise
    (D) beta-adrenergic blocking agents
    (E) all of the above

24. Which agent provides the MOST rapid effect and best therapeutic index in the treatment of asthma?

    (A) inhaled beta-adrenergic agonist medication
    (B) subcutaneous epinephrine
    (C) intravenous aminophylline
    (D) hydrocortisone
    (E) oral aminophylline

25. All of the following are characteristic physical findings in a patient with epiglottitis EXCEPT

    (A) inspiratory retractions and stridor
    (B) muffled voice
    (C) drooling
    (D) bradypnea
    (E) cyanosis

26. The MOST common cause of acute bronchiolitis in a child under 2 years of age is

    (A) cystic fibrosis
    (B) respiratory syncytial virus (RSV)
    (C) bacterial pneumonia
    (D) tuberculosis
    (E) tracheomalacia

27. All of the following are characteristic physical findings in a patient with chronic obstructive pulmonary disease (COPD) EXCEPT

    (A) decreased anteroposterior (AP) diameter
    (B) use of accessory muscles of ventilation
    (C) diminished breath sounds
    (D) hyperresonant note on percussion
    (E) decreased fremitus

28. Common cause(s) of dyspnea include

    (A) exercise
    (B) asthma
    (C) emphysema
    (D) chronic bronchitis
    (E) all of the above

29. Onset of a barking cough and mild stridor in a child who has been experiencing a low-grade fever and the prodrome of upper respiratory tract symptoms suggests the diagnosis of

    (A) epiglottis
    (B) asthma
    (C) croup
    (D) chronic bronchitis
    (E) pneumothorax

30. Treatment of pulmonary embolism may include

    (A) oxygen therapy
    (B) intravenous heparin
    (C) thrombolytic therapy
    (D) oral anticoagulant therapy continued for 3 to 6 months
    (E) all of the above

31. The MOST common cause of respiratory distress in the preterm infant is

    (A) meconium aspiration
    (B) asthma
    (C) congenital pneumonia
    (D) spontaneous pneumothorax
    (E) hyaline membrane disease

32. Complications of influenza include

(A) acute sinusitis
(B) otitis media
(C) purulent bronchitis
(D) pneumonia
(E) all of the above

33. Clubbing of the fingers is associated with

(A) acute dyspnea
(B) chronic hypoxia
(C) transient hypercapnia
(D) hypokalemia
(E) none of the above

34. Clinical findings suggestive of the presence of pneumococcal pneumonia include all of the following EXCEPT

(A) typical pulmonary signs of lobar pneumonia
(B) abundant gram-positive cocci visualized on examination of a sputum specimen
(C) marked leukopenia
(D) sudden onset with shaking chills (rigors)
(E) high fever

35. The drug of choice in treating *Mycoplasma pneumoniae* is

(A) a penicillin
(B) ampicillin
(C) an erythromycin
(D) an aminoglycoside
(E) none of the above

36. Which of the following binds hemoglobin with an affinity more than 200 times greater than that of oxygen

(A) nitrogen
(B) sulfur dioxide
(C) carbon dioxide
(D) carbon monoxide
(E) chlorine

37. Which of the following is TRUE about coughing?

(A) chronically, it may be a symptom of viral bronchitis
(B) irritation leading to a nonproductive cough can be caused by mechanical, chemical, thermal, or inflammatory means
(C) normal bronchial secretions are usually removed by coughing and expectoration
(D) syncope and rib fractures are common complications of coughs
(E) the most common cause of chronic cough is emphysema

38. All of the following might be used to determine if there is partial airway obstruction above or below the tracheal bifurcation EXCEPT

(A) stridor
(B) pulmonary function tests
(C) chest x-ray
(D) ventilation-perfusion scanning
(E) pulse oximetry

39. Pleural effusion may be caused by

(A) tuberculosis
(B) a malignancy
(C) pulmonary infarction
(D) pancreatitis
(E) all of the above

40. All of the following are TRUE concerning sarcoidosis EXCEPT

(A) It is a systemic disease characterized by granulomatous inflammation of the lung.
(B) Its incidence is highest in North American Blacks and Northern European Whites.
(C) Onset of the disease is usually in the third or fourth decade of life.
(D) The causative organism is a retrovirus.
(E) Patients may present with malaise, fever, and dyspnea of insidious onset.

DIRECTIONS (Questions 41 through 50): Each group of items in this section consists of lettered headings followed by a set of numbered words or phrases. For each numbered word or phrase, select the ONE lettered heading that is most closely associated with it. Each lettered heading may be selected once, more than once, or not at all.

Questions 41 through 45

Select the MOST probable diagnosis given this initial presentation

(A) *Streptococcus pneumoniae*
(B) *Mycoplasma pneumoniae*
(C) Legionnaire's disease (*L. pneumophilia*)
(D) *Pneumocystis carinii* pneumonia
(E) viral pneumonia

41. A 25-year-old white male presents with shortness of breath and a nonproductive cough. The patient's temperature is 103.5°F, respiration 40, and pulse 140. Physical exam reveals a thin dyspneic male in moderate respiratory distress with scattered rhonchi and peripheral cyanosis. Chest x-ray reveals a diffuse interstitial infiltrate.

42. A 45-year-old Black female with a 1-week history of clear nasal drainage suddenly develops a single shaking chill followed by fever and cough productive of thick yellow mucous. Her temperature is 103°F. Rales are noted at the right base. Chest x-ray shows a right lower-lobe pneumonia.

43. An 18-year-old female college student complains of a 3-day history of fever, headache, sore throat, left ear pain, and a productive cough of watery sputum. On exam, left bullous myringitis is noted. A chest x-ray reveals a left lower-lobe segmental pneumonia.

44. A 58-year-old male smoker returns from vacation at the beach with anorexia, malaise, and a minimal cough that is nonproductive.

The patient's wife states he has a continuous fever of 103.7°F, respirations are 22, and the pulse rate is 55. Exam reveals dry oral membranes and rales over the right base with sharp stabbing pain upon inspiration. Chest x-ray shows a bilateral lower-lobe pneumonia.

45. A 21-year-old Asian male presents with diffuse myalgias, photophobia, and a nonproductive cough. His temperature is 100.8°F, and exam reveals slight nasal congestion, expiratory wheeze, and erythema multiforme. A chest x-ray shows a scattered nodular interstitial infiltrate pattern.

Questions 46 through 50

Select the MOST probable lung disease due to an external agent

(A) asbestosis
(B) coalworker's pneumoconiosis
(C) occupational asthma
(D) pulmonary radiation fibrosis
(E) silo-filler's disease

46. Occurs in nearly all patients who receive a full course of radiation therapy for cancer of the lung or breast

47. Results in the formation of malignant mesotheliomas

48. Characteristically worst on Mondays or the first day back to work

49. Acute toxic noncardiogenic pulmonary edema caused by the inhalation of nitrogen dioxode

50. Ingestion of inhaled dust by alveolar macrophages leads to the formation of macules that appear on chest x-rays as diffuse small opacities especially prominent in the upper lung

Answers and Explanations

1. **(D)** Hemoptysis is the expectoration of blood or bloody sputum. Some important causes of hemoptysis include pneumonias, pulmonary emboli, bronchogenic carcinoma, mitral stenosis, chronic obstructive pulmonary disease (COPD), tuberculosis, and other granulomatous diseases. However, the most common cause of hemoptysis is bronchitis. *(Bennett and Plum, pp. 370–371; Stobo et al, p. 122; Tierney et al, p. 215)*

2. **(E)** Routes of bacterial inoculation of the lungs include the aspiration of oropharyngeal secretions, the inhalation of airborne microorganisms, by direct extension into lung tissue, and by septicemia. Determining the route of the infectious process may provide clues to the identity of the responsible organism. *(Bennett and Plum, p. 411)*

3. **(C)** Pleuritic chest pain is usually described as severe, sharp, knifelike pain worsened by coughing, deep inspiration, and movements of the trunk. The location of the pain tends to be identifiable on the chest wall, frequently along the intercostal nerve zones. The pain that accompanies angina pectoris often is described as squeezing. *(Bates et al, pp. 68–69; Bennett and Plum, p. 370)*

4. **(E)** The clinical manifestations of bronchogenic carcinoma can vary, and many patients are asymptomatic when the pulmonary lesion is discovered. Cough, usually productive of scant sputum is a common symptom, hemoptysis frequently occurs secondary to ulceration in the pulmonary lesion. Frequently, because of a significant smoking history, patients with carcinoma also have chronic obstructive pulmonary disease (COPD) and dyspnea with exertion. Weight loss also is a common complaint of bronchogenic carcinoma, but generally occurs with more extensive disease beyond the time frame that the neoplasm is limited to the lung. Chest pain may be due to pleural involvement, but must also suggest metastatic disease. Pulmonary infections occur distal to the bronchial obstruction and can mask the tumor. Any atypical or recurrent pulmonary infection should suggest carcinoma. Chest x-ray may demonstrate hilar and mediastinal lymph node involvement, pleural effusion, rib metastasis, elevation of a diaphragm, tracheal compression or distortion, and pericardial effusion. Although pulmonary diseases, particularly at end stages, present with similar symptoms, the entire history, physical, laboratory, and roentgenographic findings must be correlated to form the correct diagnosis. Asthma and chronic obstructive pulmonary disease usually reveal hyperinflation of the lungs and flat diaphragms. Bronchiectasis shows coarse lung markings and even honeycombing due to the abnormal dilatation of the bronchial tree. Chronic bronchitis has been used in various ways, sometimes referring to a simple smoker's cough and at other times to severe COPD. It is usually described as a productive cough that is present on most days for at least 3 months of the year. *(Bennett and Plum, pp 436–442; Tierney et al, pp. 253–258)*

5. **(C)** COPD results from some combination of chronic obstructive problems and pulmonary emphysema; both disorders are closely related to cigarette smoking. It is generally believed that emphysema results from the effect of proteolytic enzymes on lung tissue. When there is a very severe congenital deficiency of serum antiproteolytic activity, it is likely that emphysema will develop even if the subject does not smoke. This deficiency results in 0.5% to 2% of cases of COPD. The development of emphysema depends on prolonged exposure to noxious irritants, usually cigarette smoke. *(Bennett and Plum, pp. 35, 385–388; Tierney et al, pp. 228–233)*

6. **(E)** Spirometry and measurement of lung volumes provide information about the presence and severity of both obstructive and restrictive lung disease. The hallmark of obstructive disease is reduction in airflow rates. Restrictive pulmonary disease is characterized by reduction in lung volumes. *(Bennett and Plum, pp. 373–376; Tierney et al, pp. 217–218)*

7. **(D)** Pulmonary function tests are helpful in determining restrictive from obstructive pulmonary diseases but do not aid in the diagnosis of pulmonary carcinoma. Sputum cytology can yield a diagnosis in 40% to 60% of cases, and bronchoscopy with biopsy can give one a direct view of the lesion, as well as yield positive results in 75% to 80% of cases of pulmonary neoplasm. CT scan is helpful in visualizing and locating a pulmonary lesion and also is helpful in determining the existence of metastases. Ventilation-perfusion scanning is a sensitive test for the examination for regional lung function and may be helpful in the diagnosis of pulmonary carcinoma. *(Bennett and Plum, pp. 436–442; Tierney et al, pp. 253–260)*

8. **(D)** Asthma is a syndrome characterized by recurrent episodes of airway obstruction that resolve spontaneously or in response to treatment. Its cause is unknown, and it affects men and women equally. Reversible bronchospasm results in widespread airway narrowing that may be exacerbated by the presence of an infectious process. The classic clinical triad is cough, wheezing, and dyspnea. *(Bennett and Plum, pp. 376–381; Tierney et al, pp. 220–228)*

9. **(E)** The standard Mantoux test is performed by injecting 0.1 mL of purified protein derivative (PPD) intradermally on the volar surface of the forearm. The injection site should be inspected for the presence of induration 48 to 72 hours after the administration of PPD. An anergic patient will result in a false-negative reaction. *(Bennett and Plum, pp. 1683–1684; Tierney et al, pp. 246–253)*

10. **(E)** The recommendations of the Centers for Disease Control and Prevention (CDC) for the initial empiric treatment of tuberculosis (TB) in a patient who is seronegative for HIV include a variety of multidrug regimens. The CDC advises directly observed therapy for all patients found to have drug-resistant TB since noncompliance is the major cause of treatment failure and drug resistance. Treatment of extrapulmonary TB is the same as for pulmonary TB. *(Bennett and Plum, pp. 1686–1690; Tierney et al, pp. 248–252)*

11. **(C)** Foreign-body aspiration presents in children usually from ages 4 months through 6 years; frequently, there is a history of playing with small objects. The aspiration of the foreign body classically precipitates an acute episode of choking, gagging, coughing, and wheezing. The chest x-ray results in this question are classic for foreign-body aspiration. *(Hay et al, pp. 506–507)*

12. **(C)** The treatment of foreign-body aspiration is hospitalization with immediate bronchoscopy to remove the foreign body. Chest physiotherapy should not be used for fear of completely obstructing the airway. Cool-mist therapy and antibiotics would not, of course, be helpful, and intubation in this patient is not required, as the foreign body is causing only local effects. *(Hay et al, p. 507)*

13. **(C)** Air in the pleural space blocks the transmission of sound. Characteristic physical findings in a patient with pneumothorax include the presence of a hyperresonant per-

cussion note over pleural air and decreased to absent breath sounds and tactile fremitus over the area of pleural air. With a large pneumothorax the trachea may deviate to the opposite side. Prominent wheezes throughout both lung fields may be found in patients with asthma. *(Bates et al, p. 256; Way, pp. 333–334)*

14. **(C)** Spontaneous pneumothorax may occur in any age group but is most common in males 15 to 35 years of age. *(Way, pp. 333–334)*

15. **(A)** Cheyne–Stokes respiration is the most common form of periodic breathing. Periods of apnea alternate regularly with series of respiratory cycles. In each cycle, the rate and amplitude of successive respirations increase to a maximum, then decrease progressively until the series is terminated with an apneic period. Kussmaul's respiration is applied to deep, regular, sighing respirations, regardless of rate. This pattern of breathing is seen in diabetic ketoacidosis, uremia, peritonitis, severe hemorrhage, and pneumonia. Biot's breathing is an uncommon variant of Cheyne–Stokes respiration, in which periods of apnea alternate irregularly with series of breaths of equal depth. This is most often seen in meningitis. Stridulous breathing is a high-pitched whistling or crowing sound with respirations when the air passes over a partially closed glottis. This occurs with edema of the vocal cords (ie, infection), neoplasm, abscess of the pharynx, and foreign body in the pharynx. Apnea simply is the absence of respiration. *(Bates et al, p. 252)*

16. **(D)** Patients with pneumonia may present in a variety of clinical presentations. However, findings disclosed by proper physical examination of the lungs should aid in the formulation of the differential diagnosis. Vocal fremitus is increased in consolidated pneumonias and by inflammation surrounding other pulmonary lesions by transmitting bronchotracheal air vibration with greater efficiency than do the air-filled pulmonary alveoli. Consolidated pulmonary tissue has increased density than normal lung tissue, therefore yielding impaired resonance, dullness, and flatness to percussion. This consolidated tis-

sue also transmits whispered syllables distinctly, even when the pathological process is too small to produce bronchial breathing. Rales refer to sounds in the lungs from the movements of fluids or exudates in the airways. Although there are different types of rales, they sound like clicks or small bubbles and occur in bronchiectasis, pneumonia, consolidation, infarction, bronchitis, and TB. *(Bates et al, pp. 254–255)*

17. **(C)** People at risk for pulmonary embolism are those with hypercoagulable states, which may arise from the use of birth control pills, local stasis, immobilization that may be the result of an accident or illness, fractures, obesity, and congestive heart failure. Emboli that cause clinically significant pulmonary insult commonly arise in the ileofemoral and pelvic venous beds. Signs and symptoms often begin abruptly and include dyspnea, cough, anxiety, and chest pain (frequently pleuritic in nature). Hemoptysis may occur; tachycardia and tachypnea are common in this illness. A low-grade fever, hypotension, and cyanosis also are signs of pulmonary embolism. The presence of a deep venous thrombosis aids in the rapid clinical diagnosis. Radiographic evidence of consolidation may be present in cases of pulmonary embolism. *(Way, pp. 798–801)*

18. **(D)** The ventilation-perfusion scan is the most sensitive screening procedure for embolization. The perfusion of the embolized area is profoundly impaired with minimal impairment of ventilation. A negative study of good technical quality excludes angiographically detectable pulmonary embolism. Chest x-rays are abnormal in most patients with pulmonary embolization with infarction; the abnormalities are, however, often nonspecific. ECGs often are normal or may show nonspecific changes. Clinically significant embolization is almost always associated with hypoxemia; however, this may be obscured by reflex hyperventilation and hypocapnia. Pulmonary angiography allows direct visualization of the vascular tree and is the procedure of choice for establishing the diagnosis. Nonetheless, this procedure has

obvious limitations, and because of the controversy in this area, the choice of this procedure was not included in the answers. *(Way, pp. 798–801)*

19. **(C)** The term *restrictive ventilatory disorder* denotes a pattern of abnormalities in lung function. The word *restrictive* is employed to indicate a restriction of, or limitation to, the amount of gas within the lungs. The hallmark of restriction is a decrease in the vital capacity. Obstructive ventilatory disorder denotes the constellation of abnormalities that result from airway obstruction, regardless of its cause. Obstructive disorders are detected principally by the tests of the behavior of the respiratory system under dynamic conditions. The FEV_1/FVC (forced expiratory volume in 1 second divided by the forced vital capacity) is the most widely used. *(Bennett and Plum, pp. 373–376; Tierney et al, pp. 217–218)*

20. **(C)** The pneumococcus is the most common cause of community-acquired pyogenic bacterial pneumonia. Although the prevalence of penicillin-resistant pneumococci is increasing in the United States, penicillin remains the drug of choice. Penicillin-allergic patients may be treated with erythromycin or trimethoprim/sulfamethoxazole. *(Bennett and Plum, pp. 1569–1575; Tierney et al, pp. 1194–1196)*

21. **(C)** The major cell types of bronchogenic carcinoma include adenocarcinoma (30%–35%), squamous cell carcinoma (30%–35%), small cell carcinoma (20%–25%), and large cell carcinoma (about 15%). The most common histological type of breast cancer is infiltrating ductal carcinoma (70%–80%). *(Bennett and Plum, pp. 436–442, 1320–1325; Tierney et al, pp. 253–258, 617–627)*

22. **(C)** ARDS classically presents with rapid onset of tachypnea and dyspnea following the initiating event. Chest x-ray reveals diffuse patchy infiltrates that at first are interstitial and then become alveolar. Air bronchograms occur in 80% of patients. Most patients with ARDS demonstrate multiple organ failure commonly involving the kidneys, liver, gut, CNS, and cardiovascular systems. Heart size

is normal and pleural effusions are small or nonexistent. *(Bennett and Plum, pp. 454–456; Tierney et al, pp. 286–288)*

23. **(E)** All the choices may aggravate or stimulate an asthma attack. Inhaled allergens typically produce immediate Type I, IgE-mediated allergic reaction in the airway, although Type III, IgG-mediated reactions may also occur in some patients. The parasympathetic nervous system also plays a part in the asthmatic response. Cholinergic stimulation induces mediator production in the mast cell and causes contraction of bronchial smooth muscle. Vigorous exercise produces bronchoconstriction in some asthmatic patients. Furthermore, beta-adrenergic blockers as well as indomethacin, aspirin, and certain yellow coloring agents may induce asthma. Asthma-like reactions to inorganic chemicals and organic dusts are noted frequently. The role of emotional stress is difficult to assess, but clearly some subjects have exacerbations of their disease during stress. *(Bennett and Plum, pp. 376–381; Tierney et al, pp. 220–228)*

24. **(A)** Therapy for asthma can include all the choices, but inhaled beta-adrenergic agonist provides the most rapid effect and, therefore, the best therapeutic index. Use of epinephrine is contraindicated in patients with known cardiac disease and is not recommended in patients over age 50. Aminophylline, IV and oral, has a slower onset of action, and therapeutic levels must be maintained and monitored. Hydrocortisone also has a delayed onset of action, and its use should be limited if possible. *(Bennett and Plum, pp. 380–381; Tierney et al, pp. 220–228)*

25. **(D)** Epiglottitis is a medical emergency almost always caused by *Haemophilus influenzae* type B. Inflammation and swelling of the supraglottic structures develop rapidly and may lead to total airway obstruction and respiratory arrest. This process manifests clinically as stridor and inspiratory retractions, muffling of the voice, and drooling. Respiratory compromise results in an increased rate of respiration, not bradypnea. *(Hay et al, pp. 502–503)*

26. **(B)** The most common pathogen in bronchiolitis is respiratory syncytial virus (RSV). The usual course of bronchiolitis caused by RSV involves 1 to 2 days of fever, rhinorrhea, and cough, followed by wheezing, tachypnea, and respiratory distress. *(Hay et al, pp. 508–509)*

27. **(A)** The configuration of the thorax in patients with chronic obstructive pulmonary disease (COPD) usually demonstrates an increased anteroposterior (AP) diameter. Accessory muscles of ventilation are frequently used by patients with COPD. They also may exhibit diminished breath sounds throughout the lung fields, a hyperresonant note on percussion, and decreased fremitus. *(Bennett and Plum, pp. 368–369; Stobo et al, pp. 133–139)*

28. **(E)** Dyspnea involves the subjective sensation of shortness of breath. The most common pattern is seen during exercise. Other common causes are asthma, chronic obstructive pulmonary disease (COPD), including emphysema and chronic bronchitis. *(Bennett and Plum, pp. 370; Stobo et al, p. 121)*

29. **(C)** Viral croup usually includes prodrome of upper respiratory symptoms followed by the appearance of a barky cough and stridor. The tissue swelling is subglottic, and the absence of drooling tends to favor the diagnosis of viral croup rather than epiglottitis. The predominant finding is diffuse wheezing. Chronic bronchitis and pneumothorax are uncommon in children. *(Hay et al, p. 501)*

30. **(E)** The treatment of a patient with a pulmonary embolism should include bed rest, analgesics, and oxygen, as indicated. Anticoagulation should begin as soon as possible if no contraindication exists. Anticoagulation is usually performed with heparin, but in certain circumstances thrombolytics may be considered. Oral anticoagulants may be started within a few days of heparinization and are continued for 3 to 6 months. *(Way, pp. 798–801)*

31. **(E)** Hyaline membrane disease is caused by a deficiency of surfactant. The incidence of this disorder is as high as 65% at 29 to 30 weeks of gestation. *(Hay et al, p. 33)*

32. **(E)** The influenza viruses are the most important agents causing respiratory disease. Complications include acute sinusitis, otitis media, purulent bronchitis, and pneumonia. *(Stobo et al, pp. 563–564; Tierney et al, pp. 1181–1182)*

33. **(B)** Digital clubbing is present when the distal phalanx is rounded and bulbous. It accompanies chronic hypoxia associated with conditions such as lung cancer, idiopathic pulmonary fibrosis, and cystic fibrosis. *(Bates et al, p. 143; Tierney et al, p. 216)*

34. **(C)** Classically, pneumococcal pneumonia is a lobar pneumonia that presents with high fever, productive cough, occasional hemoptysis, and pleuritic chest pain. Rigors occur within the first few hours. Purulent sputum will demonstrate gram-positive diplococci 80% to 90% of the time. Rather than showing leukopenia, the peripheral white blood count may be two to three times the normal value. *(Bennett and Plum, pp. 1569–1575; Tierney et al, pp. 1194–1196)*

35. **(C)** Erythromycin is the drug of choice in treating *Mycoplasma pneumoniae*. Gastrointestinal intolerance is common, and tetracycline (unless the patient is pregnant) or doxycycline may be used as alternatives. *(Bennett and Plum, pp. 1578–1579; Tierney et al, pp. 239–240)*

36. **(D)** Carbon monoxide is the leading cause of accidental poisoning in the United States. It competes with oxygen for the binding sites on hemoglobin, exhibiting a binding affinity more than 200 times greater than that for oxygen. *(Bennett and Plum, pp. 403)*

37. **(B)** Chemical and inflammatory cough stimuli usually result in a productive response. Viral bronchitis is an acute condition. Syncope and rib fractures are infrequent complications of cough. The most common cause of chronic cough is postnasal drip. Usually airway mucus reaches the posterior pharynx via

the ciliary elevator and is then swallowed; clearing normal respiratory secretions without coughing. *(Bennett and Plum, p. 369)*

38. **(E)** The presence of partial airway obstruction below the tracheal bifurcation characteristically causes a localized wheeze over the site of obstruction and hyperinflation of the distal lung. Chest x-rays may be able to see the hyperinflation as well as the site of any foreign body or mass that is causing the obstruction. Inspiratory stridor is the hallmark of partial obstruction above the bifurcation. Pulmonary function testing reveals a relatively constant forced expiratory flow over a large portion of the FVC (forced vital capacity) in obstruction above the tracheal carina. Areas of localized decrease in airflow, as seen in obstruction below the carina, can be detected by ventilation-perfusion scanning. Pulse oximetry will not aid in localizing the obstruction. *(Bennett and Plum, pp. 368–371; Tierney et al, pp. 235–236)*

39. **(E)** Pleural effusions may be caused by a number of infectious and inflammatory processes. Pancreatitis resulting in fluid in the peritoneal space (ascites) may lead to pleural effusion as well. The five major types of pleural effusion are transudates, exudates, empyema, hemorrhagic pleural effusions, and chylous or chyliform effusions. *(Bennett and Plum, pp. 445–447; Tierney et al, pp. 288–292)*

40. **(D)** Sarcoidosis is a systemic disease of unknown cause. Patients may present with malaise, fever, and dyspnea of insidious onset. *(Bennett and Plum, pp. 431–436; Tierney et al, pp. 263–264)*

41. **(D)** *Pneumocystis carinii* pneumonia (PCP) is the most common opportunistic infection in AIDS. PCP is the initial infection in 60% of AIDS cases and occurs in 80% of patients at some time during the illness. The patient usually presents as acutely ill with an abrupt onset of tachypnea, mild cough, and cyanosis. Severe hypoxia is commonly present. Chest x-ray commonly shows diffuse interstitial infiltrates. *(Bennett and Plum, pp. 1917–1922; Tierney et al, pp. 238–245)*

42. **(A)** Streptococcal pneumonia is still the most common community-acquired pneumonia, occurring between 40% and 80% of the time in this setting. The classical onset involves a single shaking chill, fever, and cough productive of yellow-green to rusty or bloody mucous. Gram stain reveals gram-positive diplococci, and chest x-ray most typically shows a single lobar pneumonia. *(Bennett and Plum, pp. 1569–1575; Tierney et al, pp. 238–245)*

43. **(B)** *Mycoplasma pneumoniae* is a common cause of pneumonia in children and young adults, accounting for 10% to 50% of community-acquired pneumonias. Fever, headaches, and malaise precede the onset of pulmonary symptoms. Sputum is usually scant and sometimes blood-tinged. Bullous myringitis occurs in less than 25% of the cases. *(Bennett and Plum, pp. 1576–1579; Tierney et al, pp. 238–245)*

44. **(C)** Legionellosis most commonly occurs in the summer. Other factors that are associated with risk of *L. pneumophilia* include being male, middle-aged, or elderly, smoking, and alcoholism. Sputum is usually scant along with influenza-type symptoms of fever, headache, and anorexia. Pleuritic chest pain, tachypnea, and lower-than-expected pulse rate often occur. Chest x-ray shows patchy infiltrate, which progresses to lobar or segmented patterns and is commonly bilateral. *(Bennett and Plum, pp. 1583–1585; Tierney et al, pp. 238–245)*

45. **(E)** Influenza virus, adenovirus, and respiratory syncytial virus account for the majority of viral pneumonias. Coryza and sore throat, mild to moderate fever, myalgias, malaise, headache, and photophobia are common. Wheezing and dyspnea may develop as the disease progresses. Rash, conjunctivitis, and inflammation of the nasal mucosa may also be noted. Radiographs typically reveal a reticulonodular interstitial pattern. *(Bennett and Plum, pp. 1751–1756; Tierney et al, pp. 238–245)*

46. **(D)** Pulmonary radiation fibrosis occurs in nearly all patients who receive a full course of radiation therapy for cancer of the lung or breast. Most patients are asymptomatic,

though slowly progressive dyspnea occurs in some. *(Tierney et al, pp. 278–281)*

47. **(A)** Asbestosis is characterized by dyspnea and inspiratory crackles. Radiographic features include interstitial fibrosis, thickened pleura, calcified plaques on the diaphragms or lateral chest wall, and the formation of malignant mesotheliomas. *(Tierney et al, pp. 278–281)*

48. **(C)** It has been estimated that from 2% to 5% of all cases of asthma are related to occupation. Treatment consists of avoidance of further exposure to the offending agent. *(Tierney et al, pp. 278–281)*

49. **(E)** Silo-filler's disease is acute toxic noncardiogenic pulmonary edema caused by the inhalation of nitrogen dioxide encountered in recently filled silos. *(Tierney et al, pp. 278–281)*

50. **(B)** In coalworker's pneumoconiosis ingestion of inhaled dust by alveolar macrophages leads to the formation of macules that appear on chest x-ray as diffuse small opacities especially prominent in the upper lung. Simple coalworker's pneumoconiosis is usually asymptomatic. *(Tierney et al, pp. 278–281)*

REFERENCES

Bates B, Bickley LS, Hoekelman RA. *A Guide to Physical Examination and History Taking,* 6th ed. Philadelphia: Lippincott; 1995.

Bennett JC, Plum F. *Cecil Textbook of Medicine,* 20th ed. Philadelphia: Saunders; 1996.

Hay WW, Groothuis JR, et al. *Current Pediatric Diagnosis and Treatment.* Stamford, CT: Appleton & Lange; 1995.

Stobo JD, Hellmann DB, et al. *The Principles and Practice of Medicine.* Stamford, CT: Appleton & Lange; 1996.

Tierney LM, McPhee SJ, et al. *Current Medical Diagnosis and Treatment.* Stamford, CT: Appleton & Lange; 1996.

Way LW. *Current Surgical Diagnosis and Treatment,* 10th ed. Norwalk, CT: Appleton & Lange; 1994.

Internal Medicine: Infectious Diseases
Questions

Deborah Jalbert, MBA, PA-C

DIRECTIONS (Questions 1 through 14): Each of the numbered items or incomplete statements in this section is followed by answers or by completions of the statement. Select the ONE lettered answer or completion that is BEST in each case.

Questions 1 through 14

1. A patient presents with symptoms consistent with infectious mononucleosis. During your workup of this patient you would expect to find all the following EXCEPT

   (A) elevated liver function tests
   (B) hepatomegaly
   (C) lymphadenopathy
   (D) atypical lymphocytes on the differential
   (E) pharyngitis

2. Clinical manifestations of primary syphilis infection include which of the following?

   (A) diffuse macular rash
   (B) generalized lymphadenopathy
   (C) low-grade fever
   (D) painless genital ulcer
   (E) arthralgias and myalgias

3. Which of the following statements is true concerning traveler's diarrhea?

   (A) Bottled carbonated beverages can transmit infection.
   (B) Symptoms typically progress until antibiotics are given.
   (C) Amoxicillin may be given for prophylactic therapy.
   (D) Bismuth subsalicylate (Pepto-Bismol) will improve symptoms.
   (E) The most common cause is salmonella.

4. The human papillomavirus (HPV) is the causative organism for the common wart as well as genital warts. Regarding genital warts, the following are true EXCEPT

   (A) In the United States, HPV infections have been occurring at five times the rate of genital herpes since the mid-1980s.
   (B) No single treatment is effective in eradicating the virus and preventing recurrence.
   (C) The treatment of choice is cryotherapy.
   (D) The lesions can be confused with condylomata lata of secondary syphilis.
   (E) Of women with cervical dysplasia, more than 50% of male sexual contacts have HPV.

5. Which of the following is NOT characteristic of the stools seen with *Giardia lamblia* infection?

   (A) They are mushy in recurrent cases.
   (B) Blood is not present.
   (C) Mucus is not present.
   (D) There is little odor.
   (E) They tend to be greasy and float.

6. Which of the following cerebrospinal fluid analyses is an indicator of bacterial meningitis?

   (A) white blood cell count between 5 and 100
   (B) elevated protein
   (C) high glucose
   (D) predominant mononuclear cells
   (E) numerous red blood cells

7. Which of the following is NOT true regarding hepatitis D?

   (A) It can be prevented by immunizing against hepatitis B.
   (B) IV-drug users are at increased risk.
   (C) It exists only as a co-infecting disease with hepatitis B.
   (D) It is usually spread by the fecal-oral route.
   (E) Its presence in chronic active hepatitis B can indicate a poor prognosis.

8. In 1989 there was an outbreak of measles in the United States that had not been seen in recent years. As a result of this, the vaccination protocol has changed. Regarding measles prophylaxis, all of the following are true EXCEPT

   (A) In acute exposure, gamma globulin given within 6 days is preventative in most cases.
   (B) A live, attenuated virus vaccine is used in routine immunization.
   (C) An individual born before 1957 does not need to be revaccinated.
   (D) In cases where gamma globulin has been used, a follow-up live, attenuated virus vaccination should be given at least 30 days later.
   (E) In cases where outbreaks have occurred, a monovalent measles vaccine can be given as early as 6 months of age.

9. Which of the following is NOT true about the treatment of genital herpes (HSV-2)?

   (A) For initial episodes use acyclovir 200 mg PO 5 times per day for 7 to 10 days.
   (B) For recurring episodes use acyclovir 200 mg PO 5 times per day for 5 days.
   (C) For those unable to tolerate oral medications, topical acyclovir q3 hours while awake for 5 days is as effective as oral acyclovir in recurrent cases.
   (D) For initial episodes use acyclovir 400 mg PO tid for 7 to 10 days.
   (E) For suppression of recurrence, use acyclovir 400 mg PO bid, with treatment discontinued for 1 to 2 months per year to determine the frequency of recurrence.

10. Hepatitis B vaccine is recommended to all the following EXCEPT

    (A) infants born to a hepatitis B surface antigen (HBsAg)–positive mother
    (B) established hepatitis B–infected individuals
    (C) promiscuous heterosexuals
    (D) persons receiving an accidental needle-stick from HBsAg–positive blood or body fluids
    (E) health care professionals regularly exposed to blood

11. Which of the following is the MOST common etiology of bacterial meningitis in adults?

    (A) *Streptococcus pneumoniae*
    (B) *Haemophilus influenzae*
    (C) *Neisseria meningitidis*
    (D) *Staphylococcus aureus*
    (E) *Escherichia coli*

12. Which of the following is the most likely cause of diarrhea in a patient with a history of recent antibiotic use?

    (A) *Campylobacter*
    (B) *Clostridium difficile*
    (C) *Yersinia*
    (D) *Vibrio*
    (E) *Shigella*

13. Which of the following viral serologies is most definitive in diagnosing acute hepatitis B?

    (A) HBV-DNA
    (B) HBeAg
    (C) Anti-HBc (IgM)
    (D) Anti-HBs
    (E) IgG anti-HBc

14. Toxic shock syndrome is a multisystem disorder caused by which of the following organisms?

    (A) *Streptococcus pneumoniae*
    (B) *Haemophilus influenzae*
    (C) *Escherichia coli*
    (D) *Staphylococcus aureus*
    (E) *Pseudomonas aeruginosa*

DIRECTIONS (Questions 15 through 28): Each group of items in this section consists of lettered headings followed by a set of numbered words or phrases. For each numbered word or phrase, select

    (A) if the item is associated with (A) only
    (B) if the item is associated with (B) only
    (C) if the item is associated with both (A) and (B)
    (D) if the item is associated with neither (A) nor (B)

Questions 15 through 17

    (A) Kawasaki's disease
    (B) toxic shock syndrome

15. Bilateral, nonpurulent, conjunctival injection

16. Bacterial etiology believed to be the cause

17. Coronary artery involvement in some cases

Questions 18 through 20

    (A) Lyme disease
    (B) Rocky Mountain spotted fever

18. Bell's palsy is a neurological complication.

19. Doxycycline is the treatment of choice in early cases.

20. Vesicular lesions may develop as the disease progresses.

Questions 21 through 24

    (A) *Salmonella gastroenteritis*
    (B) *Shigella*

21. The disease is usually self-limited.

22. Antimicrobial treatment is unnecessary in uncomplicated cases.

23. It is associated with sexual transmission.

24. Antibiotics do not shorten the course of the illness.

Questions 25 and 26

    (A) hepatitis B
    (B) hepatitis C

25. Blood transfusions implicated as a cause

26. Associated with chronic active disease

Questions 27 and 28

    (A) gonococcal urethritis
    (B) nongonococcal urethritis

27. Diagnosis can be assisted by use of Gram stain.

28. Onset of symptoms occur within 1 week of sexual contact.

DIRECTIONS (Questions 29 through 43): Each of the numbered items or incomplete statements in this section is followed by answers or by completions of the statement. Select the ONE lettered answer or completion that is BEST in each case.

Questions 29 through 43

29. Which of the following is the most likely causative organism of bacteremia in a hospitalized patient with an intravenous line?

    (A) Beta-hemolytic streptococci
    (B) *Staphylococcus aureus*
    (C) *Bacteroides*
    (D) *Pseudomonas*
    (E) *Neisseria gonorrhea*

30. A patient presents with a sudden onset of fever, headache, and myalgias followed by a macular rash occurring initially on the wrists and ankles, then spreading to the trunk. This presentation is most characteristic of which of the following diseases?

    (A) scarlet fever
    (B) toxic shock syndrome
    (C) Kawasaki's disease
    (D) Rocky Mountain spotted fever
    (E) secondary syphilis

31. Which of the following statements is NOT true regarding herpes simplex virus, type 2 (HSV-2)?

    (A) The incubation period is 4 to 7 days.
    (B) Its recurrence rate is equal to that of herpes labialis (HSV-1).
    (C) An initial episode is less severe if there has been a prior HSV-1 infection.
    (D) There is unilateral distribution of lesions.
    (E) Acyclovir is the treatment of choice.

32. Which of the following statements is TRUE regarding *Giardia lamblia?*

    (A) It is a gram-negative rod.
    (B) It primarily affects the large intestine.
    (C) Symptoms appear within 6 to 12 hours after exposure.

    (D) It causes bloody stools.
    (E) Infected persons can be asymptomatic carriers.

33. Which of the following clinical and laboratory findings is included in the major manifestations of the revised Jones criteria for the diagnosis of acute rheumatic fever?

    (A) arthralgia
    (B) fever
    (C) elevated erythrocyte sedimentation rate
    (D) subcutaneous nodules
    (E) elevated streptococcal antibody titers

34. Which of the following is the causative organism for erysipelas?

    (A) *Streptococcus pyogenes*
    (B) *Staphylococcus aureus*
    (C) group A streptococcus
    (D) *Candida*
    (E) *Pseudomonas aeruginosa*

35. Intravenous drug users (IVDUs) are at greatest risk of developing endocarditis from which of the following organisms?

    (A) fungi
    (B) enterococci
    (C) streptococci
    (D) staphylococcus
    (E) diphtheroids

36. Hepatitis A (HAV) differs in many aspects from the other viral hepatic infections. Which of the following statements is TRUE regarding HAV?

    (A) It is transmitted through blood transfusions.
    (B) Dark urine and clay-colored stools are first noticed after jaundice occurs.
    (C) The patient can show antibodies to HAV without ever having clinically apparent disease.
    (D) The IgM antibody indicates past infection and persisting immunity.
    (E) It can become a chronic disease.

37. Which of the following is the MOST common cause of fever of unknown origin?

    (A) drug-induced causes
    (B) factitious illness
    (C) collagen vascular disease
    (D) neoplasia
    (E) infection

38. Which is the MOST definitive diagnostic test for active pulmonary tuberculosis?

    (A) tuberculin skin test
    (B) chest roentgenogram
    (C) acid-fast smear of sputum
    (D) sputum culture
    (E) blood culture

39. Which of the following is the MOST common causative organism for nongonococcal urethritis?

    (A) *Chlamydia trachomatis*
    (B) *Trichomonas vaginalis*
    (C) ureaplasma urealyticum
    (D) herpes simplex virus
    (E) *Mycoplasma genitalium*

40. Which of the following is the drug of choice for prophylactic chemotherapy of tuberculosis?

    (A) isoniazid
    (B) rifampin
    (C) pyrazinamide
    (D) ethambutol
    (E) streptomycin

41. A toddler presents with a 3-day history of conjunctivitis, coryza, nasal discharge, and a hacking cough. On examination, you notice small, irregular, grayish-white lesions on the upper buccal mucosa. The MOST likely diagnosis is

    (A) rubeola
    (B) rubella
    (C) roseola
    (D) rosacea
    (E) rotavirus

42. Which of the following is the recommended *initial* treatment of choice for a patient with known or suspected tuberculosis?

    (A) isoniazid
    (B) isoniazid + rifampin
    (C) isoniazid + rifampin + pyrazinamide
    (D) isoniazid + rifampin + pyrazinamide + ethambutol
    (E) isoniazid + rifampin + pyrazinamide + ethambutol + streptomycin

43. Which of the following drugs can cause a maculopapular rash in a patient with infectious mononucleosis?

    (A) tetracycline
    (B) erythromycin
    (C) ampicillin
    (D) sulfa
    (E) cephalosporin

Answers and Explanations

1. **(B)** Frequently, the individual with mononucleosis presents with fever, sore throat, lymphadenitis, and malaise. The spleen is enlarged in more than half of the cases. Hepatomegaly may be found in 10% to 20% of cases; however, more frequently on examination, there may be percussion tenderness over the liver, but no associated hepatomegaly. Laboratory values reveal elevated liver function tests in almost all cases. There is an increase in atypical lymphocytes noted on the differential, usually greater than 10%. *(Behrman, pp. 805–806; Berkow, pp. 2283–2285; Mandell et al, p. 1176; Rakel, pp. 109–110; Tierney et al, pp. 1163–1165; Isselbacher et al, pp. 790–793; Bennet and Plum, pp. 1776–1779; Hurst, pp. 497–499)*

2. **(D)** Syphilis is a sexually transmitted infection that remains asymptomatic in many patients throughout the course of the disease. Other than the syphilitic chancre, primary syphilis is asymptomatic. The classical chancre is a painless, solitary, indurated, and clean-based lesion. It is associated with regional adenopathy. Chancres may occur on any site used for sexual activity. *(Tierney et al, pp. 1227–1237; Isselbacher et al, pp. 726–737; Bennet and Plum, pp. 1705–1713; Hurst, pp. 422–426)*

3. **(D)** Traveler's diarrhea is most often caused by an enterotoxigenic strain of *Escherichia coli*. Bottled, carbonated beverages are considered safe to drink, as well as fruit that can be peeled. Bismuth subsalicylate (Pepto-Bismol) provides symptomatic relief. Diphenoxylate (Lomotil) and loperamide (Imodium) provide symptomatic relief but should be discontinued if symptoms persist for more than 24 hours. The symptoms resolve in 1 to 5 days and rarely last 2 to 3 weeks. Prophylactic therapy may begin the day of the trip with either doxycyline 100 mg, double-strength trimethoprim-sulfamethoxazole, norfloxacin 400 mg, or ciprofloxicin 500 mg, once daily for 3 days. However, many feel treatment should begin when symptoms develop. The same treatment may be used for symptomatic patients but in twice-daily doses for 3 days. *(Abramowicz, 1992a, pp. 41–42; Berkow, pp. 819–820; Mandell et al, pp. 856–858; Rakel, pp. 13–14; Tierney et al, p. 1127; Isselbacher et al, pp. 532–534; Bennet and Plum, pp. 1657–1658; Hurst, pp. 1603–1604)*

4. **(A)** Human papillomavirus (HPV) has at least 60 subtypes that are recognized. Approximately 10 of these subtypes are responsible for the transmission of genital warts. Some oncogenic strains also have been associated with cancer of the glans penis. Since the mid-1980s, the rate of sexually transmitted diseases (STDs) due to HPV infection has been double that for those STDs secondary to genital herpes. After contact there is an incubation period of 1 to 6 months. The lesions are soft, minute, pink, and grow rapidly. In the male the most common site is the frenulum and the coronal sulcus. Diagnosis can be made by acetowashing the affected area for 3 to 5 minutes with 5% acetic acid. The lesions can be confused with molluscum contagio-

sum and condyloma lata of secondary syphilis. The treatment of choice is cryotherapy. The most common form of treatment is topical podophyllum. Other forms of treatment are electrodessication, surgical excision, laser therapy, or topical fluorouracil. No single treatment has been found to be effective in eradicating the virus. Recurrence is frequent. *(Abramowicz, 1991, pp. 119–124; Berkow, pp. 271–272; Mandell et al, pp. 1191–1197; Rakel, pp. 782, 788; Tierney et al, pp. 133; Isselbacher et al, pp. 801–803)*

5. **(D)** The stools of one infected with *Giardia lamblia* are generally foul-smelling, greasy in appearance, and float in the water. Blood or mucus is not typically present. In chronic cases, the stools tend to be mushy. *(Berkow, p. 228; Mandell et al, p. 2113; Tierney et al, pp. 1258–1260; Isselbacher et al, pp. 910–912; Bennet and Plum, pp. 1912–1913; Hurst, pp. 1604–1605)*

6. **(B)** The cerebral spinal fluid profile typically seen in bacterial meningitis includes: 500–20,000 white blood cells, 90% polymorphonuclear leukocytes, low glucose, and high protein (100–700 mg/dL). *(Tierney et al, pp. 1196–1197; Isselbacher et al, pp. 2296–2302; Bennet and Plum, pp. 1610–1621; Hurst, pp. 309–317)*

7. **(D)** Hepatitis D, also known as the delta agent, is an incomplete RNA virus that replicates only in the presence of the hepatitis B virus (HBV). It cannot exist as an isolated infecting organism. It can be associated with a superinfection, which is more severe than infection with HBV alone. This can result in severe chronic hepatitis and cirrhosis. Hepatitis D is spread by blood products and needles. High-risk groups include IV-drug users, dialysis patients, and those receiving multiple transfusions. As hepatitis D is not pathogenic without the presence of hepatitis B, prevention can be attained by immunizing against hepatitis B. *(Berkow, pp. 900, 905; Mandell et al, pp. 1007–1008, 1213; Tierney et al, pp. 578–584; Isselbacher et al, pp. 1458–1480; Bennet and Plum, pp. 762–780; Hurst, pp. 1682–1686)*

8. **(D)** Gamma globulin given at 0.25 mL/kg within 6 days to a person exposed to rubeola

who has no previous history of vaccination or adequate antibodies for protection will be preventative. It is not effective once symptoms have developed. If indicated, a live, attenuated virus vaccine should be given at least 3 months later. Routine immunization should be done using the same type of vaccine. The first dose is given at 15 months of age, usually with the mumps and rubella vaccines. A booster vaccine also is recommended at 4 to 6 years of age (CDC guideline) or 12 years of age (American Academy of Pediatrics guideline). An individual does not need to be revaccinated if he or she was born prior to 1957, had measles previously, or has already received 2 doses of vaccine. In cases of outbreaks, a monovalent vaccine can be given initially at age 6 months or older. Routine immunization is carried out thereafter. *(Behrman, pp. 791–793; Berkow, pp. 2166–2170; Mandell et al, pp. 1279–1284; Rakel, pp. 133–125; Tierney et al, pp. 1167–1169; Isselbacher et al, pp. 825–827; Bennet and Plum, pp. 1759–1761; Hurst, pp. 485–488)*

9. **(C)** The treatment of choice for the initial episode of herpes simplex virus, type 2 (HSV-2) is acyclovir 200 mg five times per day for 7 to 10 days. Also effective is acyclovir 400 mg tid for 7 to 10 days. For recurring infections, acyclovir 200 mg five times per day for 5 days is used. This regimen for recurrence is not recommended for routine use of all recurring episodes. Preventive therapy should be considered. Treatment for prevention of HSV-2 is acyclovir 400 mg bid or 200 mg 2 to 5 times daily. Long-term use is considered safe, but treatment should be discontinued for 1 to 2 months to determine disease recurrence. Topical acyclovir offers little or no benefit in the treatment of HSV-2. *(Abramowicz, 1991, 119–124; Berkow, p. 271; Mandell et al, pp. 1150–1151; Rakel, pp. 785–786; Tierney et al, p. 1159–1161; Isselbacher et al, pp. 782–787; Bennet and Plum, pp. 1770–1774; Hurst, pp. 491–494)*

10. **(B)** Hepatitis B vaccine gives hepatitis B surface antibody response to approximately 90% of those vaccinated. The vaccine can be given before or after exposure. Pre-exposure vaccination should be given to those at risk of com-

ing into contact with hepatitis B, such as health care workers who may come into contact with infectious blood (or blood products) and promiscuous heterosexuals, as well as homosexuals. Postexposure vaccination should be given to those who have been accidentally stuck with a needle contaminated with hepatitis B surface antigen (HBsAg)–positive blood or to infants born to HBsAg–positive mothers. The vaccine is ineffective for those with currently active disease. *(Berkow, p. 903; Mandell et al, p. 1222; Rakel, p. 494; Tierney et al, pp. 578–584; Isselbacher et al, pp. 1458–1480; Bennet and Plum, pp. 762–780; Hurst, pp. 1682–1686)*

11. **(A)** In adults, the relative frequency of bacterial meningitis caused by *Streptococcus pneumoniae* is 40% to 50%, *Neisseria meningitidis* is 15% to 30%, *Staphylococcus aureus* 5% to 10%, *Haemophilus influenzae* 2% to 4%, and gram-negative bacilli 5%. The relative frequencies are age related, with haemophilus being most frequent (40%–60%) in children, and streptococci being most frequent (40%–50%) in neonates. *(Tierney et al, pp. 1196–1197; Isselbacher et al, pp. 2296–2302; Bennet and Plum, pp. 1610–1621; Hurst, pp. 312–317)*

12. **(B)** *Clostridium difficile*–induced colitis, often referred to as "antibiotic-associated colitis," is a toxin-mediated disease in which one or more toxins attach to the colonic mucosa, but rarely invade it. Growth of *C. difficile* is promoted by poorly understood antibiotic-induced alterations in the normal intestinal flora. Clinically, the patient presents with watery diarrhea and cramping abdominal pain. Leukocytes are seen on stool examination. *(Tierney et al, pp. 496–497; Isselbacher et al, pp. 637–640; Bennet and Plum, pp. 1633–1635; Hurst, pp. 340–342)*

13. **(C)** Hepatitis B surface antigen (HBsAg) is the first serologic marker of hepatitis B (HBV) infection. It usuallly occurs during the incubation period and disappears during the recovery phase. The HBV surface antibody (anti-HBs) develops after clinical recovery. It represents past HBV infection or past immunization. The HBV core antigen (HBcAg) represents the viral inner core. It is not de-

tectable in serum by conventional lab methods, but only by specialized techniques. The HBV core antibody (anti-HBc) is a marker of acute, persistent, or past infection. The anti-HBc (IgM) will be positive for 6 to 18 months after infection and establishes acute infection with hepatitis B. The anti-HBc (IgG) is the indicator of past infection. There is a "window" period in HBV, during the transition from the disappearance of HBsAg and the appearance of anti-HBs. Anti-HBc (IgM) will be the only indicator of infection during this time. The HBVe antigen (HBeAg) is found only in HBsAg–positive serum. Its presence in the serum, along with HBsAg, for more than 10 weeks correlates with ongoing viral replication and may be a predictor of chronic disease. *(Berkow, pp. 899–900; Mandell et al, pp. 1219–1221; Tierney et al, pp. 578–584; Isselbacher et al, pp. 1458–1480; Bennet and Plum, pp. 762–780; Hurst, pp. 1682–1686)*

14. **(D)** Toxic shock syndrome is believed to be caused by a strain of *S. aureus* that produces a toxin, thus causing the symptoms. Initial presenting symptoms include the sudden onset of fever, rash, pharyngitis, and nonpurulent conjunctivitis. There may also be headache, lethargy, and hypotension. *(Behrman, p. 765; Berkow, p. 139; Mandell et al, pp. 1884–1886; Tierney et al, pp. 1198–1199; Isselbacher et al, pp. 614–615; Bennet and Plum, pp. 1588–1589; Hurst, p. 404)*

15. **(C); 16. (B); 17. (A)** Kawasaki's disease is a disease of unknown etiology. It consists of an exanthem, fever, lymphadenopathy, and polyarteritis. The coronary arteries may become involved, including the formation of aneurysms. The disease also is associated with mucous membrane changes, which include pharyngeal injection, fissured lips, and injected, nonpurulent conjunctiva. *(Behrman, pp. 629–630; Berkow, pp. 2201–2202; Mandell et al, pp. 2171–2172; Tierney et al, pp. 1183–1184; Bennet and Plum, pp. 2200–2201).* Toxic shock syndrome is believed to be caused by a strain of *S. aureus* that produces a toxin, thus causing the symptoms. Initial presenting symptoms include the sudden onset of fever, rash, pharyngitis, and nonpurulent conjunctivitis. There

may also be headache, lethargy, and hypotension. There is no known coronary artery involvement. *(Behrman, pp. 629–630; Berkow, pp. 88–89; Mandell et al, pp. 2171–2172; Tierney et al, pp. 1198–1199; Isselbacher et al, p. 1678; Bennet and Plum, pp. 1588–1589)*

18. (A); 19. (C); 20. (D) Lyme disease begins with the tick bite from *Ixodes dammini* or *I. pacificans*, which transmits the spirochete *Borrelia burgdorferi*. The classic rash, erythema chronicum migrans, begins as a macular or maculopapular lesion that expands, leaving centralized clearing. This occurs within 1 month of the tick bite in most patients and can resolve spontaneously. Within 1 week to months, a second stage of the disease can occur, which includes cardiac and neurological complications. Bilateral Bell's palsy may occur, as well as severe fatigue, peripheral neuropathy, and meningitis. Early manifestations of the disease are treated with doxycycline 100 mg bid for 10 to 21 days or amoxicillin 250 mg or 500 mg for 10 to 21 days. *(Abramowicz, 1992c, pp. 95–97; Berkow, pp. 154–156; Mandell et al, pp. 1819–1825; Rakel, pp. 124–125; Tierney et al, pp. 1240–1245; Isselbacher et al, pp. 745–747; Bennet and Plum, pp. 1715–1720).* Rocky Mountain spotted fever (RMSF) is transmitted by the bite of any one of the three vectors of the genus *Dermacentor*. The Lone Star tick, *Amblyomma americanum*, also is responsible for transmitting the disease. The disease-causing organism is *Rickettsia rickettsii*. The rash of RMSF typically begins as a macular or maculopapular lesion but progresses to form petechial lesions. The lesions may coalesce to form large hemorrhagic areas. In RMSF, the treatment of choice is either chloramphenicol 50 mg/kg/day, in children over 8 years old and pregnant females or doxycycline 100 mg q12 hours. *(Berkow, pp. 174, 181; Mandell et al, pp. 1465–1470; Rakel, pp. 128–130; Tierney et al, p. 1189; Isselbacher et al, pp. 750–752; Bennet and Plum, pp. 1730–1732)*

21. (C); 22. (C); 23. (B); 24. (A) *Salmonella gastroenteritis* is usually transmitted by infected meat, poultry, eggs, egg products, and raw milk. Infections affecting the intestinal tract are manifested by watery stools, with occasional blood and mucus. The disease is usually self-limited in uncomplicated cases and does not necessarily warrant antibiotic use. Treatment with antibiotics may actually prolong the time in which *Salmonella* resides in the intestinal tract. *(Behrman, pp. 731–733; Berkow, pp. 105–106; Mandell et al, pp. 1700–1712; Rakel, p. 144; Tierney et al, pp. 1208–1210; Isselbacher et al, pp. 671–676; Bennet and Plum, pp. 1644–1646).* *Shigella* is usually transmitted by the stools of infected individuals, particularly by the fecal-oral route. There is increasing incidence in the daycare centers. Homosexuals practicing anilingus are considered a high-risk group. It can also be obtained from contaminated water and sanitation facilities. Shigellosis begins with infrequent, voluminous, watery stools. This later progresses to frequent stools with decreased volume, often containing mucus, pus, and blood. Treatment is variable. If left untreated, the disease is usually self-limited. In severe cases, antimicrobial treatment is recommended, because the disease can lead to dehydration. Infants are at greater risk for developing further complications. *(Behrman, pp. 734–736; Berkow, pp. 106–108; Mandell et al, pp. 1718–1719; Tierney et al, pp. 1210; Isselbacher et al, pp. 676–679; Bennet and Plum, pp. 1647–1648)*

25. (C) Hepatitis B infection used to make up the majority of cases associated with posttransfusion hepatitis. With the advent of blood screening by blood banks, now less than 5% of posttransfusion hepatitis cases are hepatitis B. The remainder of posttransfusion hepatitis cases are mostly hepatitis C, constituting approximately 90% of all cases. *(Berkow, pp. 900–901; Mandell et al, pp. 1214, 1220; Tierney et al, pp. 578–584; Isselbacher et al, pp. 1458–1480; Bennet and Plum, pp. 762–780)*

26. (C) Approximately 10% of hepatitis B–infected individuals will still have detectable HBsAg in their blood after 6 months. A small percentage (about 3%) of these will remain HBsAg positive for years. They may be asymptomatic carriers or develop chronic active disease. This also is confirmed by liver biopsy and failure of liver function tests to return to normal. Approximately 40% to 50%

of those with posttransfusion hepatitis C will develop chronic active disease. This, too, as in hepatitis B, is confirmed by failure of the liver function tests to return to normal and by liver biopsy. Unlike hepatitis B, the HBsAg will not be detectable in the serum. *(Berkow, p. 905; Mandell et al, pp. 1408–1410; Tierney et al, pp. 578–584; Isselbacher et al, pp. 1458–1480; Bennet and Plum, pp. 762–780)*

27. (C); 28. (A) In gonococcal urethritis (GU), the Gram stain reveals gram-negative intracellular diplococci in over 90% of the cases. This is a reliable finding in the diagnosis of GU. In nongonococcal urethritis (NGU) there are no intracellular diplococci found, but in the absence of this finding, a diagnosis of NGU can be made by exclusion, by finding at least 5 polymorphonuclear leukocytes/hpf on the Gram stain. From exposure to the onset of symptoms, GU has an incubation period of 2 to 8 days; for NGU it is 1 to 3 weeks. The discharge of GU is generally of greater quantity and purulence than NGU. There is more dysuria with GU as well. *(Berkow, pp. 254–255, 257–258; Mandell et al, pp. 942–948; Rakel, pp. 710–713; Tierney et al, pp. 1214–1215, 1225–1226; Isselbacher et al, pp. 646, 759–761; Bennet and Plum, pp. 1697–1699)*

29. (B) Bacteremia due to *S. aureus* most commonly arises from skin lesions or intravenous lines. The usual source of noscomial bacteremia is intravenous catheters. Whenever *S. aureus* is recovered from blood cultures, endocarditis, osteomyelitis, or metastatic abscesses should be considered. The appropriate therapy for uncomplicated *S. aureus* bacteremia involves removing the source (eg, intravenous line) and parenteral antibiotic therapy for 2 weeks. Recommended drug of choice is nafcillin or oxacillin, cefazolin, or vancomycin for patients with penicillin allergies or methicillin-resistant strains. *(Tierney et al, pp. 1198–1199; Isselbacher et al, p. 615; Bennet and Plum, p. 1608; Hurst, pp. 288–291)*

30. (D) Rocky Mountain spotted fever (RMSF) has a high incidence of occurrence in the South Atlantic states, with a high percentage of the cases occurring in North Carolina, Vir-

ginia, Georgia, Maryland, Tennessee, and Oklahoma. The disease is transmitted by any one of three ticks from the genus *Dermacentor*, as well as from the Lone Star tick, *Amblyomma americanum*. These ticks act as vectors of the disease-causing organism, *Rickettsia rickettsii*. Clinically, the patient presents with a sudden onset of fever, headache, and myalgias, followed in a few days with a macular or maculopapular rash that begins on the wrists and ankles and spreads to the trunk. *(Tierney et al, pp. 1198–1199; Isselbacher et al, p. 615; Bennet and Plum, p. 1608; Hurst, pp. 433–434)*

31. (D) Herpes simplex virus, type 2 (HSV-2) is the most common source of genital ulcers. It is a frequently occurring sexually transmitted disease; however, since the mid-1980s, human papillomavirus or genital warts have been occurring at twice the rate of HSV-2. Initial episodes are usually accompanied by fever, headache, malaise, and myalgia. These symptoms are usually less severe if the patient has had a prior HSV-1 infection. Lesions are preceded by itching and pain. Unlike herpes zoster virus, there is bilateral distribution. The treatment of choice is oral acyclovir. HSV-2 frequently recurs, usually at the site of the initial infection. HSV-2 has a recurrence rate of 80% to 90% within 12 months, compared to a recurrence rate of 50% for HSV-1 for the same time period. *(Berkow, pp. 270–271; Mandell et al, pp. 1144–1148, 1150–1151; Rakel, pp. 785–786; Tierney et al, pp. 1159–1161; Isselbacher et al, pp. 782–787; Bennet and Plum, pp. 1770–1774; Hurst, pp. 491–494)*

32. (E) *Giardia lamblia* is a protozoan organism spread from host to host by fecal-oral transmission. It has been associated with sexual transmission, particularly homosexuals practicing anilingus. Infected persons can be asymptomatic carriers. It primarily affects the duodenum and jejunum. Incubation period is 7 to 21 days. Malabsorption may occur, possibly from mechanical blockage of the intestinal mucosa. Regardless of frequency, the stools are free from pus or blood, but may contain mucus. *(Berkow, p. 228; Mandell et al, pp. 2110–2113; Tierney et al, pp. 373–375; Isselbacher et* *al, pp. 1046–1052; Bennet and Plum, pp. 1590–1596; Hurst, pp. 1604–1605)*

33. **(D)** Acute rheumatic fever follows a streptococcal infection and is an inflammatory syndrome involving many systems. The diagnosis of ARF is made on a combination of clinical and laboratory findings using the revised Jones criteria. The presence of two major or one major and two minor manifestations indicates a high probability of ARF. The major manifestations are carditis, polyarthritis, chorea, erythema marginatum, and subcutaneous nodules. *(Tierney et al, pp. 373–375; Isselbacher et al, pp. 1046–1052; Bennet and Plum, pp. 1590–1596; Hurst, pp. 1255–1258)*

34. **(C)** Erysipelas can be identified separately from cellulitis by its sharply demarcated painful border, often on the face or legs, with lymphedema. Patients feel ill and are febrile. Group A streptococcus is the usual cause. *(Tierney et al, pp. 129–130; Isselbacher et al, p. 562; Bennet and Plum, p. 2208; Hurst, p. 373)*

35. **(D)** *S. aureus* causes over 50% of cases of endocarditis occurring in IVDUs. In some communities these *S. aureus* strains are resistant to all B-lactam antibiotics. Enterococci and streptococci are less frequent pathogens in IVDUs. *(Tierney et al, pp. 1122–1124; Isselbacher et al, pp. 565–566; Bennet and Plum, pp. 1596–1605; Hurst, pp. 322–325)*

36. **(C)** Hepatitis A virus (HAV) is transmitted by the fecal-oral route. Compared to hepatitis B, it has a much shorter incubation period. The prodromal symptoms are varied, but include dark-colored urine and clay-colored stools prior to the onset of jaundice, which is the start of the clinical phase. The posticteric phase follows this, lasting 2 to 12 weeks. Lab indicators show a positive HAV antibody of the IgM class [anti-HA (IgM)] during an acute infection. During the disappearance of anti-HA (IgM), the anti-HA (IgG) remains as the only serological marker of past infection and persisting immunity. Passive immunization is possible through immune globulin injections. Exposure to the virus without clinically apparent symptoms can produce anti-

bodies as well. Unlike hepatitis B, there is no known chronic carrier state. *(Berkow, pp. 899, 902; Mandell et al, pp. 1387–1390; Tierney et al, pp. 578–584; Isselbacher et al, pp. 1458–1480; Bennet and Plum, pp. 762–780; Hurst, pp. 1682–1686)*

37. **(E)** The definition of fever of unknown origin (FUO) varies in regard to the degree of fever and the length of time the fever is present. A definition derived from various sources is a temperature greater than 101°F for 2 to 3 weeks without an identifiable cause, after 1 week of intensive investigation. Infections categorize about 25% to 40% of cases of FUO in adults, making this the most common cause. The remaining causes are categorized into collagen vascular diseases, such as juvenile rheumatoid arthritis or systemic lupus erythematosus; neoplasms, such as leukemia or lymphoma; and miscellaneous causes, which include factitious fever, drug fevers, and pulmonary emboli, to name a few. *(Behrman, pp. 652–653; Berkow, p. 9; Mandell et al, pp. 468, 472–477; Tierney et al, pp. 1111–1113; Isselbacher et al, pp. 85–90; Bennet and Plum, pp. 1532–1533)*

38. **(D)** The tuberculin skin test is a diagnostic test for infection with *Mycobacterium tuberculosis*, not for active disease. Sputum smears for detection of acid-fast bacilli can be obtained, but are not as sensitive as sputum cultures, which are definitive and prove disease. A chest roentgenogram is an important tool in the initial diagnostic workup. Blood cultures for mycobacteria may be useful in disseminated TB and AIDS-related TB. *(Tierney et al, pp. 1215, 1221–1223; Isselbacher et al, pp. 710–718; Bennet and Plum, pp. 1683–1689; Hurst, pp. 1043–1052)*

39. **(A)** Several organisms have been implicated in causes of nongonococcal urethritis (NGU). *Chlamydia trachomatis* can be found in 40% to 50% of cases of NGU. Ureaplasma urealyticum and *Trichomonas vaginalis* make up an additional 30% of cases. HSV-2, as well as *Corynebacterium genitalium*, can also cause NGU. *(Berkow, pp. 257–258; Mandell et al, p. 944; Rakel, pp. 712–713; Tierney et al, pp. 1225–1226; Isselbacher et al, pp. 759–761; Bennet and Plum, pp. 1697–1699; Hurst, pp. 356–360)*

40. **(A)** Isoniazid is the drug of choice of prophylactic treatment of tuberculosis. It is given in a daily dose of 300 mg for 6 to 12 months. Because of isoniazid-resistant strains of *Mycobacterium*, the Southeast Asian population may need multiple drug therapy for prophylactic treatment. The risk of developing tuberculosis is particularly high for those in close contacts of newly infected individuals and also within 2 years after the development of a positive tuberculin skin test. The risk of developing serious tuberculosis infections, including meningitis, is particularly high among infants and adolescents. *(Abramowicz, 1992b, pp. 10–11; Berkow, pp. 140–141; Rakel, p. 222; Tierney et al, pp. 1221–1223; Isselbacher et al, pp. 710–718; Bennet and Plum, pp. 1683–1689; Hurst, pp. 1043–1052)*

41. **(A)** Rubeola is a highly infectious disease. The incubation period ranges from 9 to 12 days, followed by a prodromal period where ocular symptoms are frequent. This includes mild conjunctivitis, edema of the eyelids, excessive lacrimation, as well as photophobia. Rhinorrhea and a hacking cough are usually present. Koplik spots, which are small, irregular, grayish-white lesions on the upper buccal mucosa, are pathognomonic. Last, a sudden rise in temperature to the 104°F to 105°F range occurs, accompanied by a maculopapular rash. The rash is brick-red. It is irregularly confluent and in severe cases can be petechial. It starts about 2 weeks after exposure. It occurs first to the facial area, especially to the forehead and around the ears, spreading downward as the disease progresses, eventually affecting the neck, shoulders, trunk, and upper extremities. The rash resolves in about 6 days, but persists for about 3 days in each area, disappearing in the same order of appearance. Isolation is required 7 days after exposure until 5 days after the rash has appeared. *(Behrman, pp. 791–793; Berkow, pp. 2166–2170; Mandell et al, pp. 1279–1284; Rakel, pp. 133–135; Tierney et al, pp. 1167–1169; Isselbacher et al, pp. 825–827; Bennet and Plum, pp. 1759–1761; Hurst, pp. 485–488)*

42. **(D)** Isoniazid alone for 12 months can be given prophylactically for the treatment of tuberculosis (TB), but not to treat initial uncomplicated TB. With the widespread incidence of resistance to isoniazid and other drugs, the recommended initial treatment in most communities is to use a minimum of four drugs. Adjustments in this regimen can be made after drug sensitivity testing is available. The combination of isoniazid, rifampin, pyrazinamide, and ethambutol, all taken orally, is recommended. *(Tierney et al, pp. 1221–1223; Isselbacher et al, pp. 710–718; Bennet and Plum, pp. 1683–1689; Hurst, pp. 1043–1052)*

43. **(C)** Infectious mononucleosis is caused by the Epstein–Barr virus, a herpes group virus. Clinically, there is pharyngitis, lymphadenitis, and splenomegaly. Rupture of the spleen may occur, either spontaneously or following trauma, but is rare. Elevated liver function tests are the norm. With concurrent ampicillin use, there is an associated erythematous macular or maculopapular rash in 80% to 100% of cases. *(Behrman, pp. 805–806; Berkow, pp. 2281–2285; Mandell et al, pp. 1172–1176; Rakel, pp. 109–110; Tierney et al, pp. 1163–1165; Isselbacher et al, pp. 790–793; Bennet and Plum, pp. 1776–1779; Hurst, pp. 497–499)*

REFERENCES

Abramowicz M (ed). Drugs for sexually transmitted diseases. *Med Letter.* 1991; 33: 119–124.

Abramowicz M (ed). Advice for travelers. *Med Letter.* 1992a; 34: 41–42.

Abramowicz M (ed). Drugs for tuberculosis. *Med Letter.* 1992b; 34: 10–11.

Abramowicz M (ed). Treatment of Lyme disease. *Med Letter.* 1992c; 34: 95–97.

Behrman RE (ed). *Nelson Textbook of Pediatrics*, 14th ed. Philadelphia: Saunders; 1992.

Bennet JC, Plum F (eds). *Cecil Textbook of Medicine*, 20th ed. Philadelphia: Saunders; 1996.

Berkow R (ed). *The Merck Manual of Diagnosis and Therapy*, 16th ed. Rahway, NJ: Merck; 1992.

Hurst J (ed). *Medicine for the Practicing Physician.* Stamford, CT: Appleton & Lange; 1996.

Isselbacher KJ, Braunwald I, Wilson JD, Martin FB, Fauci AS, Kasper DL (eds). *Harrison's Principles of Internal Medicine,* 13th ed. New York: McGraw Hill; 1994.

Mandell GL, Douglass RG Jr, Bennett JE (eds). *Principles and Practice of Infectious Disease,* 3rd ed. New York: Churchill Livingstone; 1990.

Rakel RE (ed). *Conn's Current Therapy.* Philadelphia: Saunders; 1993.

Tierney LM Jr, McPhee SJ, Papadakis MA (eds). *Current Medical Diagnosis and Treatment.* 35th ed. Stamford, CT: Appleton & Lange; 1996.

Internal Medicine: Cardiology
Questions

Richard E. Murphy, PA-C

DIRECTIONS (Questions 1 through 57): Each of the numbered items or incomplete statements in this section is followed by answers or by completions of the statement. Select the ONE lettered answer or completion that is BEST in each case.

Questions 1 through 57

1. Severe congestive heart failure (CHF) is characterized by

   (A) S4 gallop and jugular venous distension
   (B) low pulmonary capillary wedge pressure
   (C) S3 gallop and jugular venous distension
   (D) generalized vasodilatation
   (E) splenomegaly

2. The mechanism of action of calcium-channel blockers in the treatment of angina pectoris is

   (A) reduction of the excitation-contraction-coupling mechanism responsible for myocardial and smooth-muscle contraction
   (B) inhibition of the binding of circulating catecholamines to beta-adrenergic receptors
   (C) increase in calcium extrusion from myocardial cells
   (D) increase of diastolic filling of the left ventricle
   (E) increase in the oxygen-binding capacity of hemoglobin

3. The first pharmacological choice in the treatment of supraventricular tachycardia is

   (A) lidocaine
   (B) verapamil
   (C) digoxin
   (D) quinidine
   (E) adenosine

4. A 40-year-old male presents with a complaint of severe anterior chest pain. His examination demonstrates a blood pressure of 122/80, a loud friction rub, and diffuse ST segment elevation in all leads except for VR and V1. The most likely diagnosis is

   (A) acute myocardial infarction (MI)
   (B) rupture of the thoracic aorta
   (C) acute pericarditis
   (D) cardiac tamponade
   (E) aortic dissection

5. In atrial flutter, the following electrocardiogram changes will be present EXCEPT

   (A) atrial rate of 280 to 320 per minute
   (B) atrial rate of 150 per minute
   (C) atrial waves resembling a sawtooth pattern
   (D) 2:1 or 3:1 atrial-to-ventricular (A–V) conduction ratio
   (E) can be confused with a nodal tachycardia

6. A ventricular wall aneurysm may be caused by

   (A) diabetes
   (B) myocardial infarction (MI)
   (C) congenital malformation
   (D) high-fat diet
   (E) recurring ventricular tachycardia

7. The overall reported operative mortality rate for elective coronary bypass is

   (A) <1%
   (B) 1% to 3%
   (C) 3% to 10%
   (D) 10% to 20%
   (E) >20%

8. The most common symptom in coronary heart disease is

   (A) palpitations
   (B) claudication
   (C) shortness of breath
   (D) jaw numbness
   (E) angina pectoris

9. Aortic stenosis may present with the following signs and symptoms EXCEPT

   (A) angina
   (B) congestive heart failure (CHF)
   (C) Quincke's pulsation
   (D) systolic murmur
   (E) decreased carotid upstroke

10. Esmolol is indicated for

    (A) impending renal failure
    (B) congestive heart failure (CHF)
    (C) treatment of atrial fibrillation with slow ventricular response
    (D) control of supraventricular tachycardia and hypertension
    (E) augmentation of blood pressure

11. The following is the MOST common primary cardiac neoplasm

    (A) sarcoma
    (B) lymphoma

   (C) oat cell
   (D) left atrial myoma
   (E) myxoma

12. In acute myocardial infarction (MI), tissue plasminogen activator (t-PA) should be administered within

    (A) 4 to 6 hours after the onset of pain
    (B) 12 hours after the onset of pain
    (C) 24 hours after the onset of pain
    (D) 36 hours after the onset of pain
    (E) 48 hours after the onset of pain

13. The possible major complication of tissue plasminogen activator (t-PA) therapy is

    (A) renal failure
    (B) hemorrhage
    (C) coronary artery spasm
    (D) respiratory distress syndrome
    (E) hepatic failure

14. In a patient with a history of thromboembolism, atrial fibrillation, and diastolic murmur, the most likely diagnosis is

    (A) atrial septal defect
    (B) mitral regurgitation
    (C) aortic insufficiency
    (D) aortic stenosis
    (E) mitral stenosis

15. The most common cause of mitral valvular disease is

    (A) endocarditis
    (B) coronary heart disease
    (C) rheumatic fever
    (D) trauma
    (E) congenital malformation

16. The placement of a permanent cardiac pacemaker is indicated in the following situations EXCEPT

    (A) Mobitz type I atrioventricular (AV) block
    (B) Mobitz type II AV block
    (C) complete heart block

(D) sick sinus syndrome

(E) Stokes-Adams attacks

17. An inferior wall myocardial infarction (MI) is suggested by Q waves in leads

(A) II, III, aVF

(B) I, II, III

(C) V1–V3

(D) V4–V6

(E) I and aVR

18. The MOST common complaint of a patient presenting with an acute aortic dissection is

(A) claudication

(B) severe back pain

(C) angina

(D) palpitations

(E) shortness of breath

19. A 61-year-old male presents to the emergency department with an evolving acute myocardial infarction (MI), including stable vital signs, unrelenting chest pain for 10 hours, and ST elevations in the inferior leads. Immediate therapy should include

(A) dopamine

(B) insertion of an intra-aortic balloon

(C) oxygen and sublingual nitroglycerin

(D) insertion of a Swan–Ganz catheter

(E) t-PA

20. The earliest symptom of left-sided heart failure is

(A) orthopnea

(B) pedal edema

(C) paroxysmal nocturnal dyspnea

(D) dyspnea on exertion (DOE)

(E) fatigue

21. Ventricular end-diastolic volume reflects

(A) cardiac output

(B) preload

(C) afterload

(D) atrial contractility

(E) peripheral vascular resistance

22. The MOST likely diagnosis in a 71-year-old patient presenting with anorexia, nausea, vomiting, cardiac arrhythmias, and yellow vision is

(A) Alzheimer's disease

(B) brain tumor

(C) cocaine use

(D) procainamide toxicity

(E) digoxin toxicity

23. An absolute contraindication to thrombolytic therapy in an acute myocardial infarction (MI) is

(A) aspirin use

(B) allergy to shellfish

(C) a history of previous coronary artery bypass 10 years before

(D) a history of severe gastrointestinal bleeding

(E) a previous MI 10 years before

24. Atrial premature contractions

(A) can be seen in 60% of normal adults

(B) are frequently symptomatic

(C) usually herald ventricular arrhythmias

(D) must always be treated with medications

(E) do not reset the sinus node

25. The MOST effective treatment of atrial flutter is

(A) adenosine

(B) direct-current (DC) cardioversion

(C) digoxin

(D) quinidine sulfate

(E) propranolol

26. The MOST frequent problem with implantable automatic defibrillators is

(A) failure to defibrillate

(B) failure to pace appropriately

(C) inappropriate discharge in the absence of sustained ventricular arrhythmias

(D) chronic pain in the operative site

(E) instigation of premature ventricular contractions

27. In a witnessed cardiac arrest where ventricular fibrillation is noted on the monitor/defibrillator, the initial treatment is

    (A) precordial thump
    (B) lidocaine via central venous line
    (C) defibrillation up to three times, if necessary, beginning with 200 J
    (D) epinephrine 10 mg IV push
    (E) endotracheal intubation

28. In the presence of pulseless electrical activity (electromechanical dissociation), the following is recommended as a first-choice therapy

    (A) epinephrine at 1 mg IV every 3 to 5 minutes
    (B) atropine at 1 mg IV every 5 minutes
    (C) dopamine at 10 µg/kg/minute
    (D) isoproterenol at 1 µg/minute
    (E) epinephrine infusion at 1 µg/minute

29. Patients with Wolff–Parkinson–White (WPW) syndrome

    (A) require placement of a permanent pacemaker
    (B) do not have antegrade conduction of the atrioventricular (AV) system
    (C) are always treated with digoxin, verapamil, or beta-blockers
    (D) will have a prolonged P-R interval
    (E) will have a slurred upstroke of the QRS complex

30. All of the following are risk factors for coronary heart disease EXCEPT

    (A) high-density lipid (HDL) cholesterol ≥60 mg/dL
    (B) male ≥45 years of age or female ≥55 years of age
    (C) family history of coronary heart disease
    (D) cigarette smoking
    (E) HDL cholesterol ≤35 mg/dL

31. Reduction of cholesterol and low-density lipid (LDL) cholesterol levels is associated with

    (A) pancreatitis
    (B) increase in weight
    (C) elevation of high-density lipid (HDL) cholesterol levels
    (D) reduction of risk for cardiovascular disease
    (E) osteoporosis

32. A 55-year-old female with a history of hypertension presents to your office with exertion-induced jaw pain, nausea, and left shoulder pain of 1 hour in duration. The 12-lead ECG is normal. The most appropriate course of action is

    (A) prescribe H_2 blockers and observe
    (B) schedule the patient for an exercise stress test for the following day
    (C) repeat the ECG in 6 hours
    (D) obtain a barium swallow
    (E) admit the patient to the hospital to rule out a myocardial infarction (MI)

33. The MOST definitive test in the diagnosis of coronary heart disease is

    (A) exercise electrocardiography
    (B) dipyridamole thallium stress test
    (C) two-dimensional echocardiography
    (D) radionucleide ventriculography
    (E) coronary arteriography

34. Thromboembolism can be a complication of

    (A) aortic stenosis
    (B) aortic insufficiency
    (C) pulmonic stenosis
    (D) mitral stenosis
    (E) mitral valve prolapse

35. Hyperkalemia is manifested on the ECG by

    (A) U waves
    (B) prolonged P-R interval
    (C) tall, peaked T waves
    (D) prolonged Q-T interval
    (E) ST segment depression

36. Verapamil is contraindicated in

    (A) Wolff–Parkinson–White syndrome
    (B) atrial fibrillation
    (C) supraventricular tachycardia
    (D) the presence of a permanent pacemaker
    (E) paroxysmal atrial tachycardia

37. Digitalis toxicity is potentiated by

    (A) myocardial infarction
    (B) hypokalemia, renal impairment, quinidine
    (C) hyperkalemia
    (D) hypermagnesemia
    (E) hyperthyroidism

38. Percutaneous transluminal coronary angioplasty (PTCA) is

    (A) contraindicated in acute myocardial infarction
    (B) routinely performed for multivessel coronary heart disease
    (C) routinely successful in more than 90% of patients
    (D) without potential complications
    (E) routinely performed in any hospital emergency department

39. Most deaths following a myocardial infarction are the result of

    (A) arrhythmias
    (B) ventricular rupture
    (C) multisystem failure
    (D) stroke
    (E) respiratory arrest

40. Angiotensin-converting-enzyme (ACE) inhibitors

    (A) may reduce preload and afterload
    (B) may increase preload and decrease afterload
    (C) may decrease preload and increase afterload
    (D) have no effect on preload
    (E) have no effect on afterload

41. Which of the following statements concerning hypertension is FALSE?

    (A) A blood pressure of 160/100 mm Hg is considered the upper limit of normal.
    (B) Variations in dietary salt intake influence arterial compliance.
    (C) Hypertension is a consequence of reduced arterial compliance.
    (D) Hypertension is a consequence of increased total peripheral resistance.
    (E) In the United States, more than one half of all persons over 65 years of age are hypertensive.

42. A 6-year-old male presents to your office with a chief complaint of "cold feet" and leg cramps while running. His blood pressure is 140/80 mm Hg. The most likely diagnosis is

    (A) pheochromocytoma
    (B) primary hypertension
    (C) hyperthyroidism
    (D) coarctation of the aorta
    (E) Raynaud's phenomenon

43. A patient who has undergone a mechanical prosthetic mitral valve replacement should have an international normalized ratio (INR) that is

    (A) <1
    (B) 1 to 2
    (C) 2.5 to 3.5
    (D) 3.5 to 4.5
    (E) >4.5

44. A 26-year-old, otherwise healthy, male who suffers a syncopal episode during a basketball game should

    (A) immediately return to normal athletic activity
    (B) have carotid Doppler studies
    (C) undergo cardiac catheterization
    (D) have a 24-hour ambulatory (Holter) electrocardiogram
    (E) undergo head CT scan with contrast

45. The most appropriate approach to the management of an asymptomatic patient with mitral valve prolapse (MVP) is

    (A) cardiac catheterization
    (B) reassurance and follow-up echocardiogram in 2 to 4 years
    (C) digoxin for prevention of atrial fibrillation
    (D) anticoagulation with warfarin
    (E) beta-blocker therapy

46. A 30-year-old female presents with sudden onset of severe shortness of breath and pleuritic chest pain. Her physical examination is remarkable for jugular venous distension, a right pleural friction rub, equal breath sounds with bilateral rales, and a loud second heart sound. The next principal step in diagnosis to rule out a pulmonary embolism (PE) is to obtain

    (A) a pulmonary angiogram
    (B) a ventilation-perfusion (V/Q) scan
    (C) an arterial blood gas from the femoral artery
    (D) a 12-lead electrocardiogram
    (E) an oxygen saturation via pulse oximetry

47. An abdominal bruit in a hypertensive 50-year-old male who is otherwise healthy and asymptomatic may indicate

    (A) an abdominal aortic aneurysm
    (B) an aortic dissection
    (C) renal artery stenosis
    (D) a congenital absence of one kidney
    (E) polycystic kidney disease

48. The MOST common cause of endocarditis in the pediatric population is

    (A) *viridans streptococci*
    (B) *staphylococcus aureus*
    (C) *pseudomonas*
    (D) *pneumococci*
    (E) *enterococci*

49. The most common cause of endocarditis in a 25-year-old IV drug addict is

    (A) *staphylococcus aureus*
    (B) *staphylococcus epidermidis*
    (C) *streptococci*
    (D) *pseudomonas*
    (E) *enterococci*

50. A common complication of the use of a Swan–Ganz catheter is

    (A) pulmonary vein cannulation
    (B) arterial desaturation
    (C) air embolus
    (D) perforation of the left ventricle
    (E) arrhythmias

51. A 25-year-old female is undergoing right heart catheterization for a history of exercise intolerance, systolic murmur, and cardiomegaly. As the Swan–Ganz catheter passes through the right heart, the arterial saturation is noted to be 65% in the superior vena cava (SVC) and 81% in the right atrium. A likely diagnosis is

    (A) pulmonic stenosis
    (B) left-sided vena cava
    (C) atrial septal defect (ASD)
    (D) transposition of the great arteries
    (E) aortic stenosis

52. The MOST common cardiac defect associated with coarctation of the aorta is

    (A) aortic insufficiency
    (B) bicuspid aortic valve
    (C) persistent ductus arteriosus
    (D) ventricular septal defect
    (E) atrial septal defect

53. Deep venous thrombosis (DVT) in the calf of the leg

    (A) is more likely to produce a pulmonary embolus (PE) than a thrombus in the thigh
    (B) is more difficult to diagnose with ultrasound than in the thigh
    (C) always requires complete anticoagulation

(D) will always produce a positive venogram

(E) is less likely to produce a pulmonary embolus than a thrombus in the thigh

54. In pulmonary embolism (PE)

(A) an "abnormal" A-a oxygen gradient is always present

(B) pulmonary arteriography is required for confirmation of diagnosis

(C) neoplasm should be considered

(D) pleuritic chest pain is almost always present

(E) a CT scan should be performed prior to obtaining a V/Q scan

55. The use of heparin in the treatment of strongly suspected pulmonary embolism

(A) should be delayed until diagnosis is confirmed by V/Q scan or pulmonary angiogram

(B) is contraindicated

(C) is considered key to the prevention of additional emboli

(D) should be discontinued with the slightest increase in the platelet count

(E) helps to dissolve the embolus

56. Effects of cocaine on the myocardium include

(A) ventricular septal defect

(B) asymmetrical septal hypertrophy

(C) aneurysm formation

(D) depression of ventricular function and scattered areas of myocardial necrosis

(E) coronary vasodilatation

57. Trifascicular atrioventricular (AV) block

(A) is an indication for permanent pacemaker insertion

(B) will respond to quinidine

(C) is congenitally acquired

(D) will always result in symptoms

(E) is a result of sick sinus syndrome

DIRECTIONS (Questions 58 through 73): Each group of items in this section consists of lettered headings followed by a set of numbered words or phrases. For each numbered word or phrase, select the ONE lettered heading that is most closely associated with it. Each lettered heading may be selected once, more than once, or not at all.

Questions 58 through 61

(A) aortic stenosis

(B) mitral regurgitation

(C) both

(D) neither

58. Pansystolic murmur

59. Radiates to axilla

60. Bicuspid valve

61. Murmur reduced during Valsalva's maneuver

Questions 62 through 65

(A) increases myocardial oxygen supply

(B) decreases myocardial oxygen demand

(C) both

(D) neither

62. Atenolol

63. Diltiazem

64. Nitroglycerin

65. Intra-aortic balloon

Questions 66 through 73

(A) affects serum lipids

(B) affects serum potassium levels

(C) both

(D) neither

66. Captopril

67. Hydrocholorothiazide

68. Diltiazem

69. Furosemide

70. Clonidine

71. Digitalis

72. Lovastatin

73. Kayexalate

DIRECTIONS (Questions 74 through 80): Each of the electrocardiograms in this section is followed by possible interpretations. Select the ONE lettered answer that is BEST in each case.

Questions 74 through 80

74. (A) normal tracing
    (B) sinus bradycardia
    (C) ventricular tachycardia
    (D) old inferior wall infarction
    (E) acute inferior wall infarction

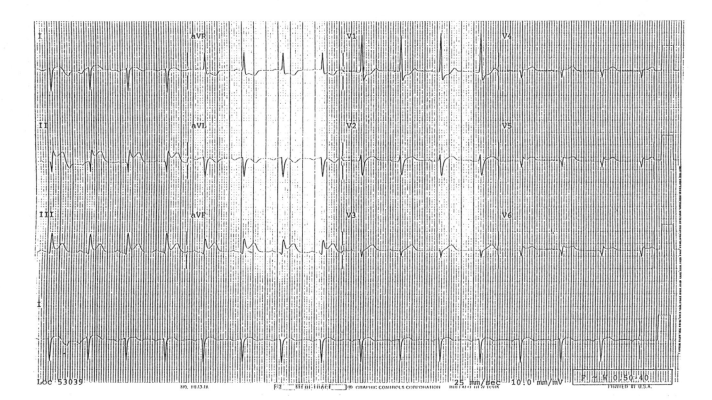

Figure 5–1. Courtesy of New England Medical Center

75. (A) normal tracing

    (B) acute inferior injury with anteroseptal ischemia

    (C) acute anteroseptal infarction

    (D) Wolff–Parkinson–White syndrome

    (E) left ventricular hypertrophy with strain

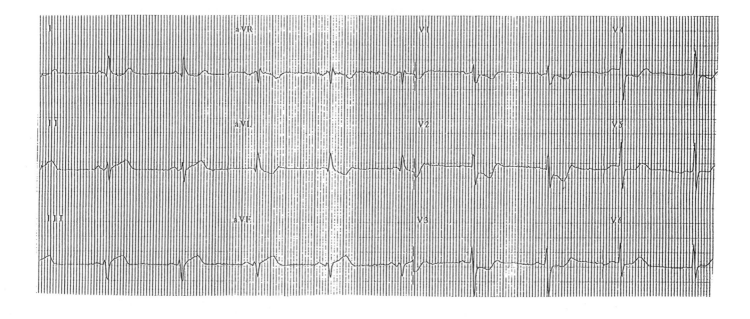

Figure 5–2. Courtesy of New England Medical Center

76. (A) normal tracing

(B) anterolateral wall ischemia

(C) old inferior wall infarction

(D) acute anterolateral wall infarction

(E) nonspecific lateral wall ST changes

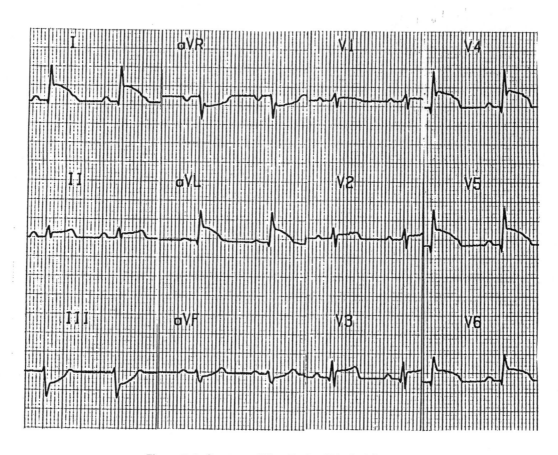

Figure 5–3. Courtesy of New England Medical Center

77. (A) normal tracing
    (B) old lateral wall infarction
    (C) left ventricular hypertrophy
    (D) complete bundle branch block
    (E) nonspecific lateral wall ST changes

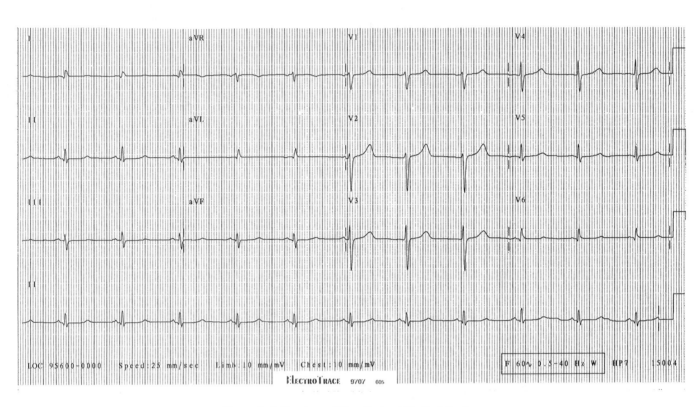

Figure 5–4. Courtesy of New England Medical Center

78. (A) normal tracing
(B) right axis deviation
(C) old inferior wall infarction

(D) acute anterolateral wall infarction
(E) premature atrial contraction

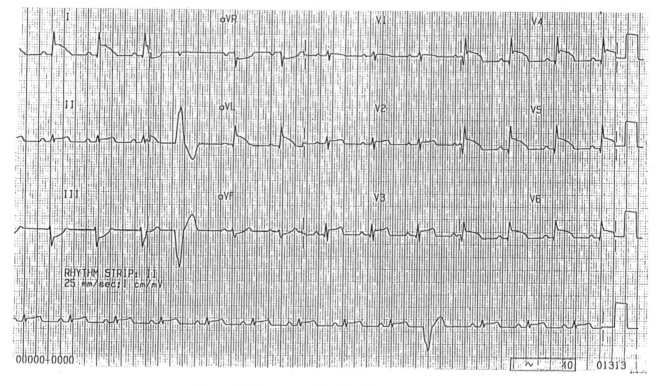

Figure 5–5. Courtesy of New England Medical Center

79. (A) normal tracing

(B) right bundle branch block

(C) sinus arrhythmia

(D) acute inferior wall infarction

(E) Wolff–Parkinson–White syndrome

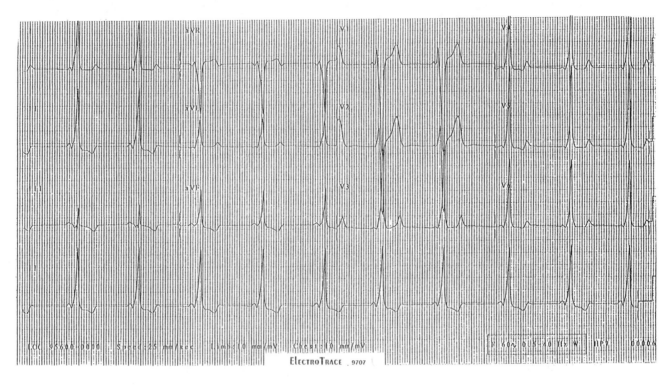

Figure 5–6. Courtesy of New England Medical Center

80. (A) premature atrial contraction (D) complete heart block
     (B) acute lateral wall infarction (E) old inferior wall infarction
     (C) Wolff–Parkinson–White syndrome

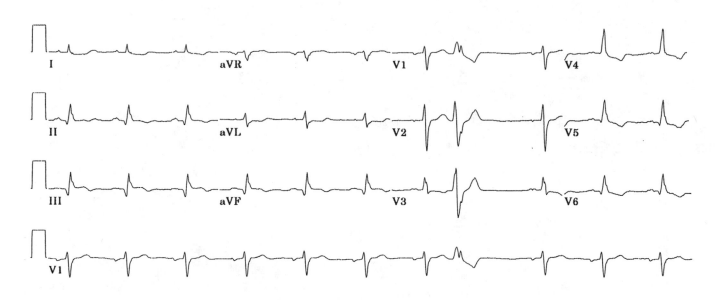

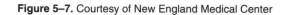

Figure 5–7. Courtesy of New England Medical Center

Answers and Explanations

1. **(C)** CHF is characterized by an S3 gallop on examination. This sound is caused by rapid blood flow into the ventricle during diastole. Jugular venous distension is caused by impedance to right ventricular filling (a result of pulmonary hypertension and high pulmonary capillary wedge pressures). *(Braunwald, p. 455)*

2. **(A)** Calcium-channel blockers are agents that block the transmembrane flux of calcium into cardiac and smooth-muscle cells. This reduces myocardial contractility, slows sinoatrial (SA) and atrioventricular (AV) node conduction, decreases coronary vascular resistance, decreases systemic vascular resistance, and increases coronary artery size. *(Herfindal and Gourley, p. 819)*

3. **(E)** Adenosine is the recommended drug of first choice in supraventricular tachycardia by terminating atrioventricular (AV) nodal reentry through its action of partial or complete AV nodal block. It is thought to act by altering calcium and potassium flux. *(Herfindal and Gourley, pp. 770–793)*

4. **(C)** Acute pericarditis is due to inflammation of the pericardium. It is manifested by chest pain, pericardial friction rub, and frequently diffuse electrocardiographic changes. Rupture of the aorta would result in profound hypotension or sudden death. Back pain is classically noted in aortic dissection, and cardiac tamponade classically presents with hypotension, jugular venous distension, and muffled heart sounds. Although an acute myocardial infarction may produce anterior chest pain and a pericardial friction rub (Dressler syndrome), the electrocardiographic changes are usually not diffuse. Therefore, myocardial infarction should be ruled out in this scenario. *(Braunwald, pp. 1481–1499)*

5. **(B)** The atrial rate in atrial flutter is classically 250 to 350/minute. Although a 1:1 A–V conduction is possible, resulting in a ventricular rate of almost 300/minute, the atrioventricular node will usually only conduct one half or one third (1:2 or 1:3 conduction, respectively) of the atrial impulses, dropping the ventricular response to either 150/minute or 100/minute. The atrial flutter waves produce a sawtooth pattern on the ECG in some leads. *(Braunwald, pp. 652–654)*

6. **(B)** Most ventricular wall aneurysms are caused by a myocardial infarction, although traumatic causes have been reported. The aneurysm is most likely to occur in the left ventricle. Ventricular tachycardia, although not a cause of the aneurysm, may result from scarring in the aneurysm. *(Braunwald, pp. 228, 1256–1257)*

7. **(B)** Although there have been reports of mortality rates as low as .2% to .3%, most multicenter trials report rates between 1.3% and 2.6% for routine elective coronary artery bypass procedures. *(Braunwald, p. 1319)*

8. **(E)** Chest pain or angina, is the most common presenting complaint of patients with coronary heart disease. Its classic descriptions, such as "vise-like," "heavy or squeezing," or "constricting" should raise a clinician's suspicion for an ischemic etiology. *(Braunwald, pp. 1290–1292)*

9. **(C)** Quincke's sign or pulsation can be seen by pressing a glass slide on the patient's lip or by transilluminating the fingertips. These visible pulsations are frequently seen in aortic insufficiency, in which there is a very wide pulse pressure caused by the incompetent aortic valve. However, aortic stenosis restricts left ventricular outflow, resulting in ventricular overload, decreased carotid pulse upstroke, poor coronary filling, and a loud systolic murmur. *(Braunwald, pp. 1049–1050)*

10. **(D)** Esmolol is a cardioselective beta-blocker that is indicated for the short-term treatment of supraventricular tachycardia and severe hypertension. *(Herfindal and Gourley, pp. 785–786)*

11. **(E)** Between 30% and 50% of primary cardiac tumors are myxomas. Approximately 75% of these are benign histologically, but can cause life-threatening consequences as they may embolize or cause significant cardiac dysfunction. *(Reynen, pp. 1610–1617; Braunwald, pp. 1467–1472)*

12. **(A)** The greatest benefit of thrombolytic therapy in myocardial infarction can be derived when it is administered in less than 4 to 6 hours after the onset of pain. Better results are seen when administered in less than 1 to 2 hours after pain onset. *(Braunwald, pp. 1215–1218; Herfindal and Gourley, pp. 846–850)*

13. **(B)** Severe, life-threatening hemorrhage is the most severe complication of t-PA use. A known history of gastrointestinal bleeding or previous cerebral hemorrhage is an absolute contraindication for its use. *(Herfindal and Gourley, pp. 1219–1220)*

14. **(E)** Mitral stenosis may produce a constellation of signs and symptoms, but dyspnea,

thromboembolism, and atrial fibrillation are common presenting problems. On physical examination a diastolic murmur is classically found; an opening snap may also be heard. *(Braunwald, pp. 1007–1012)*

15. **(C)** Rheumatic fever is the predominant cause of mitral stenosis. With the advent of antibiotics the incidence of rheumatic fever is lower in the United States than in developing nations. *(Braunwald, p. 1769)*

16. **(A)** Mobitz Type I AV second-degree heart block (also called Wenckebach) is a more benign arrhythmia and less likely to progress to complete heart block than other heart blocks. Mobitz type II, complete heart block, sick sinus syndrome, and Stokes–Adams attacks usually require the insertion of a permanent pacemaker. *(Braunwald, pp. 687–693)*

17. **(A)** Q waves usually signify infarcted myocardium. The presence of Q waves in leads II, III, aVF suggests an inferior wall infarction. *(Braunwald, pp, 127–135)*

18. **(B)** In over 90% of cases of aortic dissection, severe back pain was the presenting complaint. Its onset is sudden and dramatic. The diagnosis and treatment of aortic dissection require rapid attention to prevent death. *(Braunwald, pp. 1554–1563)*

19. **(C)** Maximizing oxygenation of the myocardium and relief of pain are primary objectives in the immediate management of this patient. Oxygen and sublingual nitroglycerin are indicated in this patient. Because of the long interval from the onset of pain, t-PA may have only questionable benefit. The patient is presently hemodynamically stable and does not require invasive interventions such as the intra-aortic balloon or Swan–Ganz catheterization. Dopamine may increase myocardial oxygen demands. *(Braunwald, pp. 1226–1232)*

20. **(D)** The earliest symptom of left-side heart failure is exertional dyspnea. The degree of exertion required to produce the dyspnea is key to the diagnosis of heart failure in a pa-

tient. Dyspnea that is produced by climbing stairs or even walking should be considered significant in elderly patients. Orthopnea and paroxysmal nocturnal dyspnea may develop later. Although pedal edema may be seen in left-side failure, it is more likely to occur in right-side failure. Fatigue is a rather nonspecific complaint and may be caused by a wide variety of ailments. (Braunwald, pp. 445–453)

21. **(B)** Preload is a direct reflection of the ventricular end-diastolic volume. As the preload increases, so does the ventricular volume just prior to ventricular contraction. Preload is affected by total blood volume, distribution of blood volume, and atrial contraction. (Braunwald, pp. 376–379)

22. **(E)** Digoxin toxicity may present with a myriad of signs and symptoms, but anorexia, nausea, vomiting, arrhythmias, and changes in visual perception are the most common. Toxicity may result in almost any single or combination of arrhythmia, and digoxin toxicity should be considered in almost any arrhythmia evaluation. (Braunwald, pp. 484, 499–501)

23. **(D)** Thrombolytic therapy is absolutely contraindicated in patients with a history of severe gastrointestinal bleeding, cerebral hemorrhage, uncontrolled hypertension, or recent head trauma. (Braunwald, pp. 1219, 1597)

24. **(A)** Atrial premature contractions (APCs) in the asymptomatic patient do not require therapy. APCs are seen in as much as 60% of normal adults. Offending causes, such as caffeine, should be identified and eliminated in patients with symptoms. When APCs precipitate other arrhythmias, treatment with calcium-channel blockers, beta-blockers, or digitalis should be considered. (Braunwald, pp. 650–652)

25. **(B)** DC cardioversion is the most commonly employed treatment for atrial flutter because it usually requires low energy levels (<50 J) to convert to normal sinus rhythm. Rapid atrial pacing, calcium-channel blockers, beta-blockers, or digitalis may be used if DC cardioversion fails. (Braunwald, p. 654)

26. **(C)** Automatic implantable defibrillators are sophisticated devices that can sense and terminate ventricular arrhythmias. These devices may inappropriately discharge in the presence of a nonventricular arrhythmia, such as sinus or supraventricular tachycardia. However, these devices have been proven effective in the treatment of recurrent ventricular tachycardia. (Braunwald, p. 734)

27. **(C)** In a witnessed cardiac arrest where a cardiac monitor/defibrillator is immediately available, defibrillation up to three times beginning with 200 J, then 200 to 300 J, and finally with 360 J for persistent ventricular fibrillation or tachycardia should be performed. A precordial thump may be used if no defibrillator is immediately available. (JAMA 1992; 268: pp. 2171–2302)

28. **(A)** An epinephrine bolus of 1 mg IV every 3 to 5 minutes is recommended as definitely helpful for pulseless electrical activity. Atropine is considered to be possibly helpful in cardiac arrest but is not a first-line choice. (JAMA 1992; 268: pp. 2171–2302)

29. **(E)** The classic electrocardiographic finding in Wolff–Parkinson–White syndrome is the "delta wave" or a slurred upsloping of the QRS complex. Verapamil and beta-blockers slow AV conduction at the AV node, but do not block the WPW accessory pathways. Digitalis has variable effects. Class IA agents, such as quinidine, and Class IC agents, such as flecainide, may slow conduction through the accessory pathway. (Braunwald, pp. 655–675)

30. **(A)** A high-density lipid cholesterol over 60 mg/dL may be protective and is considered a negative risk factor. Male gender, positive family history, tobacco use, and a low HDL cholesterol level are considered cardiac risk factors. (Ewald and McKenzie, pp. 481–483)

31. **(D)** The reduction of cholesterol and LDL cholesterol is associated with the reduction of risk for atherosclerosis and heart disease. *(Ewald and McKenzie, pp. 484–485)*

32. **(E)** Although ECG changes are highly sensitive indicators for myocardial ischemia, in the case of a nondiagnostic ECG and a strongly suggestive history for a cardiac etiology for the chest pain, continued in-hospital observation and serial ECGs and cardiac isoenzyme determinations should be performed to rule out a myocardial infarction. *(Braunwald, pp. 1202–1210)*

33. **(E)** Coronary arteriography remains the most definitive diagnostic test for coronary heart disease. The identification of the location and quantification of severity of coronary stenosis is essential in determining medical versus interventional therapy for the patient. *(Braunwald, p. 177)*

34. **(D)** Because of blood stasis in the left atrium caused by the restriction of blood flow across the stenotic mitral valve, there is a tendency for atrial clot to form, and systemic embolism can occur. Peripheral embolism may be the first symptom of mitral stenosis. Eighty percent of patients with mitral stenosis who have embolic events will have atrial fibrillation that potentiate atrial thrombus formation. *(Braunwald, p. 1010)*

35. **(C)** Potassium concentrations can affect T wave morphology in the ECG. Tall, peaked T waves may be seen when serum potassium concentrations exceed 5.7 mEq/L. U waves can be seen when potassium concentrations drop below 3.0 mEq/L. *(Braunwald, pp. 141–142)*

36. **(A)** Verapamil interferes with conduction through the atrioventricular (AV) node but may decrease the accessory pathway antegrade refractory period in conditions such as Wolff–Parkinson–White (WPW) syndrome. Verapamil is contraindicated in WPW, as it may cause ventricular tachycardia or fibrillation. *(Herfindal and Gourley, pp. 790–791)*

37. **(B)** Hypokalemia may increase the myocardial uptake of digoxin. Renal dysfunction decreases the volume of distribution and elimination of digoxin. Quinidine reduces the systemic clearance of digoxin, therefore increasing serum concentrations and potentiating toxicity. *(Herfindal and Gourley, pp. 743–745)*

38. **(C)** The angiographic success rate of PTCA in studies performed in 1990–1991 is in excess of 90%. PTCA has resulted in substantial relief of symptoms in 88% of patients. PTCA is frequently utilized in postinfarction angina. *(Braunwald, p. 1368)*

39. **(A)** Almost 50% of deaths following myocardial infarction occur within the first hour and are the result of arrhythmias. *(Braunwald, p. 1184)*

40. **(A)** ACE inhibitors affect both central and peripheral activity of the central nervous system and have a vasorelaxant effect. ACE inhibitors will reduce afterload and preload through a number of different, but interrelated, mechanisms. *(Herfindal and Gourley, pp. 739–741)*

41. **(A)** The upper limit of a normal blood pressure in an adult is 140 mm Hg (systolic) and 90 mm Hg (diastolic). *(Izzo and Black, pp. 207–209)*

42. **(D)** Upper-extremity hypertension and diminished or absent pulses in the lower extremities are classic features of coarctation of the aorta, and lower-extremity complaints are common presenting issues in children. *(Braunwald, p. 841)*

43. **(C)** Unless contraindicated by a history of hemorrhagic complications or allergy to warfarin (Coumadin), most patients who undergo mitral valve replacement with a mechanical prosthesis will require anticoagulation. The INR should be maintained between 2.5 and 3.5 and monitored on a regular basis and the dosage of warfarin adjusted accordingly. Use of the INR is preferred because of variability in thromboplastin reagents used to determine the prothrombin time in labora-

tories. The INR results in a standardization of warfarin anticoagulation. *(Chest, p. 453S)*

44. **(D)** A resting, 12-lead ECG may not detect the bradycardic or tachycardic arrhythmias that may precipitate a syncopal episode. Ambulatory monitoring for 24 hours is recommended to rule out life-threatening arrhythmias. In the absence of symptoms or ECG evidence of myocardial ischemia, cardiac catheterization is not indicated. *(Braunwald, pp. 863–875)*

45. **(B)** Because 15% of patients with mitral valve prolapse may develop progressive mitral regurgitation, regular follow-up examinations and echocardiography are indicated. In the absence of any atrial or ventricular arrhythmias, digoxin and beta-blockers are not indicated. Anticoagulation is not required for a patient in normal sinus rhythm, and cardiac catheterization not indicated in an asymptomatic patient. *(Braunwald, pp. 1029–1032)*

46. **(B)** There are some limitations to the use of a ventilation-perfusion (V/Q) scan in the diagnosis of pulmonary embolism. However, the V/Q scan remains the principal diagnostic test. Because pulmonary angiography is an invasive procedure that is not without potential complications, it should be used in cases where overwhelming clinical evidence for PE exists in the presence of a normal or low suspicion V/Q scan, or if the patient's condition deteriorates following institution of conventional therapy for PE and mechanical intervention is being considered. Although an arterial blood gas may be necessary to rule out causes other than PE, studies have shown that there is frequently no difference in the average pO$_2$ of PE and non-PE patients when confirmed at angiography. *(Braunwald, pp. 1587–1592)*

47. **(C)** Renovascular hypertension is the most common secondary form of hypertension; it is not easily recognizable, but every patient with hypertension should be carefully examined for the presence of an abdominal bruit

that might signify the presence of renal artery stenosis. Atherosclerotic disease is more likely to affect elderly males, and fibroplastic disease is more common in younger females. *(Braunwald, pp. 825–827)*

48. **(A)** *Viridans streptococci,* or group D streptococci, cause 40% to 50% of cases of endocarditis in the pediatric population. *S. aureus* cases are increasing and account for 25% of cases. *(Braunwald, pp. 1080–1097)*

49. **(A)** In the parenteral drug user population, endocarditis is most likely to be caused by staphylococci (60%). *S. aureus* accounts for 99% of all staphylococci organisms. *(Braunwald, pp. 1080–1097)*

50. **(E)** Ventricular arrhythmias, such as PVCs, or even ventricular tachycardia, as well as partial or complete heart block can be caused by the movement of the Swan–Ganz catheter through the right ventricle during insertion. *(Braunwald, p. 184)*

51. **(C)** The criteria for detection of a left-to-right intracardiac shunt is a "step-up" in arterial saturation of more than 7% from the SVC to the right atrium. The presence of a systolic murmur is common in an ASD, as the increase in right heart blood flow from the left-to-right shunt causes turbulent blood flow across the right ventricular outflow track resulting in a murmur of relative pulmonic stenosis. *(Braunwald, pp. 196–197)*

52. **(B)** A bicuspid aortic valve is the most common cardiac defect associated with coarctation of the aorta. *(Braunwald, p. 965)*

53. **(E)** There is a higher risk of pulmonary embolism when deep venous thrombosis is located proximal to the calf than in the calf. The risk of PE is approximately 30% when deep venous thrombosis remains in the calf veins. Ultrasonography is a reliable diagnostic tool for DVT in all leg veins. Venography may be nondiagnostic in the presence of clot, as the contrast may not be able to reach the deep leg veins. *(Braunwald, p. 1584)*

54. **(C)** Malignancy is a common risk factor for the creation of a hypercoaguable state. In patients with bilateral limb deep venous thrombosis (DVT) or DVT without explainable cause (ie, use of oral contraceptives, infection, or trauma), occult cancer should be ruled out. Arteriography is required only if PE is strongly suspected in the presence of a normal V/Q scan or if other lung abnormalities, such as asthma, previous thoracic surgery, or a prior PE episode, obscure the diagnosis. A normal A-a oxygen gradient does not discount the diagnosis of PE. *(Braunwald, pp. 1582–1586)*

55. **(C)** In cases of highly suspected pulmonary embolism where no history of gastrointestinal (GI) bleeding coagulopathy exists, treatment with heparin should be started pending the results of diagnostic tests. Heparin will serve only to prevent formation of additional clots and does not dissolve existing clots. Mild thrombocytopenia may occur with heparin use. *(Braunwald, pp. 1592–1596)*

56. **(D)** Cocaine has multiple effects on the myocardium, most notably transient depression of ventricular function, scattered areas of myocardial necrosis and myocarditis, and fibrosis. Cocaine also may cause coronary vasoconstriction. *(Braunwald, p. 1445)*

57. **(A)** Trifascicular block, regardless of symptoms, is an indication for permanent pacemaker placement. *(Braunwald, pp. 707–709)*

58. **(B)** A pansystolic murmur is heard in mitral regurgitation and begins immediately after S1 and continues through systole. The quality of the murmur is blowing, high pitched, and of constant intensity. The murmur of aortic stenosis is crescendo–decrescendo and begins after the onset of S1 and ends before A2. *(Braunwald, pp. 35–39, 1022–1024, 1040–1041)*

59. **(B)** The murmur of mitral regurgitation is best heard at the apex, but can radiate to the axilla and occasionally the base of the heart. The murmur of aortic stenosis is best heard at the base of the heart, but can radiate to the neck and the apex. *(Braunwald, pp. 35–39, 1022–1024, 1040–1041)*

60. **(A)** Although the mitral valve only has two leaflets, it does not per se cause mitral regurgitation. The aortic valve, normally trileaflet in shape, may become stenotic in the case of a congenitally abnormal bileaflet or bicuspid valve. A bicuspid aortic valve causes turbulent flow, resulting in fibrosis and narrowing of the aortic valve. *(Braunwald, pp. 1035–1039)*

61. **(C)** There is a decline in systemic venous return to the heart with Valsalva's maneuver. This causes decreased filling of both sides of the heart, which in turn, causes a reduction in stroke volume and systemic blood pressure. These effects reduce the turbulent blood flows across the stenotic aortic valve and regurgitant mitral valve, therefore diminishing the intensity of the murmurs of aortic stenosis and mitral regurgitation. *(Braunwald, p. 47)*

62. **(B)** Atenolol is a beta-blocker that decreases heart rate and myocardial contractility, thereby decreasing oxygen consumption. *(Braunwald, pp. 1305–1307)*

63. **(C)** Diltiazem, a calcium-channel blocker, relaxes smooth muscle, which causes coronary vasodilation that increases myocardial oxygen supply. Diltiazem will also lower systemic blood pressure, which decreases myocardial oxygen demand. *(Braunwald, pp. 1308–1311)*

64. **(C)** Nitroglycerin is a coronary vasodilator that increases myocardial oxygen supply. Its vasodilator effects also are seen in the venous circulation. By reducing both preload and afterload, it decreases myocardial oxygen consumption and increases myocardial oxygen supply. *(Braunwald, pp. 1302–1304)*

65. **(C)** The intra-aortic balloon is a mechanical device that increases coronary artery perfusion by increasing blood pressure during diastole. It also serves to decrease afterload by rapid deflation just before ventricular systole, thereby decreasing myocardial workload and oxygen consumption. *(Braunwald, pp. 535–536)*

66. **(B)** Captopril is an angiotensin-converting enzyme (ACE) inhibitor. It blocks the formation of angiotensin II, which stimulates aldosterone production. By decreasing aldosterone production, serum potassium levels may increase. Angiotensin-converting enzyme inhibitors should be used cautiously with potassium-sparing diuretics because of the potential for hyperkalemia. (*Braunwald, pp. 1933, 1935*)

67. **(C)** Hydrochlorothiazide is a diuretic and can cause an elevation of low-density lipoprotein cholesterol and a fall in serum potassium. Patients with hypokalemia may experience muscle weakness, polyuria, leg cramps, or increased ventricular ectopy. (*Braunwald, pp. 476–478*)

68. **(D)** Diltiazem is a calcium-channel blocker. It is used in the treatment of angina and hypertension. Calcium-channel agents cause a relaxation of the vascular smooth muscles in the coronaries and systemic arterial beds. Side effects include headache, dizziness, flushing, hypotension, leg edema, and gastrointestinal complaints. (*Braunwald, pp. 616–618, 1931*)

69. **(B)** Furosemide is a potent loop diuretic that inhibits the import of sodium and potassium and causes increases in K^+ and H^+ secretion. (*Braunwald, pp. 476–477, 1236*)

70. **(D)** Clonidine is an alpha-receptor agonist used in the treatment of hypertension. It does not affect serum potassium or serum lipid levels. Some side effects include dry mouth and drowsiness. (*Braunwald, pp. 852, 1932*)

71. **(D)** Although patient sensitivity to digitalis may be adversely affected by electrolyte alterations, digitalis does not directly affect the serum potassium level or have any effect on serum lipid levels. Careful monitoring of digitalis blood levels and electrolytes is imperative to avoid untoward effects and toxicity. (*Braunwald, pp. 481–484*)

72. **(A)** Lovastatin will decrease normal and elevated low-density lipoprotein (LDL) choles-

terol levels and may increase high-density lipoprotein (HDL) cholesterol concentrations. There is no effect on serum potassium. (*Braunwald, pp. 1130, 1934*)

73. **(B)** Kayexalate, a cationic–anionic exchange resin, is an agent used for the treatment of hyperkalemia. When given orally or rectally with sorbitol, it causes potassium to bind with itself by exchange with sodium in the gastrointestinal tract. Its effect is slow and should not be considered an acute treatment for life-threatening arrhythmias. It has no effect on lipid levels. (*Herfindal and Gourley, pp. 137–138*)

74. **(E)** This tracing is indicative of an acute inferior wall myocardial infarction illustrated by the ST elevations in II, III, aVF. There also is evidence of anterolateral wall infarction by ST segment elevation in leads V2–V6. (*Braunwald, pp. 111–140*)

75. **(B)** An acute inferior wall infarction is seen in this tracing with ST elevations in II, III, aVF. This tracing also demonstrates anteroseptal ischemia as evidenced by ST segment depression in V1–V5. (*Braunwald, pp. 111–140*)

76. **(D)** Acute anterolateral wall infarction can be seen in this tracing through the marked ST segment elevations in leads I, aVL, V3–V6. There also are reciprocal changes in III and aVR. (*Braunwald, pp. 111–140*)

77. **(E)** Although there is an appearance of a normal tracing, careful review demonstrates T wave flattening in lateral wall leads aVL and V6. Careful clinical correlation is warranted in situations where there are nonspecific ECG changes and historical issues that raise clinical suspicion for a cardiac etiology. (*Braunwald, pp. 111–140*)

78. **(D)** There are several marked abnormalities in this tracing, but the only applicable answer is that of an acute anterolateral wall infarction with marked ST segment elevation in I, aVL, and V4–V6. There is evidence of infe-

rior ischemia and a premature ventricular contraction. *(Braunwald, pp. 111–140)*

79. **(E)** Delta waves can be seen in almost all leads in this tracing. The short PR interval and slurred upstroke of the R wave are classically seen in Wolff–Parkinson–White syndrome. There also is evidence of early repolarization in leads V1 and V2. *(Braunwald, pp. 111–147, 150, 667–669)*

80. **(E)** Q waves in leads II, III, aVF indicate an old inferior wall infarction. There also is a premature ventricular contraction, intraventricular conduction delay, and nonspecific ST–T wave changes throughout. *(Braunwald, pp. 111–140)*

REFERENCES

Braunwald E (ed). *Heart Disease: A Textbook of Cardiovascular Medicine,* 5th ed. Philadelphia: Saunders; 1996.

Chest 1992;102(suppl): 453S.

Emergency Cardiac Care Committee and Subcommittees, American Heart Association. *JAMA* 1992; 268: 2171–2302.

Ewald G, McKenzie C (eds). *Manual of Medical Therapeutics,* 28th ed. Boston: Little, Brown; 1995.

Herfindal E, Gourley D (eds). *Textbook of Therapeutics: Drug and Disease Management,* 6th ed. Philadelphia: Williams & Wilkins; 1996.

Izzo J, Black H (eds). *Hypertension Primer.* Dallas: American Heart Association; 1993.

Reynen K. *N Engl J Med* 1995; 333(24): 1610–1617.

Internal Medicine: Endocrinology
Questions

Peter Juergensen, BS, PA-C

DIRECTIONS (Questions 1 through 11): Each group of items in this section consists of lettered headings followed by a set of numbered words or phrases. For each numbered word or phrase, select the ONE lettered heading that is most closely associated with it. Each lettered heading may be selected once, more than once, or not at all.

Questions 1 through 4

Match the following hormones with the sites where they are produced.

    (A) posterior pituitary
    (B) anterior pituitary
    (C) both
    (D) neither

1. Luteinizing hormone (LH) and follicle-stimulating hormone (FSH)

2. Thyroid-stimulating hormone (TSH) and adrenocorticotropic hormone (ACTH)

3. Antidiuretic hormone (ADH) and thyroid-stimulating hormone (TSH)

4. Corticotropin-releasing factor (CRF) and melanocyte-stimulating hormone (MSH)

Questions 5 through 7

Match the substance secreted by this section of the adrenal gland.

    (A) aldosterone
    (B) cortisol
    (C) both
    (D) neither

5. Zona glomerulosa

6. Zona reticularis

7. Zona fasciculata

Questions 8 through 11

Match the following with its cause or symptom.

    (A) nephrogenic diabetes insipidus
    (B) neurogenic diabetes insipidus
    (C) both
    (D) neither

8. Polyuria

9. Psychogenic polydipsia

10. Lithium

11. Urinary tract obstruction

DIRECTIONS (Questions 12 through 64): Each of the numbered items or incomplete statements in this section is followed by answers or by completions of the statement. Select the ONE lettered answer or completion that is BEST in each case.

Questions 12 through 64

12. A patient has a nodule on palpation over the thyroid gland. Factors indicating possible carcinoma include

    (A) a scan with a hot nodule
    (B) a scan with a cold nodule
    (C) an echo with a clean cystic mass
    (D) biopsy with chronic lymphocytic infiltration
    (E) biopsy with a granulomatous lesion

13. ACTH (corticotropin) is a potent stimulatory for

    (A) estrogen release
    (B) testosterone release
    (C) cortisol production
    (D) ammonia generation
    (E) aldactone release

14. ACTH (corticotropin) is inhibited by

    (A) high corticotropin-releasing factor (CRF)
    (B) high cortisol
    (C) low cortisol
    (D) high estrogen
    (E) adrenalectomy

15. Adequacy of levothyroxine replacement dose in primary hypothyroidism can be best determined by which of the following laboratory values?

    (A) T_3 radioimmunoassy (RIA)
    (B) reverse T_3
    (C) thyroxine-binding globulin (TBG)
    (D) T_3 stimulation test
    (E) thyroid-stimulating hormone (TSH)

16. Klinefelter's syndrome is characterized by

    (A) a tall male
    (B) a short female
    (C) an abnormal XY chromosome
    (D) an XXY male
    (E) an XXY female

17. Infiltrative ophthalmopathy secondary to thyroid dysfunction is seen with

    (A) Graves' disease
    (B) Hashimoto's thyroiditis
    (C) toxic multinodular goiter
    (D) hypothyroidism
    (E) medullary carcinoma of the thyroid

18. The major clinical features of Turner's syndrome include

    (A) baldness with short stature
    (B) gigantism alone
    (C) webbed neck, low hairline, and short stature
    (D) gigantism with low hairline
    (E) short stature alone

19. Vitamin D is essential for normal calcium homeostasis and absorption. Of the following vitamin D sterols, which is the most important for calcium absorption?

    (A) $1,25\text{-}(OH)2D_3$
    (B) vitamin D_2
    (C) vitamin D_3
    (D) $24,25(OH)2D_3$
    (E) $25\text{-}OHD_{32}$

20. Magnesium ammonium phosphate stones (struvite stones) are usually caused by

    (A) hyperparathyroidism
    (B) hyperthyroidism
    (C) renal tubular acidosis
    (D) infection
    (E) trauma

21. Parathyroid hormone can increase serum calcium

    (A) by directly stimulating the gastrointestinal (GI) tract
    (B) by stimulating nephrogenic cyclic AMP
    (C) by decreasing bone turnover

(D) by increasing serum 1,25-(OH)2D$_3$

(E) by stimulating 25-OHD$_3$

22. Single-drug therapy for pheochromocytoma should NOT include

(A) propranolol

(B) prazosine

(C) phenoxybenzamine

(D) phentolamine

(E) nitroprusside

23. The pituitary gland is located in the

(A) glenoid fossa

(B) sphenoid fossa

(C) sella turcica

(D) anterior skull

(E) median eminence

24. Release of antidiuretic hormone (ADH) from the posterior pituitary is determined by the

(A) serum osmolarity

(B) serum viscosity

(C) plasma ADH level

(D) urine osmolarity

(E) serum potassium level

25. Elevated very-low-density lipoprotein (VLDL) with normal low-density lipoprotein (LDL) is found to fit into which of the following Fredrickson classifications?

(A) type IIa

(B) type IIb

(C) type III

(D) type IV

(E) type I

26. Oral hypoglycemic agents improve glucose control in diabetic patients by

(A) improving insulin distribution

(B) enhancing beta cell function

(C) preventing gastric glucose absorption

(D) enhancing glycogenolysis

(E) preventing gluconeogenesis

27. The laboratory diagnosis of diabetes mellitus includes

(A) a fasting glucose of <140

(B) a fasting glucose of <100

(C) a fasting glucose of >140

(D) a fasting glucose of >100

(E) 2-hour postprandial glucose of >100

28. The highly characterisitic renal lesion of diabetes mellitus is called

(A) membranous nephropathy

(B) minimal change

(C) Kimmelstiel–Wilson lesion

(D) Pendred lesion

(E) focal glomerular sclerosis

29. As a patient with diabetic ketoacidosis (DKA) is being treated, the BP, pH, anion gap, and blood sugar improve except for the serum acetone level. With treatment, the acetone level increases. The MOST likely etiology for this phenomenon is

(A) laboratory error

(B) lactate being converted to acetone

(C) glucose being converted to acetone

(D) B-hydroxybutyrate being converted to acetone

(E) glycogen being converted to acetone

30. Appropriate laboratory workup for adrenal insufficiency includes

(A) a thyroid-stimulating hormone (TSH) level

(B) an adrenocorticotrophic hormone (ACTH) stimulation test

(C) a thyroid-releasing hormone (TRS) stimulation test

(D) a corticotropin-releasing factor (CRF) level

(E) a urine for ACTH level

31. TSH (thyrotropin) is stimulated by

    (A) glucagon
    (B) thyrotropin-releasing hormone (TRH)
    (C) prolactin
    (D) antidiuretic hormone (ADH)
    (E) adrenocorticotrophic hormone (ACTH)

32. Hyponatremia may be a presenting sign of

    (A) antidiuretic hormone (ADH) deficiency
    (B) Graves' disease
    (C) Cushing's syndrome
    (D) hypothyroidism
    (E) lithium therapy

33. Appropriate laboratory evaluation of Cushing's syndrome would include

    (A) random adrenocorticotrophic hormone (ACTH) level
    (B) random cortisol level
    (C) cortisol level at 4 PM
    (D) 24-hour urine for cortisol
    (E) cortisol level at 9 AM

34. Which of the following laboratory data would be most useful in the evaluation of nephrolithiasis?

    (A) urine culture
    (B) urine phosphate level
    (C) plasma to urine calcium ratio
    (D) urine citric acid level
    (E) 24-hour urine for osmolarity

35. Myxedema coma is considered a medical emergency. Which of the following would NOT be considered a precipitating factor?

    (A) cold exposure
    (B) infection
    (C) inappropriate use of Cytomel
    (D) inappropriate use of morphine
    (E) none of the above

36. Which of the following does NOT cause a rise in serum prolactin?

    (A) sleep
    (B) thyrotropin-releasing hormone (TRH)
    (C) adrenocorticotrophic hormone (ACTH)
    (D) morphine
    (E) nursing

37. Complications of therapy for diabetic ketoacidosis (DKA) may include

    (A) hyperphosphatemia
    (B) hyperkalemia
    (C) hyponatremia
    (D) hypercalcemia
    (E) hypophosphatemia

38. A 52-year-old male with new onset fasting glucose of 223 is seen in your office. Prior attempts with diet and weight loss have failed to control his hyperglycemia. He is presently on glypizide 10 mg/day. To improve this patient's glucose control, an additional option would be to

    (A) add 30 units of NPH insulin
    (B) add tolazamide
    (C) add glyburide
    (D) add metformin
    (E) add 30 units of regular insulin

39. The patient from Question 38 is seen several months later. He is now on glypizide and acrabose. Acrabose is a/an

    (A) biguanide
    (B) oral alpha-glucosidase inhibitor
    (C) sulfonylurea
    (D) pyridine compound
    (E) macrolide

40. You get a call that the patient from Question 38 is in the emergency room with a glucose of 23. Possible etiology for his hypoglycemia may include

    (A) oversensitivity to the biguanide
    (B) steroid therapy
    (C) ingestion of ascorbic acid

(D) thyroiditis

(E) uremia

41. The patient from Question 38 is on glipizide. This drug is considered to be a

   (A) first-generation sulfonylurea
   (B) second-generation sulfonylurea
   (C) third-generation sulfonylurea
   (D) biguanide
   (E) metabolite of tolbutamide

42. Insulin was added to manage the diabetes of the patient from Question 38 better. It was decided that an intermediate-acting insulin preparation would be used. The usual duration of action for this preparation would be

   (A) 6 to 8 hours
   (B) 9 to 11 hours
   (C) 11 to 14 hours
   (D) 18 to 28 hours
   (E) 30 to 38 hours

43. The glucose control for the patient from Question 38 is now worse since insulin therapy was initiated. His early morning blood sugars are high. The MOST likely cause would be

   (A) Somogyi phenomenon
   (B) dawn phenomenon
   (C) lack of sufficient insulin
   (D) insulin hypersensitivity
   (E) none of the above

44. Pathogenesis of Type 1 (insulin-dependent) diabetes mellitus (IDDM) is MOST likely caused by

   (A) increased peripheral resistance to insulin
   (B) autoimmune destruction of islet of Langerhans
   (C) absence of insulin-binding genes
   (D) pancreatitis
   (E) obesity

45. Etiology of fasting hypoglycemia does NOT include

   (A) chronic renal failure
   (B) Addison's disease
   (C) alcohol consumption
   (D) insulin-producing islet cell tumors
   (E) congestive heart failure

46. The development of microvascular complications in diabetics is due to

   (A) frequent hypoglycemia
   (B) insulin therapy
   (C) neuropathy
   (D) chronic sulfonylurea therapy
   (E) advanced glycosylation end products

47. Retinopathy is a serious complication seen in diabetics. Findings from the Diabetes Control and Complication Trial clearly demonstrate that

   (A) glycemic control will reduce incidence of retinopathy
   (B) glycemic control will not change incidence of retinopathy
   (C) strict glucose control will hasten the formation of retinopathy
   (D) nonsteroidals help retinopathy
   (E) none of the above

48. Pure calcium phosphate renal stones are MOST commonly seen with

   (A) acid urine
   (B) alkaline urine
   (C) hypoparathyroidism
   (D) allopurinol therapy
   (E) infected urine

49. Risk factors for calcium stone formation does NOT include

   (A) thiazide diuretics
   (B) hyperoxaluria
   (C) hypocitraturia
   (D) hyperuricosuria
   (E) low urine volume

50. Multiple endocrine neoplasia Type 1 (MEN Type 1) is present if a patient has

    (A) hyperparathyroidism, pancreatic tumor, medullary carcinoma of the thyroid
    (B) hyperparathyroidism, diabetes
    (C) hyperparathyroidism, pancreatic tumor, pituitary adenoma
    (D) medullary carcinoma, pheochromocytoma, hyperparathyroidism
    (E) hypoparathyroidism, pancreatic tumor

51. A 42-year-old female has random laboratory data drawn that demonstrate a serum thyroxine (T_4) of 17 µg/dL. On exam she appears to be euthyroid. The etiology for this elevated T_4 level would NOT include

    (A) high thyroid-binding globulin (TBG)
    (B) estrogen therapy
    (C) liver disease
    (D) nephrotic syndrome
    (E) pregnancy

52. For the patient in Question 51, further laboratory testing demonstrated a low radioactive iodine uptake. Possible etiologies for the low uptake with a T_4 of 17 µg/dL would be

    (A) Graves' disease
    (B) cold nodule
    (C) hot nodule
    (D) recovery from subacute thyroiditis
    (E) subacute thyroiditis

53. A serum T_3 is obtained and is high at 240 ng/dL (normal 95–190 ng/dL). Most of the T_3 in the serum is derived from

    (A) deiodination of T_4 in the periphery
    (B) direct secretion of T_3 from the thyroid gland
    (C) deiodination of T_4 in the thyroid gland
    (D) iodination of tyrosine in the periphery
    (E) none of the above

54. The patient from Question 51 is told she has Graves' disease. Graves' disease is caused by

    (A) high thyroid-stimulating hormone (TSH) levels
    (B) iodine excess
    (C) elevated thyroid-stimulating immunoglobin (TSI) levels
    (D) excessive hypothalamic thyrotropin-releasing hormone (TRH) stimulation
    (E) excessive adrenocorticotrophic hormone (ACTH) stimulation

55. Amioderone was given to the patient from Question 51 for arrhythmia. This drug may cause

    (A) hyperthyroidism
    (B) thyroid cancer
    (C) thyroiditis
    (D) thyroid nodules
    (E) suppression of the thyroid-stimulating hormone (TSH) directly

56. Therapy for chronic management of Graves' disease would NOT include

    (A) methimazole (MMI)
    (B) beta-blockers
    (C) radioactive iodine therapy
    (D) potassium perchlorate
    (E) propylthiouracil (PTU)

57. The MOST common etiology for hypothyroidism in the United States is

    (A) autoimmune thyroiditis
    (B) therapy for Graves' disease
    (C) insufficient iodine
    (D) aging of the thyroid gland
    (E) low thyroid-stimulating hormone (TSH) levels

58. Which of the following is the MOST common thyroid carcinoma

    (A) medullary thyroid carcinoma
    (B) follicular carcinoma
    (C) papillary carcinoma
    (D) anaplastic
    (E) primary thyroid lymphoma

59. Prior exposure of low-dose irradiation (ie, for acne) to the face is a risk for

    (A) hypothyroidism
    (B) hyperthyroidism
    (C) parathyroid cancer
    (D) pituitary cancer
    (E) thyroid cancer

60. The MOST common cause for a painful thyroid gland is

    (A) postpartum thyroiditis
    (B) Hashimoto's thyroiditis
    (C) deQuervain's thyroiditis
    (D) radiation thyroiditis
    (E) Graves' disease

61. Which of the following is NOT an example of metabolic bone disease seen in renal failure patients?

    (A) hyperparathyroid bone disease
    (B) aluminum bone disease
    (C) osteoporosis
    (D) osteomalacia
    (E) adynamic bone disease

62. A 67-year-old male is admitted with pneumonia and fractured hip. Therapy includes bed rest, administration of antibiotics, and subcutaneous heparin. Several days into his hospitalization, he develops hyponatremia and abdominal pain. The etiology for his abdominal pain and hyponatremia may be due to

    (A) Graves' disease
    (B) Cushing's disease
    (C) Addison's disease
    (D) toxic goiter
    (E) pheochromocytoma

63. Therapy for the patient from Question 62 would include

    (A) mineralocorticoid only
    (B) glucocorticoid only
    (C) adrenocorticotrophic hormone (ACTH) infusion
    (D) glucocorticoid and mineralocorticoid
    (E) no therapy

64. Adrenocorticotrophic hormone (ACTH) level is measured in the patient from Question 62 and found to be low at the time the serum cortisol level was also very low. Further workup demonstrates a nonfunctional pituitary. Appropriate replacement for chronic outpatient therapy would include

    (A) mineralocorticoid only
    (B) glucocorticoid only
    (C) high-sodium diet
    (D) both glucocorticoid and mineralocorticoid
    (E) thyroid hormone only

Answers and Explanations

1. **(B)** LH and FSH are secreted from the anterior pituitary. *(Felig et al, pp. 289–312)*

2. **(B)** TSH and ACTH are secreted from the anterior pituitary. *(Felig et al, pp. 289–312)*

3. **(C)** ADH is secreted from the posterior pituitary and TSH is secreted from the anterior pituitary. *(Felig et al, pp. 289–312)*

4. **(D)** CRF is released by the hypothalamus, and MSH is part of the ACTH molecule. *(Felig et al, pp. 289–312)*

5. **(A)** Layers of the adrenal gland are glomerulosa (outermost layer), fasciculata, and reticularis. The glomerulosa secretes only aldosterone. *(Felig et al, pp. 557–559)*

6. **(B)** The reticularis secretes androgens, estrogens, and cortisol. *(Felig et al, pp. 557–559)*

7. **(B)** The fasciculata makes up approximately 75% of the adrenal gland and secretes cortisol, androgens, and estrogen. *(Felig et al, pp. 557–559)*

8. **(C)** Nephrogenic diabetes insipidis and neurogenic diabetes insipidus by definition imply a polyuric state. *(Felig et al, pp. 402–414)*

9. **(D)** Psychogenic polydipsia is seen with mental disorders, and these patients drink an inordinate amount of fluid. *(Felig et al, pp. 402–414)*

10. **(A)** Lithium will cause distal tubular injury, thus making these cells insensitive to antidiuretic hormone. *(Felig et al, pp. 402–414)*

11. **(A)** Urinary tract obstruction will cause distal tubular injury, thus making those cells poorly responsive to antidiuretic hormone. *(Felig et al, pp. 402–414)*

12. **(B)** Thyroid tumors are classified into papillary, follicular, medullary, or undifferentiated. On scan they appear cold (they are usually nonfunctional). On echo they tend to be solid or exhibit evidence of blood or fragments of tissue within the cyst. Chronic lymphocytic infiltration is seen with Hashimoto's thyroiditis. Granulomatous lesions are not seen with thyroid cancer. *(Felig et al, pp. 533–539)*

13. **(C)** ACTH is mainly responsible for stimulating cortisol. ACTH does help with the stimulation of cholesterol to pregnenolone, which is the steroid needed for all subsequent steroid generation, including estrogen and testosterone. It is not a stimulator of estrogen or testosterone release. Ammonia generation as well as aldosterone release are not under ACTH control. Aldactone is a drug that blocks aldosterone. *(Felig et al, pp. 577–579)*

14. **(B)** A high serum cortisol level will inhibit ACTH release. Also, high CRF or an adrenalectomy will stimulate ACTH. High estrogen

or low cortisol levels do not inhibit ACTH release. *(Felig et al, pp. 579–580)*

15. **(E)** In primary hypothyroidism, when the TSH is elevated prior to replacement therapy following the decrease in TSH, is the most sensitive laboratory assay. The goal is to achieve a normal TSH level (unless clinically contraindictated). T_3 RIA should normalize with T_4 therapy; however, it is not sensitive enough because of the binding protein TBG. It may be of great value in diagnosis of sick euthyroid syndrome. The T_3 stimulation test does not exist. *(Felig et al, pp. 504–506)*

16. **(D)** Klinefelter's is usually caused by an extra chromosome, thus forming an XXY male with hypogonadism, usually associated with short stature and subnormal intelligence. This diagnosis needs to be entertained in a male with small firm testes, gynecomastia, and abnormal arm-to-body length. *(Felig et al, pp. 929–931)*

17. **(A)** Graves' ophthalmopathy can be seen with hyperthyroid or euthyroid Graves' disease. The etiology is unclear, but pathologically a lymphocytic and plasma cell infiltration occurs in the retro-orbital space. Because the eye lies in the socket compartment, any additional mass added to the retro-orbital space results in anterior displacement of the eye with resultant proptosis. *(Felig et al, p. 474)*

18. **(C)** Classic Turner's syndrome is a result of gonadal dysgenesis with streak gonads and they present with low hairline, low-set ears, webbed neck, broad chest, short stature, shortening of the fourth metacarpal, and commonly with renal abnormalities. They usually have a 45,X karyotype. *(Felig et al, pp. 1075–1076)*

19. **(A)** 1,25-(OH)2D$_3$ acts on the gastrointestinal tract to cause calcium absorption and in concert with parathyroid hormone help maintain normal bone homeostasis. Vitamins D_2 and D_3 are metabolized to 25-OH D_3 in the liver and then hydroxylated to 1,25-(OH)2D$_3$ or 24,25(OH)2D$_3$ in the kidney. The true func-

tion of 24,25-(OH)2D$_3$ is not clear at present, but it may be quite important in new bone formation. *(Felig et al, pp. 1445–1446)*

20. **(D)** Struvite (infection, triple phosphate) stones occur when the urine is supersaturated with magnesium, ammonium, and phosphate in the presence of urea-splitting bacteria. Proteus is the most common bacterium, although *klebsiella, pseudomonas, bacteroides*, and *staphylococcus aureus* also have been implicated. *(Felig et al, pp. 1581–1583)*

21. **(D)** Hypercalcemia of hyperparathyroidism is due to increased GI absorption of calcium mediated by 1,25-(OH)2D$_3$. Parathormone (PTH) stimulates increased 1,25-(OH)2D$_3$ formation. Remember, this is in contrast to the hypercalcemia of malignancy (either through bone metastasis or humoral causes) in which the hypercalcemia is due to bone calcium release, not increased GI absorption. Parathyroid hormone (PTH) does not stimulate 25-OHD$_3$. Nephrogenic cyclic AMP is a marker of PTH action at the kidney, but cyclic AMP does not cause hypercalcemia. *(Felig et al, pp. 1449–1474)*

22. **(A)** Prazosine, phenoxybenzamine, phentolamine, or nitroprusside can be first-line drugs in the treatment of pheochromocytoma as they are all alpha-adrenergic antagonists. Propranolol, a beta-adrenergic antagonist, should never be used alone. By only blocking the vasodilator beta receptors with propranolol, there will then be unopposed alpha stimulation resulting in vasoconstriction and a rapid rise in blood pressure. *(Felig et al, pp. 726, 740)*

23. **(C)** The pituitary gland is located at the base of the skull in a saddle-shaped cavity termed the *sella turcica*. It is divided into anterior and posterior components. Along with the hypothalamus it provides the major components to a number of autoregulatory functions of the endocrine system. *(Felig et al, p. 289)*

24. **(A)** Serum osmolarity is the most potent stimulus for ADH release. Serum osmolarity

that is greater than 285 will cause a strong stimulus for ADH release. None of the other choices linked have any influence on the ADH reflex. *(Felig et al, pp. 385–399)*

25. **(D)** Fredrickson's classification is based on the following table:

Type	Lipoprotein Abnormality
I	Chylomicrons markedly increased; VLDL and LDL are normal
IIa	LDL increased, VLDL normal
IIb	Both LDL and VLDL are increased
III	Abnormal cholesterol, normal VLDL, and increased beta-VLDL
IV	VLDL increased and LDL normal
V	Chylomicrons markedly increased, VLDL increased, LDL normal

Type IV is also commonly seen in poorly controlled diabetics. *(Grundy, p. 2045)*

26. **(B)** Oral agents enhance beta cell function and thus increase insulin release. They also improve peripheral sensitivity to insulin. Both of these actions tend to normalize blood sugar levels in the noninsulin-dependent diabetic. *(Cahill et al, p. 13)*

27. **(C)** A fasting blood sugar of >140 mg/dL on two occasions is diagnostic of diabetes mellitus. A $1/2$ hour, 1 hour, or $1\,1/2$ hour blood sugar of >200 mg can be diagnostic of diabetes during a glucose tolerance test. A 2-hour postprandial of >200 is also diagnostic of diabetes. *(Cahill et al, p. 7)*

28. **(C)** Kimmelstiel–Wilson lesions include spherical nodular hyaline masses and sclerosis of the renal glomerulus. This is characteristic of diabetes mellitus. No other disease process is known to cause this lesion. *(Felig et al, pp. 1181–1193)*

29. **(D)** As DKA worsens, especially if there is concomitant lactic acidosis, B-hydroxybucerate is more likely to be formed. B-hydroxybucerate is not measured in the acetone assay. As DKA is treated, the B-hydroxybucerate will be converted to acetone, thus giving the paradoxical rise in serum acetone as the patient improves. *(Felig et al, pp. 1197–1219)*

30. **(B)** Appropriate tests would be a serum ACTH level and an ACTH stimulation test to measure adrenal reserve. The TSH level is to evaluate the thyroid, not the adrenal gland. CRF is a research tool and is not needed, as ACTH level can be measured directly. Urine for ACTH cannot be done. *(Felig et al, p. 869)*

31. **(B)** TRH stimulates TSH. Glucagon, prolactin, ADH, and ACTH do not stimulate TSH. When T_4 and T_3 levels rise slightly above normal, they suppress TSH. *(Felig et al, pp. 445–450)*

32. **(D)** Hypothyroidism will cause an inability to secrete a water load secondary to elevated ADH level. Poor myocardial function with impaired cardiac output, often associated with hypothyroidism, will also prevent adequate free water excretion through the renal tubules. ADH deficiency and lithium therapy cause hypernatremia. Graves' disease and Cushing's disease are usually not associated with the inability to excrete a water load. *(Felig et al, pp. 492–506)*

33. **(D)** Glucocorticoid excess secondary to pituitary ACTH hypersecretion is labeled *Cushing's disease*. Cushing's syndrome has numerous etiologies (iatrogenic, tumor, etc). Laboratory workup would include a 24-hour urine for cortisol (normal <100 mg/24-hour). Random ACTH, random cortisol, and a 4 PM cortisol are of no diagnostic aid because they do not establish a cortisol excess state. ACTH has a wide daily fluctuation; cortisol is usually high in the early morning and low in the late afternoon (usual circadian rhythm). *(Felig et al, pp. 357–362)*

34. **(A)** The appropriate laboratory workup for kidney stones should include a urine culture to rule out infection as the etiology for the stone disease. Staghorn calculi in the renal pelvis are composed of struvite and are caused by infection. Urine phosphate and citric acid levels are nonexistent tests. A plasma-to-urine calcium ratio has no clinical

relevance. The urine osmolarity only tells you if antidiuretic hormone is being secreted. *(Felig et al, pp. 1565–1568)*

35. **(C)** Cytomel is a thyroid replacement hormone and thus would not precipitate myxedema coma. Cold exposure, infection, and inappropriate use of narcotics can all precipitate myxedema coma in hypothyroid patients. *(Felig et al, p. 507)*

36. **(C)** ACTH stimulates the adrenal gland to secrete cortisol. Sleep, stress, nursing, opiates, estrogen, and TRH all stimulate prolactin secretion. *(Felig et al, p. 312)*

37. **(E)** Phosphate stores are reduced in DKA, and the administration of insulin may further enhance movement of phosphate into the cell. Repletion of phosphate during therapy of DKA is usually not necessary, unless the baseline phosphate is very low. Hypokalemia is usually a complication of DKA. Hyponatremia and hypercalcemia are usually not seen with DKA. *(Felig et al, p. 1223)*

38. **(D)** Metformin (a biguanide) has recently been introduced to help diabetics with glycemic control. They seem to improve insulin sensitivity at the post receptor level. Adding 30 U of NPH or 30 U of regular insulin to 10 mg of glypizide would be too high a dose and not necessary with a fasting blood sugar of 223. Adding two other oral hypoglycemic agents would not be correct. *(Felig et al, p. 1211)*

39. **(B)** Oral alpha-glucosidase inhibitors delay digestion of ingested carbohydrates. *(Felig et al, p. 1212)*

40. **(E)** Renal failure by itself may cause hypoglycemia because the kidney is responsible for insulin degradation. Biguanides do not cause hypoglycemia as they enhance insulin sensitivity, not insulin secretion. Ascorbic acid, steroid therapy, and thyroiditis do not cause hypoglycemia. *(Felig et al, p. 1255)*

41. **(B)** Glipizide and glyburide are second-generation sulfonylurea agents. Tolbutamide, tolazimide, chlorpropamide, and acetohexamide are first-generation sulfonylurea drugs. There are at present no third-generation agents. *(Felig et al, p. 1209)*

42. **(D)** The duration of action of intermediate-acting insulin (ie, NPH) can vary from patient to patient, but usually is 18 to 28 hours. *(Felig et al, p. 1198)*

43. **(C)** The *most common* cause of early-morning hyperglycemia is insufficient insulin. The dawn and Somogyi phenomena are *rare* causes for morning hyperglycemia. Insulin hypersensitivity is not a cause. *(Felig et al, pp. 1204–1205)*

44. **(B)** The major susceptibility gene for IDDM is in the HLA region on chromosome 6p and is the most common site in familial inheritance. These genes can present antigens that can present to T cell receptors and thereby initiate a destructive autoimmune process. Increased peripheral resistance to insulin (answer A) is seen in noninsulin dependent diabetes mellitus. Pancreatitis (D) may be a cause in rare patients. Obesity is usually associated with type II diabetes mellitus. Answer (C) is nonsense. *(Felig et al, pp. 1159–1161)*

45. **(C)** Alcohol hypoglycemia is felt to be induced (not fasting) and due to malnutrition and disruption of gluconeogenesis at the liver. Fasting hypoglycemia can occur with chronic renal failure, congestive heart failure, Addison's disease, and islet cell tumors. *(Felig et al, pp. 1251–1267)*

46. **(E)** Advanced glycosylation products (AGE) is a result of glycosylation of amino acids and tissue proteins which crosslink with collagen and cause microvascular complications. Hypoglycemia and insulin therapy do not cause microvasular complications. Neuropathy is a result of microvascular disease. Chronic use of sulfonylurea threrapy is not associated with microvascular complications. *(Rose et al, pp. 1–9)*

47. **(A)** The Diabetes Control and Complications Trial has shown clear beneficial effect in re-

ducing risk of retinopathy with tight control. Nonsteroidals can cause vitreous hemorrhage. *(Felig et al, p. 1185)*

48. **(B)** Alkaline urine enhances the ability to precipitate pure calcium phosphate stones. Hyperparathyroidism also is a risk factor. Acid urine and allopurinol are not risk factors. Infected urine usually causes the formation of struvite stones. *(Felig et al, pp. 1581–1583)*

49. **(A)** Thiazide diuretics can be used as therapy for calcium stones. Hyperoxaluria and hyperuricosuria can act as nidus for calium stone formation. Citrate can act as a stone inhibitor, thus hypocitraturia may enhance stone formation. Low urine volume is a risk for stone formation. *(Felig et al, pp. 1587–1602)*

50. **(C)** Multiple endocrine tumors have been grouped into MEN Type 1 (hyperparathyroidism, pancreatic tumors, pituitary adenoma), MEN Type 2 (medullary carcinoma of the thyroid, pheochromocytoma or adrenal hyperplasia, and hyperparathyroidism), and MEN Type 3 (medullary carcinoma of the thyroid, pheochromocytoma or adrenal hyperplasia and mucosal neuromas). *(Felig et al, p. 1460)*

51. **(D)** Nephrotic syndrome will lower TBG and thus lower total T_4 levels. Estrogen therapy, pregnancy, liver disease, and high TBG will all increase T_4 values without evidence for hyperthyroidism. *(Fitzgerald, p. 163)*

52. **(E)** Subacute thyroiditis will give a low uptake during the acute phase as there is ongoing damage to the gland and it will not pick up the tracer radioactive iodine. Graves' disease, hot nodule, and the recovery phase of subacute thyroiditis are all usually associated with increased uptake. A cold nodule usually does not affect the uptake. *(Fitzgerald, p. 168)*

53. **(A)** Approximately 80% of T_3 (triiodothyronine) comes from peripheral conversion (mainly at muscle and liver) of T_4 to T_3. Approximately 20% of T_3 comes directly from the thyroid gland. In *severe* Graves' disease,

where T_3 levels are very high, a large portion of T_3 comes directly from the thyroid gland. *(Felig et al, pp. 440 and 453)*

54. **(C)** TSI are IgG immunoglobulins that attach to TSH receptors in the thyroid and stimulate the thyroid gland. Iodine excess can worsen hyperthyroidism in Graves' patients. Excess TSH or TRH does not cause Graves' disease. ACTH stimulates the adrenal gland. *(Felig et al, p. 467)*

55. **(A)** Hyperthyroidism and hypothyroidism can occur with amiodarone therapy as it contains 37% iodine. This effect can last for many months. *(Felig et al, p. 465; Fitzgerald, p. 209)*

56. **(D)** Potassium perchlorate is a competitive inhibitor of thyroid iodine transport, but is not used except for very brief times because of its toxicity. MMI and PTU are thionamide drugs to treat hyperthyroidism. Beta-blockers can be used to prevent T_4 to T_3 conversion and to alleviate hyperthyroid symptoms. Long-term treatment can include radioactive iodine. *(Felig et al, pp. 479–485)*

57. **(A)** Autoimmune thyroiditis can present with goiter (called Hashimoto's thyroiditis) or without goiter. Both forms of hypothyroidism are due to cell-mediated and antibody-induced thyroid injury. Lymphocytic infiltration and fibrosis are seen on biopsy. *(Felig et al, pp. 492–497)*

58. **(C)** The most frequent thyroid carcinoma (60% to 80%) is papillary (many times a mix of papillary and follicular). Less frequent are pure follicular followed by medullary thyroid carcinoma and anaplastic carcinoma. Primary thyroid lymphoma account for approximately 1% of all thyroid carcinomas. *(Fitzgerald, pp. 177–187)*

59. **(E)** Patients with prior head and neck irradiation have an increased risk for thyroid carcinoma that can present many years after the exposure. Similar risks occur after exposure to nuclear dust (as an example, a higher rate

of thyroid carcinoma has been seen recently after the Chernobyl nuclear accident). *(Felig et al, pp. 533–534; Kazakov et al, pp. 21–22)*

60. **(C)** DeQuervain's or subacute thyroiditis is the most common cause for thyroid pain. It is believed to be due to a viral infection. *(Felig et al, pp. 507–509)*

61. **(C)** Secondary hyperparathyroidism, adynamic bone disease, osteomalacia, and aluminum bone disease are seen with patients with renal failure or end-stage renal disease on dialysis. Osteoporosis is seen more in postmenopausal women and older men. *(Felig et al, pp. 1524–1538)*

62. **(C)** Addison's disease can present with numerous signs and symptoms, including hypotension, abdominal pain, hyperkalemia, and weakness. The patient is at risk for Addison's with heparin, which may cause adrenal infarct. *(Felig et al, p. 650)*

63. **(D)** Both glucococorticoid and mineralocorticoid therapy need to be given in a patient who has acute adrenal infarct. ACTH infusion would be useless if the adrenal glands are not functional. *(Felig et al, pp. 654–659)*

64. **(B)** If there is a lack of ACTH (secondary hypoadrenalism), the only replacement therapy required would be glucocorticoid as the adrenal gland is still intact. Thyroid hormone alone can precipitate acute adrenal crisis in patients with borderline adrenal function as it increases glucocorticoid metabolism. If glucocorticoid deficiency is documented, then start glucocorticoid therapy prior to starting thyroid hormone replacement. Renin and potassium can still stimulate the zona glomerulosa to secrete mineralocorticoid, thus there is no need to replace this hormone. *(Felig et al, pp. 654–659)*

REFERENCES

Cahill F, Arky A, et al. VI diabetes mellitus. *Sci Am.* January 1987.

Felig F, Baxter JD, et al (eds). *Endocrinology and Metabolism.* New York: McGraw-Hill; 1995.

Fitzgerald PA. *Handbook of Clinical Endocrinology,* 2nd ed. Norwalk, CT: Appleton & Lange; 1992.

Grundy M. Disorders of lipids and lipoproteins. In Stein Jay H, et al (eds), *Internal Medicine,* 2nd ed. Boston: Little, Brown; 1987.

Kazakov et al. Thyroid cancer after Chernobyl. *Nature* 1992; 359: 21–22.

Rose B. *Uptodate in Medicine,* 4th ed. CD-ROM; 1997.

Internal Medicine: Gastroenterology
Questions

Nancy Ivansek, MA, PA-C

DIRECTIONS (Questions 1 through 24): Each of the numbered items or incomplete statements in this section is followed by answers or by completions of the statement. Select the ONE lettered answer or completion that is BEST in each case.

Questions 1 through 24

1. Acute esophageal obstruction is generally seen secondary to food impaction. Treatment consists of all of the following EXCEPT

   (A) 1 mg of IV glucagon
   (B) 0.6 mg of nitroglycerin sublingually
   (C) endoscopy
   (D) barium swallow
   (E) keeping the patient NPO

2. Drug use may precipitate constipation. All of the following statements are true EXCEPT

   (A) Opiates and agents with anticholinergic activity such as antidepressants are frequently implicated.
   (B) Calcium-channel blockers may slow down bowel motility.
   (C) Aluminum hydroxide and calcium carbonate antacids are constipating.
   (D) Cholestyramine may induce constipation by binding bile salts.
   (E) Habitual use of laxatives also may be constipating because of their binding of bile salts.

3. The most common anal rectal problem affecting about half of patients over the age of 50 is

   (A) an infected pilonidal cyst
   (B) carcinoma of the anal rectal tract
   (C) perirectal abscess
   (D) hemorrhoids
   (E) fissures

4. Black or dark-colored stools may be the result of all of the following EXCEPT

   (A) gastrointestinal bleeding from the esophagus, stomach, or duodenum
   (B) friable lesions in the descending colon
   (C) ingestion of bismuth
   (D) ingestion of licorice
   (E) significant epistaxis

5. A 25-year-old black female is found to have a vitamin B deficiency and a macrocytic anemia. You have been following her several years for Crohn's disease, which is currently stable. A recent small intestinal luminal aspirate shows bacterial growth greater than 100,000 organisms/mL of a polymicrobial predominantly anaerobic nature. On physical examination today she also has guaiac-positive stools. She has no allergies to medications. Which therapy would be MOST appropriate?

    (A) tetracycline 250 mg orally 4 times daily, as well as vitamin B_{12} supplementation

    (B) tetracycline 250 mg orally 4 times daily without any vitamin B_{12} supplementation

    (C) vitamin B_{12} supplementation and cathartics used regularly for a 7-day period

    (D) vitamin B_{12} supplementation, as well as a promotility agent

    (E) tetracycline 250 mg 4 times daily, along with promotility agents and vitamin B_{12} supplementation

6. The associated gastrointestinal symptom MOST commonly found in fibromyalgia is

    (A) diverticulitis
    (B) proctitis
    (C) irritable bowel
    (D) cholelithiasis
    (E) hepatitis

7. Although variable, the signs and symptoms often associated with rectal cancer include

    (A) black tarry stools, hematochezia, and pelvic pain

    (B) black tarry stools, tenesmus, and pelvic pain

    (C) periumbilical abdominal pain, tenesmus, and black tarry stools

    (D) tenesmus, hematochezia, and pelvic pain

    (E) left lower-quadrant abdominal pain, tenesmus, and weight loss

8. Which of the following is TRUE concerning travelers' diarrhea?

    (A) The majority of cases of travelers' diarrhea are due to shigellosis.

    (B) Prophylactic antibiotics should be given to all travelers who will be visiting Central and South America.

    (C) Bismuth subsalicylate has proven effective only in the treatment of travelers' diarrhea when used in the dosing of 60 mg bid.

    (D) Bismuth subsalicylate has proven effective in both prophylaxis and the treatment of travelers' diarrhea when used in large doses at 60 mg qid.

    (E) Antibiotic resistance has not yet proven to be a problem in the treatment of travelers' diarrhea.

9. Which of the following dietary factors may cause diarrhea?

    (A) sorbitol
    (B) psyllium
    (C) methylcellulose
    (D) kaolin
    (E) pectin

10. Which of the following conditions has the anesthetic halothane been associated with?

    (A) gastritis
    (B) esophagitis
    (C) cholelithiasis
    (D) hepatitis
    (E) Gilbert's syndrome

11. A tightly packed, partially digested mass of hair or vegetable matter or other hard-to-digest matter commonly found in patients with neuropsychiatric disturbances is known as

    (A) bolus
    (B) bedsonia
    (C) bezoar
    (D) toxocariasis
    (E) asterixis

12. All of the following are true concerning the ingestion of foreign bodies EXCEPT

   (A) Sharp objects should be retrieved as quickly as possible.
   (B) In most instances, small round objects, such as coins, can probably be watched without undue worry.
   (C) Often, an object will tend to be held up at or before the ileocecal valve or at some other site of narrowing.
   (D) Objects such as toothpicks have been known to be found in the GI tract years after ingestion as granulomas or abscesses.
   (E) Because of a balloon's smooth surface, children ingesting a balloon's commonly need no follow up.

13. A patient presents to the ER with complaints of weakness, diplopia, and dry mouth, as well as nausea, vomiting, and abdominal cramps. The patient is becoming rapidly unresponsive and is having descending weakness. He appears to be having difficulty swallowing his own saliva. On history obtained from his wife, you find that he has eaten some canned peaches that had been stored in the cellar for approximately 2 years. He ate these last evening for dinner. Clinically, you decide first to

   (A) secure the patient from respiratory collapse
   (B) continue your history and physical examination
   (C) obtain a complete blood count (CBC) and neurological consult
   (D) obtain a CAT of the head without contrast because of his descending weakness
   (E) insert a nasogastric (NG) tube

14. All of the following are true concerning lactase deficiency EXCEPT

   (A) Lactase deficiency occurs normally in about 75% of adults in all groups except those of northwest European origin.
   (B) Symptoms and signs are similar regardless of the specific enzyme deficiency. The lactose tolerance test is specific for the clinical disorder of lactose intolerance and includes giving an oral dose of 50 g of lactose that causes diarrhea, abdominal bloating, and discomfort within 20 to 30 minutes.
   (C) Fructose should be avoided in children with lactose intolerance.
   (D) In lactose-free dieting, oral calcium supplementation should be given.
   (E) The diagnosis can be absolutely confirmed by the finding of low lactase activity with a jejunal biopsy.

15. Which of the following best describes hepatitis D?

   (A) The incubation period is similar to that for hepatitis A.
   (B) Hepatitis B and D infections cannot be acquired simultaneously.
   (C) There are no clinical laboratory tests available for testing for hepatitis D.
   (D) The outcome of hepatitis D is similar to that of hepatitis A.
   (E) Hepatitis D is being recognized with increasing frequency within the United States.

16. Which of the following medications are recommended in patients judged to be at high risk for bleeding from esophageal varices?

   (A) beta-blockers
   (B) calcium-channel blockers
   (C) antacids
   (D) vitamin supplements
   (E) H_2 antagonists

17. A 40-year-old female is undergoing evaluation of the abdomen for uterine enlargement, presumed to be secondary to uterine fibroids. The ultrasound report makes incidental reference of cholelithiasis. The patient gives no history of abdominal pain, nausea, vomiting, or chest discomfort. You plan to

   (A) advise the patient of the findings and refer her to a surgeon
   (B) advise the patient of the findings and refer her for an oral cholecystogram
   (C) advise the patient of the findings and of symptoms that may be suggestive of acute cholecystitis
   (D) advise the patient of the findings and suggest annual liver function studies be obtained
   (E) advise the patient of the findings and suggest she have a repeat ultrasound study on an annual basis

18. Gilbert's syndrome

   (A) is an inherited condition associated with jaundice and progressive liver dysfunction
   (B) is an inherited condition with variable elevations in circulating unconjugated bilirubin with no long-term sequela other than jaundice
   (C) is a condition attributed to alcohol intake with elevations in circulating unconjugated bilirubin and liver enzymes
   (D) is associated with elevations in conjugated and unconjugated bilirubin and lipid levels
   (E) is associated with elevations in unconjugated bilirubin. The sequelae are variable, depending on the level and duration of the bilirubin elevation

19. Early-morning nausea and vomiting are typically associated with all of the following problems EXCEPT

   (A) alcohol drinking
   (B) diabetic ketoacidosis (DKA)
   (C) addisonian crisis
   (D) uremia
   (E) pyloric channel ulcers

20. All of the following are true regarding diverticulitis EXCEPT

   (A) The patient usually complains of left lower-quadrant or suprapubic abdominal pain.
   (B) Diverticulitis usually involves the sigmoid colon.
   (C) Colonoscopy is commonly used to confirm the diagnosis, especially in patients with an atypical presentation.
   (D) Urinalysis may reflect the presence of cystitis.
   (E) A CAT scan may be used diagnostically to differentiate or rule out a perforation.

21. All of the following are true regarding dysphagia as a consequence to neurological or neuromuscular disease EXCEPT

   (A) This problem is particularly common among the very elderly.
   (B) Benzodiazepines and phenothiazines may be implicated.
   (C) Liquids are reported to be more difficult to swallow than solids.
   (D) Solid foods should be avoided because of the high incidence of aspiration.
   (E) Regurgitation of fluid into the nose may also be reported.

22. A 25-year-old male presents with cramping periumbilical to epigastric abdominal pain that began 4 to 6 hours ago. It is made worse with movement. He has no appetite and is experiencing nausea and vomiting. He denies any constipation or diarrhea. On examination the patient's temperature is 38°C. He is mildly tender in the right flank and right lower-quadrant area of the abdomen and has also rectal tenderness. Your diagnosis is

   (A) kidney stone
   (B) acute appendicitis
   (C) diverticulitis

(D) gastroenteritis

(E) prostatitis

23. Which is true regarding hepatitis B infection?

(A) The hepatitis B surface antigen (HbsAg) usually provides the first evidence of acute B infection and implies infectivity of the blood.

(B) The HbsAg usually occurs soon after the onset of symptoms.

(C) The HbsAg is positive in individuals who have chronic active hepatitis.

(D) After receiving a full series of hepatitis B vaccine, the core antigen should be positive.

(E) After receiving the hepatitis B vaccine series, the core antibody should be positive.

24. A 58-year-old male presents to the ER. His symptoms include several hours of mid-epigastric abdominal pain boring through to his back. He is also experiencing nausea and vomiting. He gives a history of ethanol abuse. On physical examination his temperature is 39°C orally and his pulse 112. On abdominal exam he appears distended, and he is extremely tender in the epigastric area. He has a bluish discoloration periumbilically. The most likely diagnosis is

(A) peptic ulcer disease

(B) alcoholic gastritis

(C) renal colic

(D) acute pancreatitis

(E) cirrhosis

DIRECTIONS (Questions 25 through 37): Each question in this section consists of two lettered headings followed by several numbered words or phrases. For each word or phrase, choose the ONE lettered heading that is closely associated with it. Each lettered heading may be selected once, more than once, or not at all.

Questions 25 through 28

Match the following cause of upper gastrointestinal (GI) bleeding with the MOST common presentation.

(A) painful

(B) painless

25. Esophageal varices

26. Mallory–Weiss tear

27. Angiodysplasia

28. Peptic ulcer disease

Questions 29 through 33

Match the following clinical features, presentations, or complications with the MOST commonly associated form of inflammatory bowel disease.

(A) ulcerative colitis

(B) Crohn's disease

29. Intestinal obstruction

30. Bloody diarrhea

31. Fistulization

32. Toxic megacolon

33. Colon cancer

Questions 34 through 37

Select the type of hepatitis described BEST by the following statements.

(A) hepatitis A

(B) hepatitis B

34. Intravenous drug use or homosexuality are risk factors.

35. It is transmitted via the fecal–oral route.

36. Gammaglobulin prophylaxis is felt to be beneficial.

37. Between 3% and 10% develop chronic active hepatitis or cirrhosis.

DIRECTIONS (Questions 38 through 45): Each of the numbered items or incomplete statements in this section is followed by answers or by completions of the statement. Select the ONE lettered answer or completion that is BEST in each case.

Questions 38 through 45

38. A 75-year-old male with a history of coronary artery disease (CAD) and chronic obstructive pulmonary disease (COPD) presents to you complaining of weight loss and crampy, dull, periumbilical pain occurring 15 to 20 minutes postprandially and lasting for hours. Stool is negative for occult blood, the complete blood count (CBC) is normal, and abdominal exam reveals only the presence of a soft abdominal bruit. The most likely diagnosis is

    (A) gallstones
    (B) mesenteric ischemia
    (C) pancreatitis
    (D) abdominal aneurysm
    (E) peptic ulcer disease

39. The most common type of small-bowel tumor is

    (A) carcinoid
    (B) lymphoma
    (C) adenocarcinoma
    (D) sarcoma
    (E) neurofibroma

40. A 30-year-old female presents to you with a 2-week history of nausea, epigastric distress, crampy abdominal discomfort, flatulence, and diarrhea. No blood has been noted in her stool, but she has lost 6 pounds. The complete blood count (CBC) drawn in your office is normal. She offers one additional bit of history—she recently returned from a camping trip. What is the most likely diagnosis?

    (A) enterotoxigenic *Escherichia coli*
    (B) giardiasis
    (C) *Campylobacter*

(D) *Salmonella*
(E) irritable bowel syndrome

41. A 55-year-old white female smoker presents to you complaining of a 10-pound weight loss, weakness, and dull upper abdominal pain radiating into her back. Physical exam is unremarkable. Lab values show a hemoglobin (Hgb) of 10, serum amylase of 90, and alkaline phosphatase of 240 (elevated). Endoscopic retrograde cholangiopancreatography (ERCP) shows a single, focal, irregular stricture of the pancreatic duct. The most likely diagnosis is

    (A) acute pancreatitis
    (B) pancreatic carcinoma
    (C) chronic pancreatitis
    (D) ampullar carcinoma
    (E) choledocholithiasis

42. Gastroparesis, or delayed gastric emptying, can be due to obstructive or nonobstructive causes. From the following list, which is the MOST common cause of nonobstructive delay?

    (A) medications such as narcotics and antidepressants
    (B) diabetes
    (C) connective tissue diseases
    (D) gastric surgery
    (E) primary chronic intestinal pseudo-obstruction

43. A 65-year-old white male is hospitalized in an intensive care setting for a serious pneumonia. He is diabetic and hypertensive. He develops recurrent spiking fever and poorly localized abdominal discomfort after initial treatment for his pneumonia. Leukocytosis is present, with a white blood cell (WBC) count of 12,000. HIDA scan is negative, and ultrasound shows a gallbladder wall measuring 7 mm with no stones seen. Your diagnosis is

    (A) acute cholecystitis
    (B) emphysematous cholecystitis
    (C) acute cholangitis

(D) acute acalculous cholecystitis

(E) ileus

44. A 23-year-old female with a history of previously diagnosed irritable bowel syndrome presents with small amounts of painful rectal bleeding on defecation. The most likely etiology for this is

(A) inflammatory bowel disease

(B) hemorrhoids

(C) anal fissure

(D) anorectal abscess

(E) rectovaginal fistula

45. Charcot's triad consists of fever, abdominal pain, and jaundice and is the clinical hallmark of

(A) chronic cholecystitis

(B) acute cholecystitis

(C) acute cholangitis

(D) acalculous cholecystitis

(E) carcinoma of the gallbladder

Answers and Explanations

1. **(D)** Pharmacological agents such as glucagon and nitroglycerin help relax the lower esophageal sphincter and may allow passage of a bolus of food. Endoscopy is used for diagnostic and therapeutic purposes by allowing extraction of an impacted foreign body. Endoscopy will allow diagnosis of occult esophageal carcinoma or strictures as the causative agent of the obstruction. If there is any question of an esophageal obstruction the patient should remain NPO. Barium swallow will increase the risk of aspiration and therefore should be avoided. *(Sachar et al, p. 16)*

2. **(E)** Opiates and other anticholinergic drugs are frequently implicated in constipation. Antihypertensive agents such as calcium-channel blockers may also slow down bowel motility, as does cholestyramine because it binds with bile salts. Aluminum hydroxide and calcium carbonate antacids can also cause constipation. The habitual use of laxatives is associated with *impaired motor activity*, and that is the reason why they are implicated in constipation. *(Goroll et al, p. 369)*

3. **(D)** Hemorrhoids are the most common anal rectal problem and affect about half of patients over the age of 50. An infected pilonidal cyst or sinus is most common in males between the ages of 16 to 30. Perirectal abscess and fissures may be more problematic in patients with Crohn's disease or immunodeficiency states. Anal rectal carcinoma is by far a less prevalent anal rectal problem than hemorrhoids. *(Goroll et al, p. 373)*

4. **(B)** Food substances such as licorice have been known to produce dark-colored stools. Pepto-Bismol or bismuth also has caused dark stools in patients. Upper gastrointestinal bleeding, as well as significant nosebleeds, can cause dark-colored stools. Friable lesions in the descending colon would more likely produce bright red blood or occult blood in the stool. *(Isselbacher et al, p. 223)*

5. **(A)** Bacterial overgrowth syndromes can be associated with Crohn's disease and will often present with a vitamin B_{12} deficiency and a macrocytic anemia. The bacterial overgrowth is defined as the demonstration of greater than 100,000 organisms/mL from small intestinal luminal aspirate. Aspirate often shows a predominance of facultative anaerobes. The treatment of choice traditionally has been tetracycline 250 mg orally 4 times daily and nutritional support to include specific vitamins required to correct deficiencies. Promotility agents and somatostatin analogs have not been demonstrated to be reliable therapeutic options. They may be considered in refractory cases. *(Conn et al, p. 495)*

6. **(C)** Fibromyalgia is a syndrome of chronic, often disabling, diffuse musculoskeletal aches and pains. Associated symptoms include irritable bowel, headaches, nonrestora-

tive sleep, fatigue, and paresthesias. *(Rakel, p. 953)*

7. **(D)** Rectal cancer often presents with tenemus, hematochezia and pelvic pain. Black tarry stools are most often associated with upper gastrointestinal (GI) bleeding. *(Conn et al, p. 514)*

8. **(D)** The majority of cases of travelers' diarrhea are caused by enterotoxigenic *Escherichia coli*. Prophylactic use of antibiotics had been in vogue, but the growing awareness of antibiotic-induced diarrhea and increasing bacterial resistance problems have been reasons for discouraging prophylaxis. Bismuth subsalicylate (Pepto-Bismol) has proven effective in both prophylaxis and for the treatment of travelers' diarrhea. The dosing requirement is 60 mg qid. Patients should be made aware that the bismuth will turn their stool black so they will not be alarmed. *(Goroll et al, p. 366)*

9. **(A)** The sorbitol commonly found in apple juice, pear juice, and sugar-free gums and mints has been found to cause diarrhea by a combination of slowing absorption and increasing small-bowel motility. The other choices listed have been used in treating diarrhea. *(Berkow and Fletcher, pp. 807–808)*

10. **(D)** Halothane-related hepatitis tends to occur after repeated exposure to the anesthetic at relatively short intervals. Hepatitis typically develops within a few days to 2 weeks after surgery. Symptoms begin with fever. Distinction from posttransfusion and viral hepatitis can be made because of both its shorter latent period and the absence of hepatitis antigens in the serum. *(Berkow and Fletcher, p. 908)*

11. **(C)** The tightly packed, partially digested conglomeration of hair or vegetable matter often is called a bezoar. It is often found in patients with neuropsychiatric disturbances and in most cases causes no symptoms. Symptoms may include postprandial fullness, nausea, and vomiting, as well as some gastrointestinal (GI) bleeding. *(Berkow and Fletcher, p. 780)*

12. **(E)** Smooth or small, round ingested foreign objects can usually be watched without undue worry that they will cause any damage to the gastrointestinal (GI) tract. Sharp objects should be retrieved because of their potential to perforate the GI tract. The most common area for compromise of the tract is just before or at the ileocecal valve or a site of narrowing. With the ingestion of balloons, you will often find an intestinal obstruction. *(Berkow and Fletcher, p. 781)*

13. **(A)** This patient presents with some rather typical symptoms of foodborne botulism. Botulism has an abrupt onset, usually within 18 to 36 hours after ingestion of the toxin, and presents often as progressive neurological symptoms. Often, the symptoms are bilateral and symmetrical. They progress with a descending weakness or paralysis. The patient will often complain of a dry mouth, diplopia, nausea, vomiting, and abdominal cramps and will demonstrate a loss of accommodation, and pupillary reflex. The patient may also develop progressive dysphasia. The major complication of this illness is respiratory failure due to diaphragmatic paralysis and pulmonary infections. Botulism may be confused with Guillain–Barré syndrome, polio, stroke, myasthenia gravis, tick paralysis, and poisonings due to curare and belladonna alkaloids. Unfortunately, the progressive paralysis prevents patients from showing visible signs of respiratory distress while their vital capacity decreases, and thus vital capacity should be checked regularly. Respiratory impairment requires management in an intesive care unit where intubation, tracheostomy, and mechanical ventilators are readily available. *(Berkow and Fletcher, pp. 817–818)*

14. **(C)** All of the statements are true except for the fact that in children, fructose can be readily absorbed even if they are lactose intolerant. *(Berkow and Fletcher, p. 826)*

15. **(E)** Hepatitis D is being recognized with increasing frequency in the United States. It has an incubation period similar to that of hepatitis B. When both hepatitis B and D infections

are acquired simultaneously, a single clinical episode of hepatitis results. There is a slightly increased risk of fulminant hepatitis if the two infections occur simultaneously. But in general, the outcome of simultaneous infection is no different than that of hepatitis B alone. A diagnosis of hepatitis D is made by demonstrating the appearance of antibody to hepatitis D or anti-HDV. Hepatitis D, or *delta* hepatitis, is caused by defective RNA and requires coinfection with hepatitis B to support its replication. Transmission is primarily by sexual contact. *(Goroll et al, pp. 320–321)*

16. **(A)** Patients judged to be at high risk for bleeding from esophageal varices are candidates for beta-blocker therapy. Therapy should be prescribed in dosages that produce a beta blockade that translates to a reduction in heart rate of about 25%. The agents can lower portal venous pressure and decrease the risk of varices bleeding by about 50%. The remaining choices will not reduce the incidence of bleeding from esophageal varices. *(Goroll et al, p. 410)*

17. **(C)** Studies in "silent" gallstones suggest that the cumulative risk for the development of symptoms or complications requiring surgery in asymptomatic gall stones is 10% at 5 years and 15% at 15 years. Patients found to be asymptomatic at 15 years were unlikely to develop symptoms. Thus, advising the patient of the findings and possible symptoms that may alert him or her to signs and symptoms of acute cholelithiasis is the only intervention necessary at this time. *(Isselbacher et al, p. 1509)*

18. **(B)** Gilbert's syndrome is an inherited condition. Individuals experience elevations in the unconjugated bilirubin, especially at times of physical stress. This abnormality produces no symptoms other than jaundice. It is not associated with liver problems or other adverse effects. *(Isselbacher et al, p. 231)*

19. **(E)** Early-morning nausea and vomiting are typically associated with metabolic etiology. Seventy-five percent of cases of diabetic ketoacidosis are accompanied by nausea and

vomiting. Emesis and nausea are found among as many as 90% of patients with addisonian crisis. Uremia may be heralded by similar symptoms. Vintage drinkers experience early morning nausea and dry heaves after excessive alcoholic intake. In pyloric channel ulcer disease, nausea and vomiting often are postprandial. *(Goroll et al, p. 344)*

20. **(C)** The patient will usually complain of left lower-quadrant or suprapubic abdominal pain accompanied by back pain. Nausea, vomiting, and dysuria or fever also are common symptoms. The urinalysis may reflect the presence of a cystitis secondary to an adjacent inflammatory reaction or a fistula. Sigmoidoscopy and colonoscopy should be avoided during the acute process to avoid perforation. *(Conn et al, p. 467)*

21. **(D)** Dysphagia secondary to neurological or neuromuscular disease may present as choking or difficulty initiating swallowing. This problem is particularly common in the elderly. Certain medications with central affects, such as benzodiazepines, Aldopa, and phenothiazines may blunt the swallowing mechanism. Individuals with dysphasia secondary to neuromuscular etiologies report that liquids are more difficult to swallow than solids and nasal regurgitation, coughing, and aspiration are common. Patients with anatomic narrowing will report more difficulty swallowing solids than liquids. *(Goroll et al, p. 339)*

22. **(B)** The maximum incidence of acute appendicitis occurs in the second and third decade of life. The initial symptoms are invariably abdominal pain of the visceral type. It is usually poorly localized to the periumbilical or epigastric area. Anorexia is so frequent that the presence of hunger should make the diagnosis of appendicitis questionable. Nausea and vomiting occur 50% to 60% of the time. On physical examination the temperature is usually normal to slightly elevated. The location of abdominal tenderness depends on where the inflamed appendix lies in the abdominal cavity. *(Isselbacher et al, p. 1434)*

23. **(A)** The HBV surface antigen is associated with the first evidence of acute B infection and implies infectivity of the blood. The surface antigen characteristically appears during incubation and usually 1 to 6 weeks before clinical or biochemical illness develops. The corresponding antibody appears only weeks or months later. In up to 10% of patients, the hepatitis B surface antigen persists for acute infection, and the hepatitis B surface antibody does not develop. These patients usually develop chronic hepatitis and are asymptomatic carriers of the disease. In individuals who have had the hepatitis B vaccine, the hepatitis B surface antibody often is utilized to ascertain whether the hepatitis B vaccine offered the individual immunity. (*Berkow and Fletcher, pp. 899–900*)

24. **(D)** The probable diagnosis is acute pancreatitis. Alcohol is implicated as the etiologic agent in many patients with acute pancreatitis. On physical examination the patient is usually febrile and tachycardic. Abdominal distention is common, as is severe epigastric tenderness. Cullen's sign, or a bluish discoloration periumbilically, is often found. (*Conn et al, pp. 496–497*)

25. **(B); 26. (B); 27. (B); 28. (A)** Esophageal variceal hemorrhage is usually massive, life-threatening, and painless. Mallory–Weiss tears are mucosal tears at the gastroesophageal (GE) junction and are generally due to vigorous retching and vomiting. These also present with painless hematemesis. Bleeding due to angiodysplasia is painless and often associated with renal disease and hereditary telangiectasia. Peptic ulcer disease is often accompanied by abdominal pain, but bleeding may be the presenting symptom in 15% of cases. (*Sachar et al, pp. 18, 32–42*)

29. **(B); 30. (A); 31. (B); 32. (A); 33. (A)** The hallmark of ulcerative colitis (UC) is bloody diarrhea. Complications of UC include toxic fulminant colitis due to deep transmural dissection of the ulcerative inflammatory process resulting in peritoneal signs, systemic toxicity, paralysis of bowel motility, and so-called "toxic megacolon." After 10 years of ulcerative colitis, there is a 20-fold increase in the risk of colon cancer, and the risk increases with the extent of the disease. Crohn's disease most frequently presents with diarrhea, abdominal pain, fever, right lower-quadrant fullness, or mass. It often results in small-bowel obstruction from edema, fibrotic stricturing, or abscess formation. Fistulization results from deep sinus tracts and transmural inflammation penetrating the bowel wall and burrowing into adjacent structures. Complications of Crohn's include kidney stone formation due to increased colonic oxalate absorption and/or increased metabolism of uric acid. Gallstone disease is increased because of impaired bile salt reabsorption from the terminal ileum. Sclerosing cholangitis also is thought to be associated with Crohn's disease. (*Sachar et al, pp. 204–210*)

34. **(B); 35. (A); 36. (A); 37. (B)** The typical symptoms of acute viral hepatitis are acute or subacute viral onset of fatigue, anorexia, right upper-quadrant discomfort, and possibly jaundice. Hepatitis A is caused by a picornavirus with incubation of 15 to 50 days and is usually asymptomatic in children. It is transmitted via the fecal–oral route. Its course is generally benign, with symptoms lasting 3 to 6 weeks. Household contacts, as well as sexual contacts, are advised to receive prophylaxis with gamma globulin IM (0.02 mL/kg). Hepatitis B is usually spread parenterally or sexually via whole blood, semen, or saliva. The usual clinical picture is similar to that of hepatitis A, though it is more often severe. Patients may develop a serum sickness pneumonia characterized by fever, urticaria, and arthralgias due to immune complex involvement. The incubation period is 1 to 6 months. About 10% of people contracting hepatitis B will become carriers. These patients may show hepatic damage ranging from persistent hepatitis to chronic hepatitis with cirrhosis. Hepatitis B vaccine is currently available for health care workers, sexual contacts, and other high-risk persons. Interferon is now being used for the treatment of hepatitis B as well. (*Chobanian and Van Ness, pp. 142–144; Sachar et al, pp. 123–127*)

38. **(B)** Mesenteric ischemia, otherwise known as abdominal angina, reflects an imbalance of blood supply and demand. Patients with significant atherosclerotic narrowing of the splanchnic arteries cannot increase blood flow to match demand during ingestion of food and thus develop abdominal pain. Clinically, patients complain of dull or crampy abdominal pain periumbilically occurring within minutes of eating and often lasting for hours. Fear of eating is common, due to the pain and, therefore, weight loss is associated. The abdominal exam is usually normal, although soft bruits may be heard. The lab studies also are within normal ranges. Angiography is the diagnostic test of choice. (*Sachar et al, pp. 224–225*)

39. **(C)** Tumors of the small bowel are rare, accounting for only 5% of benign and malignant GI tract neoplasms. Only 1% of malignant GI carcinomas are found in the small bowel. Although all of the choices listed are clearly found in the small bowel, adenocarcinomas account for nearly 50% of all small-bowel tumors. Most commonly seen in the duodenum, two thirds of the adenocarcinomas diagnosed are noted in the region of the ampulla of Vater. The exact etiology of small-bowel cancer is unknown, however there appears to be an increased incidence in patients with familial polyposis, Gardner's syndrome, and Crohn's disease. Other less common tumors of the small bowel include neurofibromatosis and Peutz–Jehgers syndrome. (*Sleisenger and Fordtran, pp. 1547–1548*)

40. **(B)** Giardiasis is the most common cause of waterborne diarrhea in the United States. Although travel history is common, as many as half of affected patients have no obvious risk factors. Incubation period is 12 to 15 days. Giardiasis is associated with nausea, flatulence, and nonbloody diarrhea. Conversely, *Salmonella* and *Campylobacter* generally invade the colonic mucosa and therefore cause bloody, mucoid diarrhea. *Campylobacter* generally causes fever and headache as well. Toxigenic *E. coli* usually has a short incubation period of 1 to 3 days and runs its course quickly. Giardiasis may be difficult to culture, but endoscopic aspiration for organisms is sometimes helpful. Treatment consists of metronidazole 250 mg tid for 5 to 7 days or quinacrine 100 mg tid for 7 days. (*Clearfield and Borowsky, pp. 206–207*)

41. **(B)** Carcinoma of the pancreas is an insidiously developing and nearly universally fatal malignancy. For most patients there are few characteristic signs or symptoms early in the course of the disease. Insidious onset of weight loss, anorexia, and abdominal pain are often seen. Pain radiating into the back suggests invasion of retroperitoneal organs or nerves. Most patients have a mild anemia from blood loss into the bowel and/or nutritional deficiency. Elevated amylase is rare; alkaline phosphatase elevation is common from either hepatic metastasis or bile duct obstruction. ERCP characteristically shows a single irregular, abrupt focal stricture of the pancreatic duct with a smooth remaining system. Biopsy will confirm endoscopic findings. (*Sleisenger and Fordtran, p. 1872*)

42. **(B)** Although all of the listed choices are clearly implicated as causes of nonobstructive gastroparesis, the most common cause is diabetes. It is thought that abnormal neural control of gastric muscular action may be a significant component in the pathogenesis of this disease. It also is felt that the resulting complication of gastroparesis may in turn be partly responsible for poor diabetic control that is frequently seen in these patients. Other causes of gastroparesis—both obstructive and nonobstructive—are postgastric surgical states (especially truncal vagotomy); pernicious anemia; psychiatric disorders, such as anorexia nervosa and bulimia; peptic ulcer disease; pyloric hypertrophy; gastric antral carcinoma; and pancreatic cancer. Treatment consists of the administration of prokinetic agents such as metoclopramide, bethanechol, and two not yet widely available agents—domperidone and cisapride. (*Sleisenger and Fordtran, pp. 244–247*)

43. **(D)** Acalculous cholecystitis is an important entity because it often progresses to gangrene and perforation. It most often occurs as a

complication of another serious illness, surgery, or other trauma. Sepsis from another condition and diabetes mellitus are common associated findings. Right upper-quadrant pain and fever are helpful, but as many as 25% of cases will have fever only. Leukocytosis is also a helpful sign but again not always present. Ultrasound findings of gallbladder wall thickening (>3 mm), and/or gallbladder enlargement, and/or pericholecystic fluid are diagnostic (without the presence of stones, of course). As many as 20% of all cases of acalculous cholecystitis will have a false-negative HIDA scan. *(Sleisenger and Fordtran, p. 1706)*

44. **(C)** Anal fissures are longitudinal defects in the anoderm, common in young and middle-aged adults, and usually caused by the trauma of passing a large, firm stool. Irritable bowel syndrome with its characteristic cycle of diarrhea and constipation can predispose a patient to the development of an anal fissure. Treatment is usually symptomatic with stool softeners, careful attention to diet, and topical creams. In more severe or nonhealing cases, surgical evaluation may be helpful. Hemorrhoids have bleeding as their cardinal symptom, but this is always painless unless the hemorrhoid is thrombosed. Inflammatory bowel diseases and anorectal abscesses usually do not have painful rectal bleeding as a presenting symptom. *(Sleisenger and Fordtran, pp. 1576–1580)*

45. **(C)** The classic presentation of acute cholangitis is fever, pain, and obstructive jaundice. The patient generally is ill appearing, often with rigors and upper abdominal tenderness.

Cholangitis is caused by bacterial infection of the bile in the bile ducts. The most common causes are choledocholithiasis, neoplasm, or stricture. Antibiotics are the initial treatment, followed by diagnostic tests to determine the cause of obstruction, then possibly decompression via endoscopic sphincterotomy, biliary stent placement, or surgery, depending on the nature of the obstruction. *(Sleisenger and Fordtran, pp. 1717–1718)*

REFERENCES

Berkow R, Fletcher AJ. *The Merck Manual of Diagnosis and Therapy*, 16th ed. Rahway, NJ: Merck Research Laboratories; 1992.

Chobanian SJ, Van Ness NM. *Manual of Clinical Problems in Gastroenterology*. Boston: Little, Brown; 1988.

Clearfield HR, Borowsky LM. *Case Studies in Gastroenterology*. Baltimore: Williams & Wilkins; 1989.

Conn HF et al. *Current Therapy; Latest Approved Methods of Treatment for the Practicing Physician*. Philadelphia: Saunders; 1996.

Goroll AH, May LA, Mulley AG. *Primary Care Medicine: Office Evaluation and Management of the Adult Patient*. Philadelphia: Lippincott; 1995.

Isselbacher KJ et al. *Harrison's Principles of Internal Medicine*, 13th ed. New York: McGraw-Hill; 1994.

Rakel RE. *Conn's Current Therapy*. Philadelphia: Saunders; 1997.

Sachar DB, Wayne JD, Lewis BS. *Pocket Guide to Gastroenterology*. Baltimore: Williams & Wilkins; 1991.

Sleisenger MH, Fordtran JS. *Gastrointestinal Disease: Pathophysiology and Management*, 4th ed. Philadelphia: Saunders; 1989.

Internal Medicine: Neurology
Questions

Ricky E. Kortyna, MHS, PA-C

DIRECTIONS (Questions 1 through 23): Each of the numbered items or incomplete statements in this section is followed by answers or by completions of the statement. Select the ONE lettered answer or completion that is BEST in each case.

Questions 1 through 23

1. A 25-year-old patient presenting with acute low-back pain, lateral thigh, and leg pain after lifting a heavy object may require

   (A) lumbar brace for compression fracture
   (B) workup for peripheral neuropathy
   (C) lumbar puncture
   (D) removal of herniated disc
   (E) rehabilitation for spinal cord injury

2. A patient who presents with ipsilateral ocular miosis, mild ptosis, and anhidrosis has findings indicative of

   (A) Horner's syndrome with parasympathetic paresis
   (B) Horner's syndrome with a sympathetic paresis
   (C) Argyll–Robertson syndrome with a parasympathetic paresis
   (D) Argyll–Robertson syndrome with a sympathetic paresis
   (E) pupillary-sparing III nerve palsy

3. To make the diagnosis of multiple sclerosis the patient should meet the following criteria EXCEPT

   (A) age between 10 and 50 years
   (B) two separate CNS lesions
   (C) two separate episodes
   (D) abnormal neurological exam
   (E) symptoms involving the gray matter

4. The differential diagnosis for Alzheimer's disease includes which of the following?

   (A) normal pressure hydrocephalus
   (B) depression
   (C) cerebral mass lesion
   (D) AIDS dementia
   (E) all of the above

5. Gingival hyperplasia may be seen with chronic administration of

   (A) phenobarbitol
   (B) phenytoin
   (C) primidone
   (D) valproic acid
   (E) clonazepam

6. The MOST common presenting symptom of a brain abscess in a 50-year-old male is

   (A) fever
   (B) nuchal rigidity
   (C) seizures
   (D) focal deficit
   (E) headache

7. A patient presents with a chief complaint of a left visual field cut involving both eyes. The anatomic source of the lesion is

   (A) right optic nerve
   (B) left optic nerve
   (C) optic chiasm
   (D) left optic tract
   (E) right optic tract

8. The MOST common primary brain tumor in adults is

   (A) pituitary adenoma
   (B) chordoma
   (C) meningioma
   (D) glioblastoma
   (E) hemangioma

9. A Glasgow Coma Score of 15 means the patient

   (A) is neurologically intact
   (B) is brain dead
   (C) has nonreactive pupils
   (D) has a severe motor deficit
   (E) is nonverbal

10. The MOST common cause of bacterial meningitis in the adult is

    (A) anaerobes
    (B) *Haemophilus influenzae*
    (C) *Staphylococcus aureus*
    (D) *Streptococcus pneumonia*
    (E) *Listeria monocytogenes*

11. Which of the following would be associated with Alzheimer's disease?

    (A) focal neurological finding
    (B) sudden, stepwise progression of symptoms
    (C) depressed state preceding memory disturbance
    (D) nutritional deficiency
    (E) none of the above

12. The MOST common neurological eye finding in the adult diabetic is

    (A) III nerve palsy
    (B) VI nerve palsy
    (C) lid lag
    (D) exophthalmos
    (E) nystagmus

13. The MOST common symptom in a patient with spinal cord metastasis is

    (A) paresthesia
    (B) pain
    (C) numbness
    (D) urinary retention
    (E) focal weakness

14. A child with hip girdle weakness will use his hands to "climb up" his legs to the upright position. This phenomenon is known as which of the following signs?

    (A) Gower's
    (B) Plower's
    (C) Moro's
    (D) Keller's
    (E) Simon's

15. Pontine hemorrhage is associated with

    (A) bilateral dilated pupils
    (B) bilateral pinpoint pupils
    (C) anisocoria
    (D) unilateral fixed pupil
    (E) unilateral pinpoint pupil

16. The MOST likely diagnosis in a patient whose cerebrospinal fluid (CSF) reveals a glucose of 20 and a protein of 400 with a white blood cell (WBC) count of 1,200 with 90% polys is

    (A) acute bacterial meningitis
    (B) partially treated bacterial meningitis
    (C) neoplastic meningitis
    (D) aseptic meningitis
    (E) cryptococcal meningitis

17. With long-term Ménière's disease, which of the following may NOT be reversible?

    (A) tinnitus
    (B) vertigo
    (C) fullness in the ears
    (D) hearing loss
    (E) pressure in the ears

18. The classic triad for normal pressure hydrocephalus consists of

    (A) gait disorder, tremors, dementia
    (B) gait disorder, dementia, incontinence
    (C) tremors, dementia, tinnitus
    (D) dementia, gait disorder, seizures
    (E) seizures, dementia, field cuts

19. Levodopa is effective in treating Parkinson's disease because it

    (A) increases dopamine in the corticospinal tract
    (B) decreases dopamine in the basal ganglia
    (C) increases dopamine in the basal ganglia
    (D) decreases dopamine in the corticospinal tract
    (E) has no effect on dopamine

20. Tertiary syphilis may have all of the following EXCEPT

    (A) tabes dorsalis
    (B) optic atrophy
    (C) meningovasculitis
    (D) Marcus–Gunn pupils
    (E) Argyll–Robertson pupils

21. Pancoast tumors may effect which nerve root?

    (A) C2
    (B) C8
    (C) T4
    (D) L4
    (E) T8

22. A patient with lumbar canal stenosis may complain of all of the following symptoms EXCEPT

    (A) leg pain
    (B) gait fatigue
    (C) bowel incontinence
    (D) leg heaviness
    (E) pain relief with sitting

23. Drugs used to prevent migraine include all of the following EXCEPT

    (A) beta-blockers
    (B) sumatriptin
    (C) calcium-channel blockers
    (D) antidepressants
    (E) anticonvulsants

DIRECTIONS (Questions 24 through 28): Each group of items in this section consists of lettered headings followed by a set of numbered words or phrases. For each numbered word or phrase, select the ONE lettered heading that is most closely associated with it. Each lettered heading may be selected once, more than once, or not at all.

Questions 24 through 28

For each of the following sets of signs/symptoms choose the neurological process MOST likely responsible.

    (A) myelopathy
    (B) radiculopathy
    (C) peripheral neuropathy
    (D) myopathy
    (E) none of the above

24. Pain, numbness, weakness confined to a nerve root distribution

25. Trunk and proximal limbs involved early in course

26. Sphincter involvement

27. Begins in the distal aspect of the extremities

28. Diplopia is a cardinal feature

DIRECTIONS (Questions 29 through 40): Each of the numbered items or incomplete statements in this section is followed by answers or by completions of the statement. Select the ONE lettered answer or completion that is BEST in each case.

Questions 29 through 40

29. Episodic headaches associated with ipsilateral lacrimation and rhinorrhea are

    (A) traction headaches
    (B) muscle contracture headaches
    (C) delusional headaches
    (D) cluster headaches
    (E) nonmigrainous migraine headaches

30. The biceps deep tendon reflex tests which nerve root?

    (A) C4
    (B) C5
    (C) C6
    (D) C7
    (E) C8

31. In the Brown–Sequard syndrome there is all of the following EXCEPT

    (A) ipsilateral loss of position and vibration
    (B) crossed loss of pinprick and temperature
    (C) loss of touch below the lesion
    (D) preservation of touch below the lesion
    (E) A and D only

32. A patient who enters the emergency department with a complaint of the "worse headache of my life" and the findings of a cranial nerve III palsy indicate

    (A) subgaleal hemorrhage
    (B) subarachnoid hemorrhage
    (C) subdural hemorrhage
    (D) cerebellar hemorrhage
    (E) epidural hemorrhage

33. The hallmark of neurological Lyme disease is

    (A) mononeuritis multiplex
    (B) VII nerve palsy
    (C) myositis
    (D) meningitis
    (E) radiculitis

34. Signs of hydrocephalus in a newborn include all of the following EXCEPT

    (A) distended scalp veins
    (B) decreased level of consciousness
    (C) Macewen's sign
    (D) bulging anterior fontanelle
    (E) spasticity and clonus of the legs

35. In a child with febrile "seizures" which test should always be considered as part of the workup?

    (A) brain CT
    (B) brain MRI
    (C) lumbar puncture (LP)
    (D) EEG
    (E) electromyograph (EMG)/nerve conduction velocity (NCV)

36. Signs of a basilar skull fracture include all of the following EXCEPT

    (A) cerebrospinal fluid (CSF) rhinorrhea
    (B) CSF otorrhea
    (C) Battle's sign
    (D) Raccoon's sign
    (E) Macewen's sign

37. A patient with a shagreen patch, sebaceous adenomas, seizures, and mental retardation has

    (A) linear nevus syndrome
    (B) neurofibromatosis
    (C) von Hippel–Landau disease
    (D) tuberous sclerosis
    (E) Sturge–Weber syndrome

38. Headaches that indicate a brain tumor may have all of the following characteristics EX-CEPT

    (A) wake patient at night
    (B) worse in AM, improve throughout the day
    (C) worse with coughing
    (D) worse with defecation
    (E) have an aura

39. Blindness is a potential complication of

    (A) Takayasus' arteritis
    (B) Behçet's disease
    (C) polyarteritis nodosa
    (D) temporal arteritis
    (E) Sjögren's syndrome

40. Tardive dyskinesia is seen with large doses of

    (A) paraldehyde
    (B) buspirone
    (C) ethylene glycol
    (D) phencyclidine
    (E) phenothiazides

Answers and Explanations

1. **(D)** This patient has symptoms classic of nerve root compression from a herniated disc causing a lumbar radiculopathy (nerve root pain). On examination, the patient may have reflex abnormality, weakness, or decreased sensation within a dermatomal/myotomal distribution. The straight leg testing maneuver is frequently positive. Compression fracture is unlikely in a 25-year-old without a pathological cause. Peripheral neuropathy is not related to trauma. There are no symptoms of spinal cord injury (eg, gait or incontinence), and lumbar puncture would add no useful diagnostic or therapeutic information. *(Youmans, pp. 2678–2679)*

2. **(B)** A Horner's syndrome is caused by a sympathetic paresis. The pupil dilates more slowly (or less completely) in the dark and is associated with miosis, mild ptosis, and anhidrosis. Common causes of a Horner's syndrome include obstetrical/perinatal trauma, malignancy, cervical spine injury, thyroid disease, or thoracic outlet syndrome. *(Youmans, pp. 554–555)*

3. **(E)** Multiple sclerosis (MS) afflicts at least 250,000 Americans. It is thought to be an autoimmune disease. Women are affected more often than men by a 2:1 ratio. The peak incidence is between the ages of 20 and 30 years, and it rarely affects people under 10 or over 60 years of age. The hallmark of MS is dissemination of lesions in time and space; in other words, the symptoms cannot be explained by a single neurological lesion. The

physical exam must show at least one objective abnormality. It involves the white matter almost exclusively. *(Samuels and Feske, pp. 350–353; Rowland, p. 825)*

4. **(E)** The diagnosis of Alzheimer's is one of exclusion. Potentially reversible causes of dementia need to be ruled out. The differential diagnosis of Alzheimer's includes normal pressure hydrocephalus, alcohol abuse, depression, cerebral mass lesion, AIDS dementia, and stroke. *(Adams and Victor, pp. 959–966)*

5. **(B)** Side effects from chronic use of phenytoin (Dilantin) include gingival hyperplasia and hirsutism. Dose-related toxicity includes ataxia, lack of coordination, diplopia, tremor, and horizontal nystagmus. Phenytoin is teratogenic. Other drugs that may cause gingival hyperplasia are diltiazem and dihydropyridines. *(DiPalma et al, p. 308)*

6. **(E)** The most common symptom of a brain abscess is headache (75%). The other symptoms may occur, but at a lower frequency: fever (30%), nuchal rigidity (20%), seizures (40%), and focal deficit (65%). *(Samuels and Feske, pp. 371–373; Rowland, pp. 136–137)*

7. **(E)** Because fibers originating in the nasal half of the retina cross at the chiasm and temporal fibers do not cross, a lesion in the *right* optic tract will block *right* temporal and *left* nasal fibers. This produces a *left* homonymous hemianopsia. (Remember that visual

stimuli are transmitted to the retina reversed.) *(Greenberg et al, pp. 121–129)*

8. **(D)** The most common primary brain tumor is glioblastoma. Approximately 60% of the primary brain tumors are glioma, 20% are meningioma. Pituitary adenomas, chordomas, and hemangiomas occur much less frequently. The most common brain tumors are metastatic tumors that occur at about 24,000 cases per year, the same as all primary brain tumors combined. *(Samuels and Feske, p. 810; Rowland, p. 313)*

9. **(A)** A Glasgow Coma Scale of 15 means the patient is neurologically intact. A result of three or less is seen with brain death. The scale is divided into three sections: eye opening (4 points), motor response (6 points), and verbal response (5 points). The more complex the response, the greater the number of points given. For example, no response for eye opening is given one point and spontaneous opening is given four points. The sum of eye, motor, and verbal gives a scale of 3 to 15. *(Samuels and Feske, p. 144; Rowland, p. 422)*

10. **(D)** The most common cause of bacterial meningitis in the adult is *S. pneumoniae*. It accounts for nearly 40% of all cases. Anaerobes are extremely rare causative agents of meningitis. *Haemophilus, Staphylococcus,* and *Listeria* combined account for nearly 20% of cases. *(Samuels and Feske, p. 366)*

11. **(E)** Alzheimer's disease is characterized by progressive dementia, increased loss of memory and intellect, speech disturbances, and shuffling gait. A focal neurological finding suggests a neurological lesion. The stepwise progression of symptoms suggests multiinfarct dementia which may be treated with anticoagulants to halt progression. Depression can mask dementia, but patients with Alzheimer's are actually unaware of their condition and not likely to be depressed. Nutritional deficiencies, such as vitamin B_{12} deficiency, may lead to symptoms of dementia but can be treated with supplementation. *(Adams and Victor, pp. 959–966)*

12. **(A)** The most commonly affected cranial nerve in diabetics is the III nerve. The VI nerve may also be affected, but less so than III. Lid lag, exophthalmos, and nystagmus are not seen as a result of diabetic neuropathy. *(Samuels and Feske, p. 510)*

13. **(B)** Pain is the most common symptom of spinal cord metastasis. The pain is frequently well-localized back pain but may be radicular. The pain may precede neurological deficit by several weeks, and the goal is to institute treatment prior to the onset of weakness. *(Adams and Victor, pp. 1104–1108)*

14. **(A)** Gower's sign is the correct answer. A patient with hip girdle weakness who arises this way probably has Duchenne muscular dystrophy. The Moro reflex is done by holding the infant in a semi-upright position and allowing him to fall backward partway to the examination table; the child should extend his arms and flex his thumbs. Failure to do this indicates pathology. Plower's, Keller's, and Simon's are fictitious names. *(Behrman et al, p. 1478, 1479)*

15. **(B)** Pontine hemorrhage is associated with bilateral pinpoint pupils. Other causes of pinpoint pupils include opiate overdose and drugs used to treat glaucoma. Bilateral dilated pupils that are not reactive may be caused by anticholinergic agents, glutethimide, amitriptyline, antiparksinsonian drugs, and profound hypoxia. Parasympathetic lesions, such as oculomotor compression from herniation, may cause unilateral dilation and loss of reaction to light, as may a seizure. *(Samuels and Feske, p. 282; Rowland, pp. 21, 22; Bates, p. 194)*

16. **(A)** CSF glucose may be low in any of the meningitides listed. Protein as high as 400 is a good indication of acute bacterial meningitis, although it can be that high in cryptococcal or neoplastic meningitis. However, the WBC clearly identifies acute bacterial meningitis. Counts greater than 500 are rare in other diseases and 90% polys excludes the other diagnoses. *(Weiner and Goetz, p. 17; Adams and Victor, pp. 604–605)*

17. **(D)** Hearing loss may not be reversible in Meniere's. Vertigo, fullness, and pressure in the ear are transient, occurring only during attacks. Tinnitus may persist between attacks but tends to intensify during the attack. The hearing loss is usually most severe in the low frequencies. *(Samuels and Feske, p. 88; Rowland, p. 18)*

18. **(B)** The classic triad for normal pressure hydrocephalus (NPH) includes gait disorder, dementia, and incontinence. The gait disturbance generally occurs first. However, as gait disturbances are fairly common in the elderly, NPH is often not considered. Abulia, or slowness of thought and action, is characteristic of NPH. Urinary incontinence occurs later in the course of the disease. Remember, that with NPH, papilledema is absent. *(Samuels and Feske, p. 139; Rowland, p. 297)*

19. **(C)** Levodopa increases dopamine levels in the basal ganglia. However, as Parkinson's disease progresses, the ability of levodopa to continue to raise levels decreases, thus making treatment a challenge. *(DiPalma et al, p. 315)*

20. **(D)** Tertiary syphilis is associated with Argyll–Robertson pupils, not Marcus–Gunn pupils. Argyll–Robertson pupils do not react to light, but do react to accommodation. Marcus–Gunn pupils show a better constriction to indirect response than to direct light. Tabes dorsalis, optic atrophy, and meningovasculitis may all be seen in tertiary syphilis. *(Samuels and Feske, p. 381; Rowland, pp. 200–208)*

21. **(B)** Pancoast tumors may extend into the brachial plexus and therefore affect C8. The patients complain of pain under the upper portion of the scapula and pain and numbness of the inner portion of the arm. There is weakness of C8 and T1 innervated muscles. Other tumors that may extend into the brachial plexus include lymphomas, melanomas, and breast cancers. *(Samuels and Feske, p. 499)*

22. **(C)** Patients with lumbar canal stenosis frequently complain of leg pain and heaviness, and gait fatigue. They find relief of the pain with sitting or lying down. These symptoms, although caused by neural compromise, so mimic vascular disease that the term *neurogenic claudication* often is used. Diagnosis is performed via a CT with attention to bony windows. *(Samuels and Feske, p. 464; Rowland, p. 460)*

23. **(B)** Sumatriptin is used in the acute treatment of migraine. Beta-blockers, calcium-channel blockers, antidepressants, and anticonvulsants have all been used to prevent migraine. *(Samuels and Feske, p. 1115)*

24. **(B); 25. (D); 26. (A); 27. (C); 28. (E)** Myelopathy is a disorder of the spinal cord. Motor function is affected from the site of the lesion distally. There is a sensory level suggesting the location of the lesion or a "suspended" sensory level on the trunk (eg, shawl distribution). Reflexes are usually hyperactive, the Babinski sign is positive and the urethral and anal sphincters are affected.

Peripheral neuropathy is a lower motor neuron disease distal to the nerve roots. There is a flaccid weakness, reflexes are hypoactive, and sensory findings are confined to the distribution of the peripheral nerve(s). Distal extremities are affected first. Sphincters are rarely involved.

Myopathy (muscle disease) involves the trunk and proximal musculature initially. There is a flaccid weakness; no sensory abnormality; reflexes are initially unaffected, then become hypoactive; and there is no sphincter disturbance.

Radiculopathy is a disorder of the nerve root. Pain, numbness, weakness, and reflex change are confined to a specific dermatome/myotome. *(Youmans, pp. 3, 2678–2679)*

29. **(D)** Episodic headaches associated with ipsilateral lacrimation and rhinorrhea are cluster headaches. This form of headache generally starts around age 30, and about 10% of patients have a family history. The clusters, periods when the patient is susceptible to headaches, occur cyclically, generally with a 2-month window of susceptibility followed by a year of remission. Other symptoms include ipsilateral forehead sweating, miosis,

and ptosis. Prophylactic treatment consists of verapamil and/or ergotamine. *(Samuels and Feske, pp. 1129–1131; Rowland, pp. 842, 843)*

30. **(B)** The biceps deep tendon reflex tests C5. C4 is tested via the deltoid reflex, C6 via the brachioradialis reflex, and C7 the triceps reflex. There is no gross reflex for C8 as it innervates the hand. *(Hoppenfield, p. 55)*

31. **(C)** With hemisection of the cord, the Brown–Sequard syndrome, there is loss of position and vibratory sense below the level of the lesion ipsilaterally and loss of pinprick and temperature contralaterally. Touch remains intact. *(Samuels and Feske, p. 33; Rowland, pp. 442, 443)*

32. **(B)** A patient entering the emergency department with a complaint of "the worse headache of my life" must be assumed to have had a subarachnoid hemorrhage. A III nerve palsy will be seen with an aneurysm of the internal carotid artery at the junction of the posterior communicating artery. It is the acuity and severity of the headache that are the distinguishing characteristics. *(Samuels and Feske, p. 285; Rowland, p. 276)*

33. **(D)** The hallmark of neurological Lyme disease is meningitis. However, all of the symptoms listed may occur. These symptoms occur during the second stage of Lyme disease. *(Samuels and Feske, p. 384; Rowland, p. 210)*

34. **(B)** Signs of hydrocephalus in an infant include distended scalp veins, bulging anterior fontanelle, and spasticity and clonus of the legs. Percussion of the skull gives a "cracked pot" sound—Macewen's sign. There is no change in the level of consciousness as the sutures have not fused and the skull may grow in size in response to an intracranial mass. *(Behrman et al, p. 1489)*

35. **(C)** An LP must be considered in a child with a febrile seizure to rule out meningitis as a cause of the seizure. The other studies are not of immediate help and should not be considered as part of the initial workup. *(Behrman et al, p. 1455)*

36. **(E)** Signs of a basilar skull fracture include CSF rhinorrhea, CSF otorrhea, Battle's sign (ecchymosis overlying the mastoid), Raccoon's sign (bilateral ecchymosis and swelling of the upper eyelids), and hematotympanium. Macewen's sign is a term that refers to a "cracked pot" sound heard when percussing the skull of a hydrocephalic infant. *(Behrman et al, p. 1521)*

37. **(D)** Tuberous sclerosis, a phakomatosis, is unique for having the following findings on physical exam: hypopigmented areas on the trunk and extremities likened to an "ash leaf," a roughened raised lesion with an orange peel consistency overlying the lumbosacral lesion (the shagreen patch), sebaceous adenomas of the face and cheek, and retinal tumors. There also may be associated mental retardation, seizures, intraventricular tumors, and renal hamartomas or polycystic kidneys. *(Behrman et al, pp. 1510, 1511)*

38. **(E)** Features of a headache associated with a brain tumor includes headache that wakes the patient at night or early in the morning and decreases throughout the day. During REM sleep there is an increased amount of blood flow to the brain. The combination of increased blood flow with a mass lesion causes either direct or transmitted pressure on the cerebral arteries, venous sinuses, dura, and cranial nerves—thus the headache. Coughing and defecation also increase intracranial pressure. An aura is seen with migraine. *(Samuels and Feske, p. 813; Rowland, p. 315)*

39. **(D)** Blindness is a potential complication of temporal arteritis. Temporal arteritis is associated with headache, an elevated sedimentation rate of >50, and the affected temporal artery may be prominent, nodular, tender, and noncompressible. Other signs include temporal tenderness, jaw claudication, polymyalgia rheumatica, malaise, fever, and weight loss. Unilateral visual loss occurs secondary to central retinal artery occlusion and affects 14% to 37% of the patients. *(Samuels and Feske, p. 310; Rowland, p. 955)*

40. **(E)** Tardive dyskinesia may be seen with the administration of phenothiazines. It is probably caused by an imbalance of acetylcholine and dopamine leading to an increased dopaminergic activity. There is no direct relationship between dose and symptomatology. The syndrome consists of a variety of rhythmic involuntary movements most commonly involving the face, tongue, and lips. *(DiPalma et al, p. 281)*

REFERENCES

Adams RD, Victor M. *Principles of Neurology,* 5th ed. New York: McGraw-Hill; 1993.

Bates B. *A Guide to Physical Examination and History Taking,* 4th ed. Philadelphia: Lippincott; 1987.

Behrman RE, et al (eds). *Nelson Textbook of Pediatrics,* 14th ed. Philadelphia: Saunders; 1992.

DiPalma JR, DiGregorio GJ, Barbieri EJ, Ferko AP. *Basic Pharmacology in Medicine,* 4th ed. West Chester: Medical Surveillance; 1994.

Greenberg DA, Aminoff MJ, Simon RP. *Clinical Neurology.* Norwalk, CT: Appleton & Lange; 1993.

Hoppenfield S. *Physical Examination of the Spine and Extremities.* Norwalk, CT; Appleton-Century-Crofts; 1976.

Rowland L (ed). *Merritt's Textbook of Neurology,* 9th ed. Baltimore: Williams & Wilkins; 1995.

Samuels MA, Feske S (eds). *Office Practice of Neurology.* New York: Churchill Livingstone; 1996.

Weiner W Jr, Goetz CG (eds). *Neurology for the Non-Neurologist,* 2nd ed. Philadelphia: Lippincott; 1989.

Youmans JR (ed). *Neurological Surgery,* 3rd ed. Philadelphia: Saunders; 1990.

Internal Medicine: Rheumatology
Questions

Henry W. Stoll, PA-C

DIRECTIONS (Questions 1 through 16): Each of the numbered items or incomplete statements in this section is followed by answers or by completions of the statement. Select the ONE lettered answer or completion that is BEST in each case.

Questions 1 through 16

1. A 42-year-old man presents with low-grade fever, fatigue, arthralgias, and myalgias. He noted a peculiar erythematous rash on his lower leg last week after clearing out a brush pile. The rash enlarged over the course of several days and had a clear center before finally fading away. After hearing this history, you would be suspicious of the possibility of

   (A) systemic lupus erythematosus (SLE)
   (B) rheumatoid arthritis (RA)
   (C) Lyme disease
   (D) polymyalgia rheumatica
   (E) psoriatic arthritis

2. All of the following laboratory and radiologic findings are consistent with the diagnosis of osteoarthritis EXCEPT

   (A) normal to slightly elevated sedimentation rate
   (B) joint space narrowing, osteophytes, and subchondral sclerosis
   (C) clear synovial fluid on joint aspiration
   (D) elevated antinuclear antibody test (ANA)
   (E) normal rheumatoid factor (RF)

3. Radionuclide bone scanning would be a particularly helpful test for making the diagnosis of

   (A) rheumatoid arthritis (RA)
   (B) systemic lupus erythematosus (SLE)
   (C) herniated intervertebral disc
   (D) metastatic bone lesions
   (E) polymyalgia rheumatica

4. Signs and symptoms associated with psoriatic arthritis include all of the following EXCEPT

   (A) urethritis
   (B) pain and stiffness of the distal interphalangeal joints
   (C) scaling plaques of the elbows and knees
   (D) pitting of the fingernails
   (E) "sausage" appearance of fingers and toes

5. A history of widespread musculoskeletal pain, pain to palpation in at least 11 of 18 specific sites, fatigue, stiffness, and non-restorative sleep are characteristic for

   (A) fibromyalgia
   (B) polymyalgia rheumatica
   (C) bursitis
   (D) tendinitis
   (E) osteoarthritis (OA)

6. Osteoarthritis (OA) is primarily a disorder of

   (A) synovial inflammation
   (B) autoimmune attack on the joints
   (C) crystalline deposits in joint fluid
   (D) postviral inflammation
   (E) cartilage destruction

7. All of the following lab findings are consistent with the diagnosis of rheumatoid arthritis EXCEPT

   (A) positive rheumatoid factor
   (B) elevated sedimentation rate
   (C) group II (inflammatory) synovial fluid analysis
   (D) mild hypochromic, normocytic anemia
   (E) elevated uric acid

8. A 40-year-old female presents with a history of acute onset of right-knee pain, chills, and sweats. Her temperature is 103.0°F. The right knee is erythematous and swollen with an effusion, and x-rays reveal only soft-tissue swelling. Arthrocentesis reveals 80,000/μL leukocytes with 90% polymorphonuclear cells, but no crystals. Gram stain is positive for gram-positive cocci. The patient's symptoms and physical and laboratory findings are most consistent with

   (A) gouty arthritis
   (B) osteoarthritis
   (C) gonococcal arthritis
   (D) bacterial septic arthritis
   (E) Lyme disease

9. The majority of clinical and pathological findings in rheumatoid arthritis (RA) are a result of chronic inflammation of

   (A) synovial membranes
   (B) epiphyseal disc
   (C) articular cartilage
   (D) periosteal membrane
   (E) subchondral bone

10. Which of the following tests is most useful in assessing the response to treatment of rheumatoid arthritis?

    (A) hemoglobin and hematocrit
    (B) sedimentation rate
    (C) rheumatoid factor
    (D) synovial fluid exam
    (E) white blood cell (WBC) count

11. All of the following are used in the treatment of rheumatoid arthritis (RA) EXCEPT

    (A) gold salts
    (B) colchicine
    (C) nonsteroidal anti-inflammatory drugs (NSAIDs)
    (D) methotrexate
    (E) aspirin

12. Patients with rheumatoid arthritis (RA) can present with many types of deformities of the hand. Hyperextension of the proximal interphalangeal (PIP) joint, in conjunction with flexion at the distal interphalangeal (DIP) joint, constitutes what deformity?

    (A) Dupuytren's contracture
    (B) mallet finger
    (C) swan neck deformity
    (D) boutonniere deformity
    (E) trigger finger

13. Ossification of the annulus, fibrosis of the intervertebral disc, and longitudinal ligament (bamboo spine) appearing on x-ray are classically associated with which of the following diseases?

    (A) systemic lupus erythematosus (SLE)
    (B) osteoarthritis (OA)
    (C) degenerative disc disease
    (D) ankylosing spondylitis
    (E) post-traumatic changes from a compression fracture

14. A 52-year-old man presents with severe right-ankle pain for 2 days and no other complaints. During the exam, the joint is erythematous and warm, and an effusion is noted. The patient is afebrile; his white blood cell count is 9,000, with normal differential; his blood urea nitrogen (BUN) and creatinine levels are within normal limits. Synovial fluid analysis shows 40,000/μL leukocytes with 50% polymorphonuclear cells, with presence of negatively birefringent, needle-like crystals. Uric acid level is 9.6 mg/dL (normal is 2.5 to 8 mg/dL). The most likely diagnosis is

    (A) rheumatoid arthritis
    (B) osteoarthritis
    (C) pseudogout
    (D) gouty arthritis
    (E) bacterial septic arthritis

15. An 82-year-old man presents with a 1-month history of bilateral pain and weakness in his shoulders. He has no prior history of trauma, overuse, arthritis, or musculoskeletal problems. Physical exam is unremarkable except for difficulty raising his arms above shoulder height. An erythrocyte sedimentation rate (ESR) is significantly elevated, but other lab tests are essentially normal. His MOST likely diagnosis is

    (A) fibromyalgia
    (B) polymyalgia rheumatica
    (C) temporal arteritis
    (D) bursitis
    (E) rheumatoid arthritis (RA)

16. A 10-year-old child presents with acute onset of right-knee pain, inflamed conjunctiva, mild burning with urination, and a history of fever and diarrhea 1 week prior. The MOST likely diagnosis is

    (A) juvenile rheumatoid arthritis (JRA)
    (B) joint sepsis
    (C) Reiter's syndrome
    (D) ankylosing spondylitis
    (E) systemic lupus erythematosus (SLE)

DIRECTIONS (Questions 17 through 26): Each group of items in this section consists of lettered headings followed by a set of numbered words or phrases. For each numbered word or phrase, select the ONE lettered heading that is most closely associated with it. Each lettered heading may be selected once, more than once, or not at all.

Questions 17 through 21

Match the following diseases with the most appropriate description and physical findings.

   (A) A multisystem disease characterized by persistent inflammatory synovitis, usually symmetrical and polyarticular, with morning stiffness. The proximal interphalangeal (PIP) and metacarpophalangeal (MCP) joints are frequently involved.
   (B) A multisystem disorder characterized by fibrotic infiltration of the skin and various organ systems. Raynaud's phenomenon, fibrosis of the skin (scleroderma), and hypomotility of the esophagus are common.
   (C) The earliest changes in this disease are frequently found in the sacroiliac joints of young men. The disease is strongly associated with histocompatibility antigen HLA-B27.
   (D) It may affect any joint, usually limited to one or few joints, and laboratory investigation is usually unremarkable.
   (E) It may involve virtually any organ system; common features include fatigue, fever, weight loss, and skin rashes (particularly malar rashes over both cheeks).

17. Progressive systemic sclerosis (PSS)

18. Rheumatoid arthritis (RA)

19. Systemic lupus erythematosus (SLE)

20. Ankylosing spondylitis (AS)

21. Osteoarthritis (OA)

Questions 22 through 26

Match each of the following patients with low-back pain with their MOST likely diagnosis.

(A) A 34-year-old man noticed onset of low-back pain after lifting a heavy box. He has some tenderness, paravertebral muscle spasm, and limitation of motion, but no radicular pain or neurological findings. He has a temperature of 100.8°F and a history of IV drug use.

(B) A 78-year-old woman with marked thoracic kyphosis presents with back pain after a simple fall in her home. She has point tenderness at about the T10 level and some paravertebral muscle spasm. Her range of motion is limited by both age and pain, but there are no neurological findings and she is afebrile.

(C) A 38-year-old overweight man has low-back pain after a weekend of gardening. He has limited range of motion and marked paravertebral muscle spasm, but is afebrile and has a normal neurological exam.

(D) A 72-year-old man with unexplained weight loss develops unrelenting back pain that does not respond to rest. His back and neurological exams are relatively normal and he is afebrile.

(E) A 42-year-old man complains of low-back pain that radiates down the side of his right leg. His knee and ankle reflexes are intact, but there is an area of numbness between his right first and second toes, and his right big toe is weak on dorsiflexion. His pain can be reproduced by straight leg raising.

22. Lumbar strain

23. Herniated disk

24. Vertebral osteomyelitis

25. Vertebral compression fracture

26. Vertebral metastasis

Answers and Explanations

1. **(C)** Low-grade fever, fatigue, myalgias, and arthralgias can be caused by a variety of rheumatological and nonrheumatological disorders. This patient's history of outdoors exposure followed by a rash should suggest an exposure of some sort—in this case, to a tick bite. The characteristic rash of Lyme disease, known as *erythema migrans,* starts as an erythematous macule or papule. It expands outward, often has a clear center, and resolves spontaneously. The rash of SLE is usually on the face and is often worse with sun exposure. Psoriatic arthritis is usually associated with the typical chronic erythema and plaques of psoriatic skin disease. Polymyalgia rheumatica is typically a disease of adults older than 55. *(Noble, p. 1196)*

2. **(D)** The laboratory investigation in osteoarthritis (OA) is mostly helpful in excluding other joint disease. There is no single diagnostic test for OA. Rheumatoid factor and antinuclear antibody (ANA) tests are negative; the erythrocyte sedimentation rate is usually normal to slightly elevated in patients with generalized or erosive OA. Synovial fluid exam reveals clear, straw-colored fluid with a low leukocyte count. The peripheral white blood cell count is usually normal. A roentgenographic exam usually shows narrowing of the interosseous joint space resulting from destruction of articular cartilage, osteophytes at the margins of affected joints, and subchondral sclerosis. *(Noble, p. 1096)*

3. **(D)** Bone scan abnormality is due to increased osteoblastic activity. Therefore, radionuclide bone scanning is useful in searching for neoplastic, reactive, reparative, or metabolic processes affecting bone. Occult fractures, metastatic disease, and osteomyelitis are examples of clinical problems where bone scans may reveal pathology not immediately evident on plain films. *(Ravel, pp. 390–391)*

4. **(A)** Psoriatic arthropathy is a common disease, that occurs in about 20% of individuals with psoriasis, particularly in those patients with psoriatic nail disease. It is associated with a synovitis generally indistinguishable from rheumatoid arthritis (RA). Arthritis of the distal interphalangeal joints of the hands is one potential pattern. Dactylitis, or sausage digits, of the fingers and toes is another. In some individuals there can be erosive, inflammatory joint changes that are usually polyarticular and occasionally can be severe, even mutilating. Psoriasis classically presents with plaques over the elbows and knees, but can appear over the thorax as well. Pitting of fingernails with lifting and flaring can be associated with psoriasis, though urethritis is not. The combination of urethritis and arthritis should suggest Reiter's syndrome. *(Noble, pp. 1154–1155)*

5. **(A)** Fibromyalgia is a generalized musculoskeletal pain syndrome characterized by diffuse soft-tissue pain associated with physical findings of multiple tender points. The American College of Rheumatology in 1990 established criteria for the diagnosis of fibromyalgia, which include pain on palpation of at least 11 specific tender point sites. Symptoms of fatigue, morning stiffness, and nonrestorative sleep are common. Physical exam and laboratory workup are usually negative. Other possibilities in the differential diagnosis, such as hypothyroidism or various rheumatologic diseases, can usually be identified or excluded on the basis of specific physical or lab abnormalities. *(Noble, pp. 1126–1128)*

6. **(E)** OA is a degenerative disease of cartilage that increases steadily with age. Trauma, obesity, and altered joint anatomy are contributing factors. Synovial inflammation is the hallmark of RA. SLE is a prototypical autoimmune disease. Crystalline deposits in synovial fluid is the cause of inflammation in gout and pseudogout. A number of viruses may cause arthritis and arthralgias, but viruses are not implicated in the pathogenesis of OA. *(Tierney et al, pp. 751–752)*

7. **(E)** Elevated uric acid is usually associated with gout. Rheumatoid factor may be absent in the first year of symptoms, but is eventually positive in the majority of patients with RA. Sedimentation rate is a sensitive, but nonspecific, indicator of inflammation that is usually elevated in active RA. Synovial fluid is obtained by arthrocentesis and classified into Group I (noninflammatory), Group II (inflammatory), and Group III (septic) categories. RA is a classic cause of Group II synovial fluid. RA is one of several causes of a mild hypochromic or normochromic, normocytic anemia known as the "anemia of chronic disease." *(Tierney et al, p. 768)*

8. **(D)** This patient presents with an acute onset of fever and a monoarthritis. There are no x-ray findings consistent with bony pathology or an intra-articular foreign body. There is a markedly elevated synovial white count.

There are no urate crystals in the synovial fluid to support a diagnosis of gouty arthritis. Lyme disease is usually recognized clinically by an early, expanding, erythematous skin lesion (erythema chronicum migrans). One would not expect to find fever and an elevated synovial white count with osteoarthritis. These findings are most consistent with the diagnosis of bacterial septic arthritis. The Gram stain reveals gram-positive cocci, which would be consistent with *Staphylococcus* or *Streptococcus* infections, which cause the great majority of cases of septic arthritis in adults. *Neisseria gonorrhea* are gram-negative diplococci. Septic arthritis is a medical emergency. Failure to diagnose this condition rapidly has the potential to cause permanent damage to the involved joint. Septic arthritis typically affects one joint or a few asymmetric joints. Patients with septic arthritis usually present with an acute onset of pain, fever, erythema, and swelling of the affected joint; systemic signs of infection are common. Weight-bearing joints (most commonly the knee) and the wrist are most commonly involved. *(Tierney et al, pp. 790–791)*

9. **(A)** The classic presentation of RA is the result of chronic inflammation of synovial membranes. It is the formation of chronic granulation tissue (pannus) resulting from chronic synovitis that produces hydrolytic enzymes. These enzymes are capable of eroding articular cartilage, subchondral bone, ligaments, and tendons. *(Tierney et al, p. 767)*

10. **(B)** The erythrocyte sedimentation rate (ESR) is elevated in most patients with RA and roughly parallels the disease activity. Therefore, it becomes a useful parameter for assessing response to therapy. WBC counts are most often normal; only about 25% of patients are considered to have leukocytosis. Rheumatoid factor is not present in everyone with RA, especially in the first year of symptoms. There is some correlation between the degree of anemia and the initial severity of the illness in RA, but it does not correlate with disease activity. Synovial fluid analysis is helpful in establishing the initial diagnosis of RA, but is too invasive to justify as a rou-

tine follow-up test, unless one needs to rule out bacterial infection. *(Ravel, pp. 369–370)*

11. **(B)** Colchicine is a traditional agent used in the acute or chronic treatment of gout. Aspirin and other NSAIDs are traditional first-line treatment for pain and inflammation in RA. Earlier use of more aggressive disease-modifying antirheumatic drugs (DMARD), such as methotrexate and gold salts, is now advocated by many rheumatologists to prevent joint damage. *(Noble, pp. 1102–1104)*

12. **(C)** A hyperextension of the PIP joint in conjunction with flexion of the DIP joint describes a swan neck deformity. This deformity usually occurs in the index and middle fingers due to contraction of the interosseous and flexor muscles and tendons. Dupuytren's contracture is caused by thickening and shortening of the palmar and sometimes the plantar fascia. A mallet finger deformity is usually the result of a traumatic injury in which the extensor tendon of the distal phalanx is ruptured. Boutonniere deformity is also common in RA, but is a flexion deformity of the PIP joint and extension of the DIP joint. A trigger finger refers to flexor tendon sheath inflammation in association with the development of a tendon nodule, giving rise to a "locking" of the digit in flexion. *(Noble, p. 1100)*

13. **(D)** "Bamboo spine," as described in the question, is seen most frequently in patients with ankylosing spondylitis. SLE has no classical radiographic pattern; however, 15% of patients with SLE develop deforming arthritis, and 5% to 8% develop aseptic necrosis. Osteoarthritis radiographically reveals joint space narrowing, subchondral sclerosis, and osteophyte formation. Degenerative disc disease also shows joint space narrowing, and osteophyte formation and spondylolisthesis may be present. Post-traumatic changes from compression fractures usually involve anterior wedging of the vertebral body. *(Tierney et al, p. 788)*

14. **(D)** The patient presents with a monoarticular arthritis involving the ankle joint. The laboratory investigation reveals an elevated uric acid level, and synovial fluid exam shows the urate crystals classically seen in gouty arthritis. Acute, gouty arthritis tends to affect the lower extremities, particularly the metatarsal phalangeal (MTP) joint (75% of patients), but is also frequently seen in the tarsal joints and ankle. Bacterial septic arthritis is easily ruled out, as the patient has no fever, and one would expect a synovial white cell count in the range of 50,000 to 200,000. In rheumatoid arthritis, a monoarticular presentation is unlikely. Normal x-ray and presence of urate crystals in the joint fluid make the diagnosis of osteoarthritis remote. Pseudogout presents similarly to gout, but exam of the synovial fluid would show the rod-shaped crystals of calcium pyrophosphate. *(Tierney et al, pp. 753–755)*

15. **(B)** Polymyalgia rheumatica affects older adults (> age 50) and presents with pain and stiffness in the shoulder and/or pelvic girdle areas. Patients may also have nonspecific signs of fever, malaise, and weight loss. Anemia and an elevated sedimentation rate are the usual lab findings. It responds to low-dose steroids. Temporal arteritis is a closely related disease that also affects the elderly and is marked by an elevated ESR, but the presenting complaints are headache, scalp tenderness, and possible vision loss. It also responds to steroids. Blindness is a potential outcome of untreated temporal arteritis. Fibromyalgia usually affects a younger population and presents with widespread musculoskeletal pain and fatigue. Subacromial bursitis and acute tendinitis are part of the differential diagnosis of shoulder pain, but without a history of trauma or overuse are unlikely in this patient; the ESR would also not be elevated. RA can appear at any age, and an elevated ESR would be consistent with this diagnosis, but bilateral shoulder pain alone would be unusual. *(Tierney et al, pp. 783–784)*

16. **(C)** Reiter's syndrome has a classic triad of urethritis, conjunctivitis, and arthritis. It usually follows a venereal infection (*Chlamydia*) or dysentery (*Salmonella, Shigella, Campylobacter*, or *Yersinia* may be implicated). Many cases are associated with HLA-B27. There can be involvement of ligaments and tendons, along with joint involvement. It can manifest itself in skin lesions (keratoderma blennorrhagicum), which can be misdiagnosed. No cure exists for Reiter's syndrome, and symptomatic management includes the use of NSAIDs and steroid eye drops for recurrent uveitis. For patients with progressive disease, sulfasalazine, methotrexate, or other second-line agents may be effective. *(Noble, pp. 1150–1153)*

17. **(B)** PSS is a multisystem disorder characterized by inflammation, fibrosis, and degeneration of the integument. These problems are associated with similar changes and prominent vascular lesions in the gastrointestinal tract, synovium, heart, lung, and kidneys. Raynaud's phenomenon, fibrosis of the skin (scleroderma), and hypomotility of the esophagus are common. *(Tierney et al, pp. 777–778)*

18. **(A)** RA is a multisystem disease characterized by persistent inflammatory synovitis that is usually symmetrical, polyarticular, and associated with morning stiffness. RA is often associated with extra-articular involvement of other organ systems. Organs frequently affected include the skin, eye, cardiovascular system, respiratory system, spleen, and nervous system. *(Noble, pp. 1098–1100)*

19. **(E)** SLE is an acute and chronic inflammatory process of unknown etiology that may involve virtually every organ system. The clinical presentation of SLE is highly variable, and common features include fatigue, fever, weight loss, and the classic butterfly rash. Polyarthralgias and polyarthritis are the most common manifestations of SLE, occurring in 95% of patients. *(Tierney et al, pp. 774–775)*

20. **(C)** AS usually presents during young adulthood in a male-to-female ratio of 3:1. The earliest changes in this disease are frequently found in the sacroiliac joints. There is an association with histocompatibility antigen HLA-B27. Inflammatory ocular disease, particularly acute anterior uveitis, occurs in approximately one quarter of those patients with AS. *(Noble, pp. 1148–1149)*

21. **(D)** OA is the most frequently encountered disorder of connective tissue affecting the joints in humans. It is a disease of both the articular cartilage and the subchondral bone. It may affect any joint, but is usually limited to one or a few. There are no specific laboratory features of osteoarthritis. *(Noble, pp. 1093–1096)*

22. **(C)** The history and physical exam in this patient are consistent with simple lumbar muscle strain, especially given the absence of fever or neurological findings. *(Noble, pp. 1033–1034)*

23. **(E)** Radicular pain and a positive straight leg raising test are hallmarks of nerve root impingement caused by a herniated intervertebral disc. Loss of big toe dorsiflexion and numbness in the web space between the first and second toes are consistent with a herniation at the L4–5 level. Herniation at the L5–S1 level often produces a diminished or absent ankle reflex, while herniation at the L3–4 level results in a diminished or absent knee reflex. *(Noble, pp. 1033–1034)*

24. **(A)** The worrisome elements in this patient's presentation are the fever and the history of IV drug abuse. These would be suggestive of osteomyelitis. *(Noble, pp. 1033–1034)*

25. **(B)** Elderly women are at risk for vertebral osteoporosis, suggested here by the marked thoracic kyphosis. They can suffer consequent compression fractures after even minor trauma. *(Noble, p. 1031)*

26. (D) Elderly patients with unexplained weight loss should be investigated for possible cancer. The history of unrelenting back pain unresponsive to rest is not typical for simple muscular strain or disc syndromes. Cancers that frequently metastasize to bone include prostate, thyroid, breast, lung, and kidneys (mnemonic: "P.T. Barnum loves kids"). *(Noble, pp. 1033–1034; Ravel, p. 585)*

REFERENCES

Noble J (ed). *Textbook of Primary Care Medicine,* 2nd ed. St. Louis, MO: Mosby–Year Book; 1996.

Ravel R. *Clinical Laboratory Medicine,* 6th ed. St. Louis, MO: Mosby–Year Book; 1995.

Tierney LM, et al. *Current Medical Diagnosis and Treatment,* 36th ed. Stamford, CT: Appleton & Lange; 1997.

Internal Medicine: Hematology/Oncology
Questions

Ronald P. Grimm, BHS, PA-C

DIRECTIONS (Questions 1 through 5): Each group of items in this section consists of lettered headings followed by a set of numbered words or phrases. For each numbered word or phrase, select the ONE lettered heading that is most closely associated with it. Each lettered heading may be selected once, more than once, or not at all.

Questions 1 through 5

Most chemotherapeutic agents share some common toxicities such as nausea and vomiting, neutropenia, hair loss, and painful mouth sores. However, a few agents have special toxicities that target a specific organ or system and require these to be monitored during treatment. Match the side effects listed below with the drug that is MOST commonly associated.

- (A) bleomycin (Blenoxane)
- (B) cisplatin/carboplatin (Platinol, CDDP/Paralatin)
- (C) cyclophosphamide (Cytoxan, CTX)
- (D) doxorubicin (Adriamycin, Rubex)
- (E) 5-fluorouracil (5-FU)
- (F) vincristine (Oncovin, VCR)

1. Cardiomyopathy

2. Renal insufficiency

3. Pulmonary fibrosis

4. Peripheral neuropathy

5. Hemorrhagic cystitis

Questions 6 through 11

Tumor markers may be used to aid in the diagnosis of certain cancers. Although they should not be considered diagnostic of certain cancers but an indicator that a certain tumor may be present, these same markers also may be used to follow the progression of disease or evaluate how well treatments are progressing. Tumor markers can also be used for screening purposes. Match the primary tumor below with the MOST appropriate tumor marker. Use each answer only once.

- (A) ovary
- (B) carcinoid
- (C) myeloma
- (D) bone
- (E) hepatocellular
- (F) pancreas

6. AFP (alpha-fetoprotein)

7. CA 125

8. CA 19-9

9. Immunoglobulins (Bence–Jones protein)

10. 5-HIAA (5-hydroxyindoleacetic acid)

11. Alkaline phosphatase

DIRECTIONS (Questions 12 through 35): Each of the numbered items or incomplete statements in this section is followed by answers or by completions of the statement. Select the ONE lettered answer or completion that is BEST in each case.

Questions 12 through 35

12. Obtaining a biopsy and pathological diagnosis is an essential step in the evaluation of cancer. The histological type of a tumor can be an important prognostic factor, as well as a determinant in planning treatment. Regarding lung cancer, in which of the following histological subtypes would chemotherapy be the initial choice of therapy versus surgery?

    (A) squamous cell
    (B) adenocarcinoma
    (C) small cell
    (D) mesothelioma
    (E) cystic adenoid carcinoma

13. A 33-year-old Filipino female is found to have anemia during a pre-employment physical examination. She is asymptomatic except for occasional fatigue. Her past medical history is unremarkable except for a history of having to receive iron during each of two normal pregnancies. She uses no medication and denies alcohol use. She also denies any gynecological or gastrointestinal symptoms. Physical examination (including a stool hemoccult) and vital signs are normal. Complete blood count (CBC) confirms a mild decrease in hemoglobin (10.7 g/dL) and hematocrit (34.8). Her mean corpuscular volume (MCV), however, is very low (68 fl). Erythrocyte sedimentation rate, serum ferritin, serum iron, and total-iron-binding capacity (TIBC) are all normal. What is the MOST likely explanation for this patient's anemia?

    (A) early iron deficiency
    (B) anemia of chronic disease
    (C) occult hemorrhage
    (D) thalassemia
    (E) folate deficiency

14. The complete blood count (CBC) picture of iron deficiency anemia and anemia of chronic disease may occasionally look very similar. Which of the following distinguish anemia of chronic disease from iron deficiency anemia?

    (A) increased mean corpuscular volume (MCV)
    (B) decreased total iron-binding capacity (TIBC)
    (C) increased reticulocyte count
    (D) decreased serum ferritin
    (E) increased platelet count

15. A 64-year-old male who smokes two packs of cigarettes per day is seen in the ER for evaluation of increased weakness and mild paresthesia of his lower extremities. He is unable to stand without assistance. He notes progressive back pain for the 4 months. Three months ago he saw a physician assistant for the low-back pain and was given an nonsteroidal anti-inflammatory drug (NSAID) that did not relieve his pain. Over the past 7 days he has resorted to taking three tablets of his wife's Tylenol #3, every 3 hours to help lessen his pain. He denied any falls, trauma, fever, chills, myalgias, or arthralgias. What is the most likely diagnosis?

    (A) herniated lumbar disc
    (B) renal failure secondary to NSAID use
    (C) Guillain–Barré syndrome
    (D) cord compression secondary to metastatic carcinoma
    (E) constipation secondary to narcotic use

16. All of the following clinical signs and symptoms may be seen with thrombocytopenia EXCEPT

    (A) bleeding into the knee joint
    (B) prolonged bleeding occurring immediately after minor tissue injury
    (C) petechiae
    (D) bleeding controlled by local pressure
    (E) gastrointestinal bleeding

17. All of the following hemostatis disorders are associated with a prolonged partial thromboplastin time (PTT) EXCEPT

    (A) disseminated intravascular coagulation (DIC)

    (B) heparin anticoagulation

    (C) von Willebrand's disease

    (D) hemophilia A

    (E) immune thrombocytopenic purpura (ITP)

18. Initial therapy of idiopathic thrombocytopenic purpura (ITP) most commonly consists of

    (A) splenectomy

    (B) immunosuppressive agents

    (C) vitamin B_{12} injections

    (D) IV gamma globulin

    (E) corticosteroids

19. Transfusion of fresh frozen plasma (FFP) is the therapy of choice in controlling acute bleeding episodes in all the following coagulopathies EXCEPT

    (A) hemophilia B

    (B) factor XI deficiency

    (C) vitamin K deficiency

    (D) hemorrhagic diathesis of liver disease

    (E) hemophilia A

20. All of the health problems below are commonly associated with homozygous sickle cell anemia EXCEPT

    (A) cholelithiasis

    (B) congestive heart failure (CHF)

    (C) aseptic necrosis of the femoral head

    (D) gout

    (E) hepatic infarct

21. All of the following statements regarding polycythemia vera (PV) are true EXCEPT

    (A) erythropoietin levels are increased in PV

    (B) PV can progress to myelofibrosis

    (C) PV can progress to other hematological neoplasms

    (D) splenomegaly is commonly seen in PV

    (E) pruritis and hyperuricemia are common findings in PV

22. All of the following statements regarding chronic lymphocytic leukemia (CLL) are true EXCEPT

    (A) CLL and diffuse well-differentiated lymphocytic lymphoma are both neoplasms of B-cell origin and are so similar that they follow essentially the same clinical course.

    (B) CLL, which presents with massive splenomegaly, lymphadenopathy, and lymphocytosis, has a median survival time of 5 years.

    (C) Combination chemotherapy for CLL is routinely initiated at the time of diagnosis in an attempt to achieve decreased tumor load and possible remission as early in the disease process as possible.

    (D) A Coombs'-positive hemolytic anemia occurs in up to 20% of patients with CLL.

    (E) Patients who demonstrate anemia and/or thrombocytopenia at the time of diagnosis of CLL have a 2-year median survival.

23. A prolonged bleeding time is NOT found in which of the following clinical settings?

    (A) aspirin ingestion

    (B) von Willebrand's disease

    (C) thrombocytopenia

    (D) hemophilia A

    (E) none of the above

24. Which of the following side effects commonly occurs as a complication of radiation therapy for cancer?

    (A) infertility

    (B) neutropenia and thrombocytopenia

    (C) diarrhea

    (D) painful swallowing

    (E) all of the above

25. In treating chronic cancer pain, which of the following is NOT indicated for long-term control of pain due to cancer?

    (A) nonsteroidal anti-inflammatory drugs (NSAIDs)
    (B) nortriptyline (Pamelor)
    (C) meperidine (Demerol)
    (D) morphine
    (E) fentanyl patch (Duragesic Transdermal)

26. Two men, X and Y, 53 and 57 years old, are seen in the office for routine physical exams. Patient X had a prostate-specific antigen (PSA) level of 2.0 during his last exam. Patient Y had a PSA of 7.2 during his last exam. Both had normal rectal exams on previous exam and today's exam. The PSA results done last week are: patient X's PSA was 2.0 and now is 4.0; patient Y's PSA was 7.2 and now is 7.3. Which of the following is true?

    (A) Neither have high risk for cancer of the prostate based on PSAs.
    (B) Patient X has no risk of cancer of the prostate based on normal PSA values.
    (C) Patient Y has a high risk of cancer of the prostate based on high PSAs.
    (D) Patient X has risk of prostate cancer based on recent increase of PSA.
    (E) Both patients are at high risk for cancer of the prostate based on PSAs.

27. Screening tests have greatly reduced the incidence of death due to cancer and help to prolong survival. Which of the following answers are NOT considered routine screening tests for carcinoma?

    (A) Pap smear (cervical cancer)
    (B) chest x-ray (lung cancer)
    (C) mammography (breast cancer)
    (D) hemoccult stool screening (colon cancer)
    (E) none of the above (all are recommended for routine cancer screening)

28. A 68-year-old female insulin-dependent diabetic with oat cell carcinoma (small cell) of the lung without known metastases is undergoing treatment for her cancer. She is tolerat-ing her regimen well; however, she is not able to resume the good eating habits she had prior to diagnosis of cancer. She is not hungry. The best treatment option is

    (A) psychiatric consult and antidepressants
    (B) nasogastric feeding tube
    (C) total parenteral nutrition (TPN)
    (D) high-dose megestrol acetate (Megace)
    (E) prednisone

29. Regarding the anemia associated with folate deficiency, which of the following is NOT true?

    (A) The mean corpuscular volume (MCV) is elevated.
    (B) Alcholics are at increased risk for this disorder.
    (C) Associated neurological symptoms, such as peripheral neuropathy, are common.
    (D) The complete blood count (CBC) picture may be similar to that seen in vitamin B_{12} deficiency.
    (E) Folate requirements are increased in pregnancy.

30. Treatment of the underlying disease-precipitating factor is essential to successful management of disseminated intravascular coagulation (DIC). Common situations triggering this disorder include

    (A) bacterial sepsis
    (B) disseminated malignancy
    (C) catastrophic obstetrical event
    (D) massive trauma
    (E) all of the above

31. Which of the following is NOT associated with vitamin B_{12} deficiency?

    (A) anticonvulsant therapy
    (B) partial gastrectomy
    (C) strict vegetarian diet
    (D) Crohn's disease
    (E) fish tapeworm

32. A 60-year-old male is admitted to the hospital with recent changes in his sensorium.

With the exception of hypertension, he has been in good health. Preliminary labs show a calcium of 14.9 (moderately elevated) and a slightly lower-than-normal albumin. A chest x-ray shows a mass in the right lower lobe highly suggestive of primary carcinoma. Which of the following is the LEAST likely to be used in the treatment of the hypercalcemia of malignancy?

(A) furosemide (Lasix)
(B) D$_5$ 0.45 NS IV fluids at 150 cc/hr
(C) calcitonin (Calcimar/Miacalcin)
(D) pamidronate (Aredia)
(E) plicamycin (Mithramycin)

33. Problems common to multiple myeloma include

(A) pathological fractures
(B) hypercalcemia
(C) spinal cord compression
(D) hyperviscosity syndrome
(E) all of the above

34. Which of the following statements about chronic myelogenous leukemia (CML) is True?

(A) Initially single-agent therapy is used to reduce symptomotology and leukocytosis.
(B) Presentation of CML commonly includes splenomegaly, leukocytosis, and symptoms of hypermetabolism.
(C) The Philadelphia chromosome (Ph1) is present in 80% to 90% of CML patients.
(D) The majority of CML patients progress to a blastic phase that can be either myeloid or lymphoid.
(E) All of the above.

35. You are called to see a 47-year-old male who was admitted to your service in the hospital 48 hours ago. He smokes three packs of cigarettes a day, has abused alcohol, and has recently been diagnosed with adenocarcinoma of the lung with metastases to his brain and skeleton. He has received radiation to three bony sites and whole-brain radiation. The patient is now difficult to arouse. His respirations are seven per minute and pupils are pinpoint and equal. His exam earlier that day was normal. You remember that his MS Contin (morphine sulfate-controlled release) was increased from 30 mg q12 hours to 90 mg q8 hours to control his pain better. You feel that he is overdosed on the MS Contin and promptly give IV naloxone (Narcan). Within five minutes he is improving to baseline. You decrease the MS Contin and hold the next dose due at this time. Five hours later you are again called as this patient has recurrent symptoms. You reassess him. He has not received any further doses of MS Contin or morphine solution (for breakthrough pain). You hastily make a list of possibilities. Which of the following is the MOST likely scenario?

(A) embolic stroke
(B) brain metastases and the effects of radiation to the brain
(C) morphine overdose
(D) hypoxia secondary to tumor and long-term tobacco abuse
(E) hypercalcemia

Answers and Explanations

1. **(D); 2. (B); 3. (A); 4. (F); 5. (C)** Cardiomyopathy or myocarditis-pericarditis is associated with doxorubicin used in doses above 550 mg/m². Clinical manifestations include signs and symptoms of congestive heart failure (CHF), ECG changes, and arrhythmias. Many oncologists assess ejection fraction by multiple gated acquisition (MUGA) scan before and after doxorubicin therapy, especially in older patients. Cisplatin is associated with a cumulative renal insufficiency manifested by rising blood urea nitrogen (BUN) and creatinine. The risk of renal insufficiency is greatly reduced by adequate IV hydration and use of Lasix diuresis prior to administration of the drug. Cisplatin/carboplatin may also cause ototoxicity and other signs of peripheral neuropathy. With aggressive chemotherapy using cisplatin/carboplatin more long-term peripheral neuropathies are seen. Bleomycin causes pneumonitis and pulmonary fibrosis, especially when the total dose exceeds 400 units. Cough and dyspnea are common symptoms. Pulmonary function abnormalities include decreases in total lung volume, forced vital capacity, and DLCO. Bleomycin has also been associated with a fatal anaphylaxis-like reaction. For this reason, test doses of 2 units of the drug are often given prior to beginning therapy. Vincristine very commonly produces peripheral neuropathy manifested by some combination of paresthesias, decreased deep tendon reflexes (DTRs), muscle weakness, or cranial nerve dysfunction. Paralytic ileus may also occur. Hemorrhagic cystitis (occasionally massive) has been reported with cyclophosphamide therapy, especially when used in high doses. Adequate hydration and the occasional use of Mesna may prevent this complication. Ifosfamide, which is related to cyclophosphamide, is also associated with hemorrhagic cystitis. *(Holland et al, pp. 891–902)*

6. **(E); 7. (A); 8. (F); 9. (C); 10. (B); 11. (D)** Tumor markers can be used in the following areas; screening, diagnosis, and monitoring response to treatment or monitoring course of the cancer. Alpha-fetoprotein is a marker for hepatocellular carcinoma (monitors course of disease and treatment monitoring) and cancers involving yolk sac elements (testicular-germ cell tumors). Beta hCG (monitors diagnosis, prognosis, and treatment and course of disease) may also be used in testicular carcinoma. Ovarian cancer is monitored by CA 125, and high values indicate a poor prognosis. Pancreatic, colorectal, and gastric carcinoma can be followed by CA 19-9 (follows course of disease and monitors response to treatment) and CEA (carcinoembryonic antigen). The CEA tumor marker may also be used to monitor prognosis and response to treatment of gastrointestinal and pancreatic cancer. Breast cancer can also be monitored (course of disease or response to treatment) by CEA. Prostate cancer is monitored by PSA (prostate-specific antigen). But its use in screening is sometimes controversial. Bence–Jones proteins can be used to diagnose and help in prognostic indications for

multiple myeloma. 5-HIAA is indicative of carcinoid in the midgut and is useful in diagnosis. Bone cancer can be identified by alkaline phosphatase and is useful in diagnosis, prognosis, and monitoring course of disease or treatment regimens. Liver metastasis can also be monitored by alkaline phosphatase and lactate dehydrogenase (LDH). Other major tumor markers are thyroglobulin-thyroid, VMA (vanillylmandelic acid)-neuroblastoma, and calcitonin-medullary thyroid. *(Haskell, pp. 532–537)*

12. **(C)** Small-cell lung cancer (also called oat cell) represents approximately 20% of all lung cancers. It is an aggressive disease that is rapidly fatal if not treated in a timely fashion. Fortunately, tumor regression occurs in about 75% of patients treated with combination chemotherapy and radiation therapy. The other neoplasms are treated with surgery or radiation therapy. Their response to chemotherapeutic agents has been disappointing. *(Holland et al, pp. 1782–1791)*

13. **(D)** This clinical picture is most consistent with beta-thalassemia. The combination of Oriental race and an MCV disproportionately low to the level of anemia is a tipoff to the diagnosis. Diagnosis may usually be confirmed by demonstrating an elevated hemoglobin A_2 on hemoglobin electrophoresis. An MCV less than 75 fl is unusual with iron deficiency anemia. The normal serum iron and ferritin also rule out this diagnosis. While anemia of chronic disease may present with a microcytic picture, there is often a history of underlying chronic infection, renal disease, endocrine disease, or malignancy. In addition, patients with anemia of chronic disease usually have low serum iron with normal or increased serum ferritin. The erythrocyte sedimentation rate is very often increased with anemia of chronic disease. Hemorrhage should be evident from history and physical. In addition, microcytic anemias resulting from hemorrhage are usually due to iron deficiency. Folate deficiency produces a macrocytic anemia. *(Williams et al, pp. 585–590, 598–599)*

14. **(B)** Unlike iron deficiency, which characteristically exhibits an increased TIBC, anemia of chronic disease has a decreased TIBC. Apparently this is due to decreased transferrin synthesis, which occurs in many chronic conditions. Anemia of chronic disease may have a decreased MCV; however, it most commonly presents as a normocytic anemia. Decreased reticulocyte count and normal or increased serum ferritin are also typical of anemia of chronic disease. Platelet counts are usually not affected. *(Williams et al, p. 490–511, 518–524)*

15. **(D)** There is no history of strain or injury, and both legs are symptomatic, decreasing the chances that this gentleman has a herniated lumbar disc. Although renal failure can cause back pain, it does not cause paresthesia in both legs. NSAIDs are probably not the cause of this pain. Guillain–Barré can present as a distal weakness progressing proximally. There is no history of viral illness. This patient had generalized weakness and paresthesias. Although constipation (from the heavy narcotic use) may give him back pain, it would not cause weakness and paresthesias. Cord compression and back pain are frequently overlooked in early stages. Persistent back pain should always warrant a follow-up physical with evaluation for loss of sphincter tone and any other neurological deficits. CT scan or MRI are sometimes needed to confirm diagnosis. Initial treatment consists of emergency (stat) radiation/oncology consult, possible neurosurgery consult, and decadron. Doses of 10 to 20 mg of decadron IVP are given initially, then 4 to 10 mg IVP is administered q6 hours. *(Holland et al, pp. 3117–3122)*

16. **(A)** Hemarthrosis almost always indicates a coagulation factor deficiency rather than a problem with formation of the primary hemostatic platelet plug. The remaining clinical signs are not unusual with thrombocytopenia or disorders of platelet function. *(Williams et al, pp. 1169–1191, 1415, 1417, 1550–1551)*

17. **(E)** The PTT is prolonged in disorders affecting the intrinsic coagulation cascade (factors XII, XI, IX, and VIII), as well as from defects in the common coagulation pathway. Hemophilia A (factor VIII deficiency) is the most common intrinsic pathway disorder encountered clinically. DIC is associated with the consumption of multiple coagulation factors. The effects of heparin result partly from its interference with the synthesis of many of the intrinsic and common pathway factors. In addition, because factor VIII requires von Willebrand's factor to be functionally active, von Willebrand's disease often is associated with a mildly increased PTT. ITP affects the formation of the primary hemostatic plug and is not associated with coagulation factor deficiency. *(Williams et al, pp. 1278, 1295–1296, 1420, 1470)*

18. **(E)** A significant percentage of patients with ITP will normalize their platelet counts on high-dose prednisone, which is tapered after several weeks of therapy. If there is no response to this treatment regimen, or relapse occurs during or after tapering the steroids, splenectomy is usually considered. This is effective in significantly raising platelet counts in a high percentage of patients. Immunosuppressive agents (drugs such as cyclophosphamide, azathioprine, and vincristine) are generally considered only when both of the above have failed, because of serious potential toxicities. IV gamma globulin is used for temporary phagocytic blockade in situations such as impending surgery or ITP in late pregnancy. Its value is limited because improvement is usually limited to approximately 4 weeks' duration. Vitamin B_{12} is of no value in treating ITP. *(Williams et al, pp. 1290–1298)*

19. **(E)** The therapy of choice in hemophilia A (factor VIII deficiency) is infusion of partially purified factor VIII concentrate when available, or cryoprecipitate if it is not (this contains 50% of the factor VIII of FFP in 10% of the volume). Hemophilia B (factor IX deficiency) and factor XI deficiency must be differentiated from hemophilia A, because cryoprecipitate and factor VIII concentrate do not supply these factors effectively, whereas FFP does. FFP, rather than vitamin K, is the therapy of choice for acute bleeding in vitamin K deficiency (as well as oral anticoagulant overdose) because it immediately supplies the diminished prothrombin factors (II, VII, IX, X, and proteins C and S) needed for hemostasis. Purified prothrombin complexes are avoided because these entail a high risk of thrombotic events. Administration of vitamin K (parenterally) requires 8 to 10 hours to permit normal factor synthesis. The hemorrhagic diathesis of liver disease involves vitamin K deficiency, decreased production of multiple coagulation factors, and increased production of coagulation inhibitors. Only FFP can immediately supply enough of the deficient factors to control acute hemorrhage, although vitamin K administration may be helpful in long-term management. *(Williams et al, pp. 1649–1659)*

20. **(D)** Gout has no specific association with sickle cell anemia. Cholelithiasis is commonly associated with sickle cell anemia because of the icterus that occurs secondary to chronic hemolysis and must always be kept in mind when evaluating the sickle cell patient with abdominal pain (ie, one cannot automatically assume that such pain is due to sickle cell crisis). Chronic anemia and hypoxemia often lead to a chronic hyperdynamic cardiac state and later to CHF. Skeletal infarction can readily lead to aseptic necrosis of the femoral head. Hepatic infarcts are common and can lead to significant hepatic parenchymal damage. *(Williams et al, pp. 616–628)*

21. **(A)** In *secondary* polycythemia, erythropoietin is increased in an effort to compensate for chronic hypoxia (as in chronic pulmonary disease, high-altitude dwelling, congenital heart disease, Pickwickian syndrome, increased methemoglobin or sulfhemoglobin states), or due to conditions such as Cushing's syndrome and tumors (particularly renal). In PV, erythropoietin is *decreased* or absent, leukocyte alkaline phosphatase is increased, B_{12} is within normal limits or increased, and hyperuricemia, thrombocytosis, and leukocytosis are common. Clinical features, mostly due to increased blood viscos-

ity, may include plethora, headaches, gout, fatigue/malaise, pruritis, edema, thrombotic or bleeding events, splenomegaly, and acne rosacea. Approximately 30% of patients with PV go on to develop myelofibrosis, and up to 15% may develop leukemias (or, less commonly, lymphomas). Intermittent phlebotomy is a safe mode of therapy. Myelosuppression is recommended in the advent of symptomatic thrombocytosis, rapidly enlarging spleen, or symptoms of hypermetabolism. This can be achieved with radioactive P32 every 3 months as needed, or chemotherapeutic agents such as melphalan, busulfan, chlorambucil, or hydroxyurea. There is fear that myelosuppressive therapy may increase the risk of later leukemia or lymphoma, so phlebotomy alone is usually tried as initial therapy. (*Williams et al, pp. 714–723*)

22. **(C)** Chronic lymphocytic leukemia is a disease that usually appears in the fourth or fifth decade of life or later and is characterized by increased mature-appearing lymphocytes in the peripheral blood, associated with spleen, node, and bone marrow infiltration by a B-cell neoplasm. It is clinically indistinguishable from diffuse, well-differentiated, lymphocytic lymphoma. It is a relatively indolent disease that often presents with massive hepatosplenomegaly, peripheral lymphocytosis, and occasionally with lymphadenopathy, with surprisingly few symptoms. It is often picked up on routine exam or complete blood count (CBC). Stage A—lymphocytosis ± mild lymphadenopathy—has a median survival of more than 7 years. Stage B—lymphocytosis, larger lymphadenopathy, and hepatosplenomegaly—has a median survival of 5 years. Stage C—Stage B findings plus anemia and/or thrombocytopenia—has a 2-year median survival. No potentially curative therapy regimen has been found. Single alkylating agents, such as low-dose daily or pulse high-dose chorambucil, or pulse cyclophosphamide, are indicated to palliate hemolytic anemia, symptomatic organomegaly or lymphadenopathy, or systemic symptoms (such as fever, weight loss, fatigue, night sweats). Steroid therapy may be of value in instances of hemolytic anemia, which occurs

in about 20% of CLL patients, or autoimmune thrombocytopenia (differentiated from thrombocytopenia secondary to neoplastic marrow invasion by presence of antiplatelet antibodies and increased megakaryocytes in the marrow). Splenectomy may be helpful if such problems fail to respond to steroids, but is not otherwise indicated. Radiation therapy may control localized symptomatic disease; interferon is of no value. Hairy cell leukemia, another adult lymphoid leukemia (seen predominantly in males over 40 years old) must be differentiated from CLL, as interferon *is* very effective in such patients with progressive disease, and alkylating agents are poorly tolerated. As in the other leukemias, infection is a major problem in patients with progressing disease; thus, early diagnosis of infection and initiation of appropriate therapy are essential. (*Williams et al, pp. 1017–1033*)

23. **(D)** The bleeding time is a sensitive screening test for defects in primary hemostasis—the formation of an adequate platelet plug. Aspirin interferes with platelet aggregation, and von Willebrand's disease affects platelet adhesion. With thrombocytopenia, the risk of minor spontaneous hemorrhage increases when the platelet count falls below 50,000. More serious bleeding occurs at platelet counts below 20,000. With hemophilia A, primary hemostasis is not affected, and the bleeding time is normal. The defect in hemophilia A prevents the formation of an adequate fibrin clot (secondary hemostasis). (*Williams et al, pp. 1281–1360, 1458–1480, 1551–1552*)

24. **(E)** Ionizing radiation affects cells that are actively replicating. In addition to neoplastic cells, this includes normal hematopoietic stem cells in the bone marrow, the mucosal lining of the mouth and gastrointestinal tract, gonadal germ cells, and hair follicles. Pulmonary fibrosis, cataracts, and secondary malignancies (especialy leukemia) can also complicate radiation therapy. (*Holland et al, pp. 294–296, 716–717*)

25. **(C)** Morphine and fentanyl are mainstays of treatment of chronic pain in cancer patients.

NSAIDs can be either initiated at the start of treatment for pain or added to morphine. Trisalicylate (Trilisate) is used commonly. It comes in pill and liquid forms and is usually well tolerated from the gastric standpoint. Trilisate does not cause thrombocytopenia in normal dosing. Nortriptyline, imipramine (Tofranil), and amitriptyline (Elavil) are excellent adjuvants in decreasing neuropathic pain. Meperidine used in chronic pain management accumulates metabolites (with long half-life) that produce central nervous system irritability (seizures may be difficult to treat). Although meperidine is often chosen to lessen spasm at the sphincter of Oddi rather than morphine, tests show that in actuality, they are about equal. Fentanyl can make sphincter of Oddi spasms potentially worse. High-dose steroids may also be used in pain management but should be reserved for the final 2 or 3 weeks of a patient's life. A new antiseizure medication, gabapentin (Neurontin) also has been noted to be an effective adjuvant medicine in the treatment of neuropathic pain. Studies are ongoing and are promising at this date. *(DeVita et al, pp. 2428–2431; Haskell, pp. 235–236)*

26. **(D)** PSA values between 4.0 and 10.0 are usually a result of benign conditions. Patient Y probably has much less chance of prostate cancer with no change in his PSA level from 1 year ago. Men who are later found to have cancer of the prostate have a rise in PSA of greater than or equal to 0.75 ng/mL/year. Patient X had doubled his PSA and must be considered at higher risk for cancer of the prostate. Further evaluation and follow-up are warranted. *(Haskell, p. 552)*

27. **(B)** Screening recommendations vary among the American Cancer Society, National Cancer Institute, and Canadian and European cancer organizations. But there is agreement that the chest x-ray should not be part of the routine cancer screening at the present time. In large series of patients, evaluating screening sputum and chest x-ray showed no significant reduction in mortality from lung cancer even in high-risk patients. *(Haskell, pp. 14–17).*

The American Cancer Society recommends routine screening for skin cancer (complete skin exam), breast cancer (breast self-exam and mammography), cervical cancer (Pap and pelvic exam), prostate (digital rectal exam and prostate specific antigen), colon cancer (fecal occult and sigmoidoscopy). Time intervals between exams and ages of patients to be examined can be variable among the various cancer organizations. See recent guidelines for updated recommendations. *(Haskell, p. 16)*

28. **(D)** It has been difficult to find a "magic pill" to enhance appetite in cancer patients. One medicine that has consistently helped patients in small studies is Megace. It enhances appetite significantly even in advanced cancer. Megace is a progestational agent used to treat advanced breast cancer. It must be given in high doses and usually given in liquid form (rather than have a patient take 10 to 20 pills per day). It is given in doses of 400 to 800 mg per day. Disadvantages are high cost and some occasional edema of the lower extremities. Formation of blood clots may potentially be a hazard, but there has been little evidence to suggest this. The patient is not obviously depressed, and antidepressants will offer little. Feeding tubes are a good choice, but many patients dislike the social issues surrounding them and too frequently refuse to leave them in. TPN would require marshaling forces to be maintained at home. Prednisone is also a good appetite stimulant, but side effects for long-term use probably make this a less than optimal choice. Giving steroids to this diabetic would not be in her best interest. *(Loprinzi et al, pp. 8–12; Haskell, pp. 225–226)*

29. **(C)** The anemia of folate deficiency is associated with an increased MCV and is indistinguishable from the CBC picture of vitamin B_{12} deficiency. Dietary deficiencies in the alcoholic can lead to folate deficiency. B_{12} deficiency is associated with demyelinating neuropathies manifested by paresthesias, decreased vibratory sense, ataxia, or dementia. Folate deficiency is not associated with neu-

rological disease. This can be used clinically to differentiate folate deficiency from B$_{12}$ deficiency. (*Williams et al, pp. 473–481*)

30. **(E)** Management of DIC has several components: (1) Control of major symptoms. Administration of fresh frozen plasma, cryoprecipitate, and/or platelets to replace depleted blood components and prevent exsanguination, and heparin when thrombosis and/or incipient gangrene are evident. (2) Treatment of the triggering disorder. Broad-spectrum antibiotic therapy after appropriate cultures are obtained in suspected sepsis, prompt delivery of fetus and placenta in the event of abruptio placenta, extraction of a retained dead fetus, surgical intervention after trauma, and aggressive antitumor therapy (if possible) in the setting of malignancy, etc. (3) Heparin prophylaxis where (2) is not rapidly manageable and chronic DIC is likely, for example, in acute promyelocytic leukemia, unresectable or disseminated malignancy, when surgical intervention must be postponed, and fat or amniotic fluid embolus. (Automatic initiation of heparin therapy, other than in the above situations, is controversial.) (*Williams et al, pp. 1497–1511*)

31. **(A)** General causes of vitamin B$_{12}$ deficiency include: gastric malabsorption due to diminished or absent intrinsic factor after partial or total gastrectomy or in pernicious anemia; intestinal malabsorption, as in Crohn's disease, blind loop syndrome, chronic pancreatitis, fish tapeworm, strict vegetarian diet (B$_{12}$ is found only in animal products); and abnormal metabolism, which can be congenital or acquired (secondary to nitrous oxide exposure). Therapy consists of B$_{12}$ intramuscularly (there are several dose/frequency regimens). Anticonvulsant therapy can cause a macrocytic anemia due to *folate* deficiency. Lead poisoning causes a hypochromic anemia by interfering with hemoglobin synthesis, and some degree of hemolysis. (*Williams et al, pp. 475–481*)

32. **(B)** Calcitonin, which inhibits reabsorption of calcium in bone, increases filter calcium by

decreasing tubular reabsorption of calcium; Pamidronate, which inhibits bone reabsorption and increases urinary secretion of calcium; and Plicamycin, an antineoplastic agent that may lower calcium levels by inhibiting the effects of parathyroid hormone upon osteoclasts, are all medicines used to lower high serum calcium levels and can be most effective. Furosemide can facilitate the loss of calcium by diuresis. However, the key to treatment of hypercalcemia is hydration with normal saline (not D$_5$ 0.45 NS). The saline load on the distal loop increases the amount of calcium excreted in urine. Furosemide also will facilitate loss of calcium at this level. Note that thiazide diuretics should be avoided because it may induce renal calcium absorption in exchange for sodium. (*Haskell, p. 255*)

33. **(E)** Multiple myeloma is a malignant neoplasm of the plasma cell, usually producing a monoclonal immunoglobulin increase (seen on protein and/or urine electrophoresis). This disease tends to create multiple osteolytic lesions (best demonstrated on skeletal survey rather than bone scan) that are often very painful and can lead to pathological fractures, increased osteoporosis, hypercalcemia, and spinal cord compression. The excessive protein production can cause CNS symptoms due to hyperviscosity (confusion, paresthesias, somnolence, headache, and hemiplegia or coma when severe), amyloid deposition in (and failure of) multiple organs, and proteinuria/nephrotic syndrome. Tumor invasion of the bone marrow can cause depression of WBC, RBC, and/or platelets, hypogammaglobulinemia, and markedly increased susceptibility to infection. Cryoglobulin production and platelet dysfunction are common, and renal failure can occur as a result of amyloidosis, urate nephropathy, and other disorders. Radiation therapy may be of great value in controlling painful bone symptoms or impending cord compression. Chemotherapy is used to treat the systemic disease, usually consisting of pulse therapy with an alkylating agent (melphalan, cyclophosphamide, or chlorambucil) plus a steroid, and can achieve

remission (although not cure). Allopurinol helps minimize hyperuricemia, and good hydration assists clearance of calcium and light protein chains. Plasmapheresis may be appropriate in severe hyperviscosity syndrome, and prompt assessment and treatment of infection is essential. *(Williams et al, pp. 1109–1123)*

34. **(E)** Chronic myelogenous leukemia (CML) is a neoplasm of the multipotent hematopoietic stem cell that most commonly is found in middle-aged patients. The chronic phase is characterized by an elevated total WBC, predominantly granulocytic (but it is not uncommon to have increased eosinophil and/or basophil counts), with less than 5% blasts in blood and marrow, low or absent leukocyte alkaline phosphatase (LAP), and presence of a specific chromosome marker called the Philadelphia (Ph1) chromosome (a translocation of chromosomes 22 and 9) in 80% to 95% of patients. These studies are valuable in differentiating CML from leukemoid reactions (such as LAP, no Ph1 chromosome), myelofibrosis (such as normal LAP, no Ph1 chromosome), and other myeloproliferative disorders. Presentation often includes splenomegaly, leukocytosis with anemia (platelet counts are variable), hypermetabolism (weight loss, fever, hyperuricemia, sweating), and arthralgias; lymphoadenopathy may be present, and thrombohemorrhagic events may occur. Single-agent theapy (busulfan, cyclophosphamide, melphalan, or hydroxyurea) may be used to decrease the leukocytosis and symptomatology. It does not clear the Ph1 chromosome abnormality from the marrow—it simply diminishes tumor load enough to remove the immature cells from the blood. It has not been demonstrated that conventional combination chemotherapy improves survival, although promising results are being achieved with intensive chemotherapy and radiation therapy followed by HLA-matched bone marrow transplantation early in the chronic phase. Allopurinol decreases the hyperuricemia, which often otherwise increases on initiation of chemotherapy. Splenectomy is helpful only in relieving symptoms of hypersplenism and does not change the overall course of the disease. Approximately 50% of patients will accelerate to a blastic phase or crisis, resembling acute leukemia within 3 to 4 years, and almost all patients ultimately continue on to this state. Blastic crises may be myeloid in origin in two thirds of cases, and lymphoid in one third, consistent with the stem cell level of disease process. The blastic phase is usually very resistant to treatment, including bone marrow transplantation, and most patients die within 6 weeks of diagnosis of conversion to this phase, although the lymphoid cases may briefly respond. *(Williams et al, pp. 298–309)*

35. **(C)** The history reveals that the patient had an inappropriate increase in his dose of MS Contin (from 30 mg q12 hours to 90 mg q8 hours). Most drug increases in pain management should be only in the range of 25% to 50% over a 24-hour period. (This patient had over a 400% increase in medication.) Because MS Contin is sustained release, another wave of medication was released and the patient again became overdosed. Reoccuring overdosage symptoms are common in treating MS Contin overdosages. Giving naloxone is appropriate if respirations become below 8 per minute or if there is any respiratory compromise. The pinpoint pupils indicate the medicine is working (maybe too well). Care should be given when administering naloxone as it can precipitate a morphine withdrawal. A safe way to administer naloxone is to mix one amp in a 10-cc syringe of saline and administer the solution in 1-cc increments until proper level of alertness is obtained. This method allows you to titrate the patient and still maintain good pain control and avoid a withdrawal reaction. *Note:* MS Contin is given every 8 or 12 hours, never every 6 hours. It should not be used as a PRN medication. Morphine solution is the drug of choice for breakthrough pain in patients who can take medications by mouth. Hypercalcemia would not improve with naloxone and is usually insidious. Hypoxia would nor-

mally make the respiratory rate increase. Stroke and brain metastases do not usually present in this fashion. *(Ellison, pp. 409–419; Haskell, pp. 324–238)*

REFERENCES

DeVita VT, Heilman SL, Rosenberger SA (eds). *Cancer Principle and Practice of Oncology,* 4th ed. Philadelphia: Lippincott; 1993.

Ellison NM. Pharmacologic management: The opioid analgesics. *Hem/Onc Annals.* 1994; 12: 409–419.

Haskell CM (ed). *Cancer Treatment,* 4th ed. Philadelphia: Saunders; 1995.

Holland JF, Frei E, Bast RC, et al (eds). *Cancer Medicine,* 4th ed. Philadelphia: Lea & Febiger; 1997.

Loprinzi CL, Ellison NM, Goldberg RM, et al. Alleviation of cancer anorexia and cachexia: Studies of the Mayo Clinic and the North Central Cancer Treatment Group. *Sem Oncol.* 1990; 17: 8–12.

Williams WJ, Beutler E, Erslev AJ, et al (eds). *Hematology,* 5th ed. New York: McGraw-Hill; 1995.

CHAPTER 6

Pharmacology
Questions

Doris Rapp, PharmD, PA-C

DIRECTIONS (Questions 1 through 28): Each of the numbered items or incomplete statements in this section is followed by answers or by completions of the statement. Select the ONE lettered answer or completion that is BEST in each case.

Questions 1 through 28

1. The treatment of choice of dermatophytosis involving the hair and nails is

    (A) selenium sulfide
    (B) griseofulvin
    (C) clotrimazole
    (D) haloprogin
    (E) tolnaftate

2. The first-line drugs presently used against tuberculosis include

    (A) isoniazid, streptomycin, and ethambutol
    (B) isoniazid, ethambutol, rifampin, streptomycin, and pyrazinamide
    (C) isoniazid, streptomycin, cycloserine, rifampin, and ethionamide
    (D) isoniazid, ethambutol, and cycloserine
    (E) isoniazid, viomycin, and cycloserine

3. All of the following are true of H-1 antagonists EXCEPT

    (A) They block the action of histamine that results in increased capillary permeability.
    (B) They inhibit gastric secretions.

    (C) They inhibit the vasoconstrictor effects of histamine on respiratory smooth muscle.
    (D) They inhibit most responses of smooth muscle to histamine.
    (E) They suppress the "flare" component of the action of histamine.

4. When strict adherence to dietary changes is insufficient to lower an elevated cholesterol, the drug of first choice in further treatment is

    (A) a bile acid-binding resin, such as cholestyramine
    (B) nicotinic acid
    (C) HMG Co-A reductase inhibitor (eg, lovastatin)
    (D) fibric acid derivative (eg, gemfibrozil)
    (E) probucol

5. When propranolol is to be used in the treatment of sinus tachycardia, the presence of another disease may be a relative contraindication or at least a precaution to its use. All the following are considered such precautions EXCEPT

    (A) congestive heart failure
    (B) asthma
    (C) hypertension
    (D) type I diabetes mellitus
    (E) AV block

6. Which of the following micronutrients is considered to have the narrowest therapeutic index?

 (A) zinc
 (B) molybdenum
 (C) selenium
 (D) manganese
 (E) magnesium

7. All of the following beta-adrenergic agonists are classified as beta$_2$-specific EXCEPT

 (A) albuterol
 (B) isoproterenol
 (C) terbutaline
 (D) pirbuterol
 (E) bitolterol

8. All of the following statements are true regarding the use of acyclovir in the treatment of herpes simplex EXCEPT

 (A) Acyclovir ointment is used for the treatment of HSV-1 only.
 (B) The infusion of IV acyclovir should be given slowly over 1 hour to prevent renal tubular damage.
 (C) Headache and gastrointestinal discomfort are the most frequent adverse reactions to continuous acyclovir administration.
 (D) The dosage for chronic suppressive therapy is 200 mg three to five times per day.
 (E) Absorption of oral acyclovir is unaffected by food.

9. Mr. Brown has developed itching, crusted lesions in his beard area. New lesions develop each time he shaves. A bacterial culture from a lesion showed *Staphylococcus aureus* (coagulase positive) and beta-hemolytic *Streptococcus*. Mr. Brown is allergic to penicillin. The appropriate course of therapy would be to start the patient on

 (A) Burow's compresses and topical steroids
 (B) topical antibiotics and wait for the report of antibiotic sensitivity
 (C) Burow's compresses, topical steroids, and dicloxacillin 250 mg four times a day
 (D) Burow's compresses, topical steroids, and erythromycin 250 mg four times a day
 (E) Burow's compresses and wait for report of antibiotic sensitivity

10. An aminoglycoside antibiotic, such as gentamicin, would be LEAST effective against

 (A) *Streptococcus pneumoniae*
 (B) *Pseudomonas aeruginosa*
 (C) *Staphylococcus aureus*
 (D) *Staphylococcus epidermidis*
 (E) *Escherichia coli*

11. Excessive doses of which vitamin may cause infantile idiopathic hypercalcemia?

 (A) vitamin A
 (B) vitamin B$_{12}$
 (C) vitamin C
 (D) vitamin D
 (E) vitamin E

12. Weekly complete blood count (CBC) monitoring must be performed in a patient taking

 (A) carbamazepine
 (B) risperidone
 (C) olanzapine
 (D) clomipramine
 (E) clozapine

13. Prophylactic antibiotics are recommended within 2 hours of making an initial surgical incision. A patient is scheduled for a routine appendectomy. Which of the following procedures is the procedure of choice for this situation?

 (A) cefazolin, 1.0 g IV at induction of anesthesia
 (B) penicillin G, 1,000,000 U IV at induction of anesthesia
 (C) cefoxitin 2.0 g IV at induction of anesthesia

(D) doxycycline 300 mg PO at induction of anesthesia

(E) ampicillin 2.0 g IV and clindamycin 600 mg IV at induction of anesthesia

14. Topical glucocorticoids are used for

(A) treatment of inflammation and itching
(B) treatment of keloids
(C) tretment of burns
(D) treatment of herpes
(E) treatment of dermatophytosis

15. A new patient is referred to your office by her hometown pharmacist. She has requested the refill of two prescriptions from out of state: digoxin 0.25 mg daily, and furosemide 40 mg three times a day. You immediately recognize the potential for a problem which is

(A) hypovolemia; administer IV solution and terminate furosemide use
(B) hyperkalemia and digitoxicity; terminate both drugs until labs are ordered
(C) hypokalemia; order serum potassium and add supplements if value is low
(D) drug-seeking behavior; alert the local authorities
(E) an impending MI; send to the ER

16. Which of the following calcium-channel antagonists block calcium channels in cardiac cells at clinically used doses?

(A) nifedipine
(B) felodipine
(C) diltiazem
(D) nicardipine
(E) amlodipine

17. The major dose-limiting toxicities of foscarnet are

(A) headache and fever
(B) abnormal liver function tests (LFTs)
(C) nausea and vomiting

(D) nephrotoxicity and hypocalcemia
(E) leukopenia and thrombocytopenia

18. You have cultured *Chlamydia trachomatis* from the cervix of a 23-year-old female who is allergic to doxycycline. You would treat her with a(n)

(A) sulfonamide
(B) macrolide
(C) penicillin
(D) aminoglycoside
(E) tetracycline

19. Phenobarbital and phenytoin are effective for generalized motor seizures. Which drugs are effective for absence seizures?

(A) ethosuximide/valproic acid
(B) phenobarbital/carbamazepine
(C) valproic acid/phenytoin
(D) diazepam/ethosuximide
(E) phenytoin/carbamazepine

20. A frightened mother phones you stating that her 5-year-old has ingested about 20 of her synthroid 0.1-mg tablets. What is your advice to the mother?

(A) Observe the child closely; should any symptoms occur, call back for instructions.
(B) Your child will go to sleep and sleep soundly for several hours; check on her periodically.
(C) Have the child eat some bread to "bind up" the drug particles and bring her to the emergency department.
(D) Induce emesis by using syrup of ipecac and bring her to the emergency department.
(E) In a growing child, excess synthroid is of little consequence as her metabolic rate is already very fast.

21. A 5-year-old was brought to the emergency department. The mother states her daughter ingested 20 of her synthroid 0.1-mg tablets about 1 hour ago. The child convulsed at home and is now comatose, has lost the gag reflex, has bibasilar rales, and a temperature of 101°F. Labs reveal a glucose of 50 mg%. Which of the following procedures are considered medically incorrect for this patient?

    (A) begin an IV solution of D_5W
    (B) administer an antithyroid drug
    (C) maintain ventilation and administer oxygen
    (D) administer a digitalis glycoside and glucocorticoids
    (E) administer cholestyramine

22. Which of the following can interfere with interpretation of ovulation prediction kits?

    (A) phenytoin
    (B) amitriptyline
    (C) nitrofurantoin
    (D) oral contraceptives
    (E) ibuprofen

23. Drugs useful in the treatment of breast cancer include all of the following EXCEPT

    (A) Nolvadex
    (B) Cytoxan
    (C) Megace
    (D) Platinol
    (E) Arimidex

24. All of the following topical antibacterial agents are useful in treating acne vulgaris EXCEPT

    (A) benzoyl peroxide
    (B) clindamycin
    (C) metronidazole
    (D) erythromycin
    (E) erythromycin/benzoyl peroxide

25. A single, 25-year-old woman was admitted to the hospital with classic symptoms of pelvic inflammatory disease (PID). The pa-

tient had been sexually active, using an intra-uterine device (IUD) for contraception. A laparoscopy with subsequent cultures grew *Haemophilus influenzae*, *Chlamydia trachomatis*, and *Bacteroides oralis* from the endometrium, and *Trichomonas vaginalis* from the vagina. The most appropriate therapy would include

    (A) doxycycline/metronidazole
    (B) ampicillin/clindamycin
    (C) metronidazole/ampicillin
    (D) erythromycin/doxycycline
    (E) doxycycline/ampicillin

26. Intestinal cramping, nausea, vomiting, and diarrhea are significant side effects associated with the ingestion of this drug

    (A) tacrine (Cognex)
    (B) ramipril (Altase)
    (C) dexfenfluramine (Redux)
    (D) zidovudine (Retrovir)
    (E) fluoxymesterone (Halotestin)

27. Which of the following adverse reactions is NOT a contraindication to further administration of pertussis-containing vaccines?

    (A) fever of 40.5°C or greater within 48 hours
    (B) hypotonic-hyporesponsive episode within 48 hours
    (C) persistent inconsolable crying lasting 3 or more hours
    (D) a swollen area of 2 cm at the injection site within 48 hours
    (E) a severe acute neurological illness within 7 days

28. The discomfort of oral ulcerations caused by herpes simplex virus-1 (HSV-1) may be relieved by all EXCEPT

    (A) holding and swishing diphenhydramine elixir in the mouth for several minutes
    (B) holding and swishing diphenhydramine elixir mixed with an equal amount of Kaopectate concentrate in the mouth for several minutes

(C) applying lidocaine hydrochloride 2% viscous to the lesions

(D) swishing warm salt water in the mouth for several minutes

(E) Avoidance of pressure and spicy foods

DIRECTIONS (Questions 29 through 50): Each group of items in this section consists of lettered headings followed by a set of numbered words or phrases. For each numbered word or phrase, select the ONE lettered heading that is most closely associated with it. Each lettered heading may be selected once, more than once, or not at all.

Questions 29 through 32

For each drug, select its most common usage.

(A) fluphenazine (Prolixin)
(B) oxybutynin (Ditropan)
(C) tamoxifen (Nolvadex)
(D) triazolam (Halcion)
(E) astimazole (Hismanal)

29. Allergic rhinitis

30. Psychotic disorders

31. Neurogenic bladder

32. Insomnia

Questions 33 through 36

For each condition, select the drug MOST useful in its treatment.

(A) hypertension
(B) peptic ulcer disease
(C) asthma
(D) nausea
(E) diabetes mellitus

33. Glyburide (Micronase)

34. Promethazine (Phenergan)

35. Enalapril (Vasotec)

36. Famotidine (Pepcid)

Questions 37 through 40

(A) sedation
(B) excitation
(C) both
(D) neither

37. Terfenadine (Seldane)

38. Flurazepam (Dalmane)

39. Methyldopa (Aldomet)

40. Diphenhydramine (Benadryl)

Questions 41 through 45

(A) bronchodilation
(B) vasodilation
(C) both
(D) neither

41. Ipratropium (Atrovent)

42. Salmeterol (Severent)

43. Nitroprusside (Nipride)

44. Amrinone (Inocor)

45. Nimodipine (Nimotop)

Questions 46 through 50

Match the following serotonergic drugs to their clinical uses

(A) buspirone
(B) sumatriptan
(C) ondansetron
(D) cisapride
(E) fluoxetine

46. Chemotherapy-induced emesis

47. Depression

48. Anxiety

49. Gastrointestinal (GI) disorders

50. Migraine headaches

Answers and Explanations

1. **(B)** The treatment of dermatophytosis if hair and nails are involved requires systemic therapy with griseofulvin. The topical agents do not enter hair and nails in sufficient concentration to eradicate infection. *(Hathaway et al, p. 382)*

2. **(B)** Isoniazid, ethambutol, rifampin, streptomycin, and pyrazinamide are the first-line drugs presently utilized for the chemotherapeutic treatment of tuberculosis. Isoniazid is the most commonly used drug for tuberculosis. This should not be used for active tuberculosis as a single agent, as this favors the resurgence of drug-resistant TB. Cycloserine is a second-line agent generally reserved for highly resistant *M. tuberculosis*. Significant side effects include central nervous system (CNS) dysfunction, as well as psychotic reactions. Streptomycin, like other aminoglycosides, may damage the eighth cranial nerve and induce nephrotoxicity. Ethionamide is used in treating resistant tuberculosis. It can cause peripheral neuropathy and psychiatric disturbances. All patients must be well monitored with appropriate laboratory tests. *(Hardman et al, pp. 1156–1163; Tierney et al, pp. 1201–1203; Mandell et al, pp. 350–354)*

3. **(B)** Specific H-2 receptor antagonists (cimetidine, ranitidine, etc) are used to suppress gastric secretion and in the treatment of peptic ulcers. H-1 antagonists (antihistamines) will cause the responses in A, C, D, and E. *(Hardman et al, p. 588)*

4. **(A)** Atherosclerosis in this disorder is due to long-standing elevation in plasma low-density lipid (LDL) levels, so every attempt should be made to bring the LDL level into normal range. Bile acid-binding resins should be added first, as these resins prevent the reabsorption of bile acids. The liver responds by converting additional cholesterol into bile acids. The long-term effect of the resins may be limited, however, because the liver may enhance cholesterol synthesis. The addition of nicotinic acid may help to block this compensatory increase in cholesterol synthesis. The HMG Co-A reductase inhibitors may be used in this disorder but have more severe side effects and are even more effective when given in combination with a bile acid-binding resin. The fibric acid derivatives are useful in patients with hypertriglyceridemia and chylomicronemia. Probucol also lowers LDL levels but will significantly decrease HDL as well. It, too, is more effective when added to a bile acid-binding resin. *(Hardman et al, pp. 884–894)*

5. **(C)** Propranolol is a nonselective, beta-adrenergic receptor blocking agent. Blocking of beta receptors in the heart may worsen cardiac failure when sympathetic stimulation is often a vital component supporting circulatory function. Beta-receptor blockade in the lungs can lead to bronchoconstriction. Further, beta blockade may mask certain premonitory signs and symptoms (those that are adrenergically mediated) of acute hypoglycemia, thus making insulin dosage more

difficult and predisposing the patient to the possibility of hypoglycemic attacks. *(Hardman et al, pp 232–237)*

6. **(C)** Twenty to forty micrograms daily of selenium as selenious acid is recommended for maintenance, and up to 100 ng/day for 4 weeks is needed for repletion. It is noted to be a toxic trace element. Suggested maintenance doses of the other trace elements are zinc, 15 mg/day; molybdenum, 20 to 120 ng/day; and manganese, 2.5 to 5.0 mg/day. *(Hardman et al, pp. 1523–1529)*

7. **(B)** Isoproterenol activates $beta_1$- and $beta_2$-receptors and is associated with cardiac side effects, namely tachycardia. Albuterol, Terbutaline, Pirbuterol, and Bitolterol are B_2 receptor specific, especially at low doses. This means they will produce bronchodilation with few if any effects on the heart. *(Hardman et al, p. 664)*

8. **(A)** Acyclovir ointment appears to have some value in reducing healing time and duration of pain in HSV-1 and HSV-2 initial infections. Its overuse can lead to resistant strains of the herpesvirus. It does not reduce the risk of recurrent lesions. *(Hardman et al, pp. 1197–1198; Katzung, pp. 676, 677, 876)*

9. **(D)** *S. aureus* (coagulase positive) and beta-hemolytic *Streptococcus* organisms cause the majority of skin infections. These organisms may invade through breaks in the stratum corneum, through the hair follicles, or through the bloodstream. Both organisms are sensitive to erythromycin, certain penicillins, and cephalosporin antibiotics. Systemic therapy is combined with topical therapy. Compresses with Burow's solution are used for impetigo. As long as systemic antibiotics are being used, topical steroids may be applied to reduce inflammation and speed restoration of the stratum corneum barrier. Solid clinical evidence shows that topical steroids enhance the rate of recovery and do not spread infection. Topical antibiotics are not needed when systemic antibiotics are employed. *(Hardman et al, p. 1605; Tierney et al, pp. 88, 98)*

10. **(A)** Aminoglycosides have limited action against gram-positive bacteria. *Streptococcus pneumoniae* and *Streptococcus pyogenes* are highly resistant. They do exhibit some activity against *Staphylococcus* species but should be used in combination with other antibiotics in the treatment of such infections. Gram-negative bacilli vary in their susceptibility to aminoglycosides, but tobramycin in particular is relatively effective against *Pseudomonas* and *E. coli*. *(Hardman et al, pp. 1031–1037, 1107–1108)*

11. **(D)** The absorption of calcium is influenced by vitamin D. Excessive doses of vitamin D are manifested as hypercalcemia with numerous clinical consequences, such as demineralization of bones, renal calculi, and metastatic calcifications in soft tissues. In addition, hypercalcemia is associated with weakness, vomiting, diarrhea, and lack of muscle tone. Vitamins A, B_{12}, and C are not required for calcium absorption. *(Hardman et al, pp. 1529–1536)*

12. **(E)** The incidence of bone marrow suppression approaches 1% in patients taking clozapine, independent of the dosage taken. Therefore weekly CBC determinations are required. Carbamazepine may cause hematologic abnormalities, but weekly CBC determinations are not required. The primary side effects associated with risperidone are extrapyramidal reactions at high doses and the potential for cardiovascular abnormalities. Clomipramine is associated with anticholinergic side effects primarily. *(Hardman et al, pp. 402–417)*

13. **(C)** For maximal effectiveness, antimicrobial activity must be present at the wound site at the time of its closure. Thus, the drug should be given immediately preoperatively or even intraoperatively. The antibiotic also must be active against the most likely contaminating microorganisms. With a nonperforated appendix, cefoxitin 2.0 g IV preoperatively and every 6 hours for three doses provides sufficient coverage. In a perforated appendix, coverage should be continued for 3 to 5 days. *(Hardman et al, pp. 1050–1053; Mandell et al, p. 2254)*

14. **(A)** Glucocorticoids may worsen burns, herpes, and fungal infections. They are effective in treating keloids but not when applied topically. A standard recommendation for the use of topical steroids is in relief of inflammation and itching, especially those associated with an allergic disorder. *(Hathaway et al, pp. 1067–1068)*

15. **(C)** The potential problem is hypokalemia caused by furosemide. A serum potassium level should be taken. Hypokalemia can lead to the potentiation of the digitalis glycosides and to digitalis toxicity. The preventive measure is to use potassium supplements along with the diuretic. If the measured potassium is not very low, recommending foods high in potassium, including fresh fruits and vegetables, may be useful in preventing hypokalemia and may obviate the need for potassium supplements. *(Hardman et al, pp. 819–824)*

16. **(C)** Verapamil, diltiazem, and bepridil block calcium channels in cardiac cells at clinically used doses. All others preferentially block calcium channels in vascular smooth muscle, and as a result, an accelerated heart rate is often seen and is attributed to sympathetic activation. *(Hardman et al, p. 854)*

17. **(D)** Increases in serum creatinine occur in up to one half of patients taking foscarnet but are reversible in most patients when the drug is stopped. Rapid infusion, prior renal insufficiency and dehydration along with concurrent nephrotoxic drugs are risk factors. Foscarnet is highly ionized at physiologic pH, and metabolic abnormalities are very common, especially a decrease in serum ionized calcium. *(Hardman et al, p. 1200)*

18. **(B)** Erythromycin and azithromycin are recommended drugs of second choice in treating chlamydial cervicitis. A sulfonamide is a third-line drug. Penicillins and aminoglycosides are not indicated at all, and the patient is allergic to doxycycline; therefore, a tetracycline would be contraindicated. *(Hardman et al, pp. 1040–1041)*

19. **(B)** Absence seizures differ considerably from generalized seizures. They occur mostly in children; the attacks are of short duration and consist of syncope or temporary clouding of consciousness during which the individual may stare blankly or exhibit minor movements of the head and limbs. Ethosuximide and valproic acid are generally used to control absence seizures. Diazepam is used in status epilepticus. *(Hardman et al, pp. 461–470; Hathaway et al, pp. 688–689)*

20. **(D)** Obviously, this would represent a huge overdose with a central nervous system (CNS) stimulant. The child requires immediate medical attention. Use of ipecac syrup to induce vomiting is advocated as long as the child is alert enough to protect her airway. If not, gastric lavage may be used to remove the poison and subsequently the use of activated charcoal to bind the medication. The addition of 70% sorbitol to the activated charcoal will act as a cathartic and increase gastrointestinal (GI) motility. Because thyroxin is a CNS stimulant, it is unlikely the child would go to sleep and sleep it off. She may become comatose, however, because of hypoglycemia, hyperpyrexia, and cardiac problems. *(Hardman et al, pp. 1390–1394; Saunders and Ho, pp. 730–738)*

21. **(B)** Because the child is comatose, ventilation must be maintained. She may have congestive heart failure as evidenced by the bibasilar rales. Therefore, digitalis glycosides may be of benefit to improve cardiac motility and slow down the tachycardia. D_5W will provide dextrose, which is needed to maintain her serum glucose. Larger concentrations of dextrose, such as D_{50} may be needed if a significant hypoglycemia exists. Further, cholestyramine may be administered to interfere with thyroxine absorption. The addition of glucocorticoids will inhibit the peripheral conversion of T_4 to T_3. Administration of an antithyroid is not indicated as it inhibits the bodily formation of thyroid hormones by interfering with the incorporation of iodine into thyroglobulin. In this case, the child took exogenous thyroxine. *(Hardman et al, pp. 1397–1401)*

22. (D) Ovulation is the release of an egg from the ovary. This event is caused by a sudden surge in the level of luteinizing hormone (LH). Ovulation prediction tests try to determine this initial surge so that intercourse can follow to maximize the chances for fertilization. The progestin component of oral contraceptives produces feedback suppression of the hypothalamic-pituitary axis but primarily affects LH. This would inhibit growth of the expelled follicle, but in most cases the follicle is not released because of the action of the estrogen component. Dilantin, Elavil, Macrodantin, and Motrin do not interfere with ovulation. *(Hardman et al, p. 1375)*

23. (D) Cisplatin (Platinol) has significant activity in testicular, ovarian, bladder, head and neck, and lung carcinomas. It produces nephrotoxicity and ototoxicity, as well as marked nausea and vomiting. Nolvadex, Megace, Cytoxan, and Arimidex are routinely used to treat breast cancer. *(Hardman et al, pp. 1229, 1237–1271; Isselbacher et al, pp. 1843–1844)*

24. (C) Metronidazole is approved for the topical treatment of acne rosacea, a chronic eruption characterized by flushing, persistent erythema, and telangiectasia with inflammatory papules and pustules. *(Hardman et al, p. 1605)*

25. (A) Sexually transmissible agents of importance in PID are *Neisseria gonorrhoeae* and *Chlamydia trachomatis*. Treatment of nongonococcal PID requires an antibiotic directed at the agents of nongonococcal urethritis, combined with an antianaerobic agent, such as a combination of doxycycline and metronidazole. Doxycycline will cover *Chlamydia*. Metronidazole will cover the *Trichomonas* and *Bacteroides*. If there is a treatment failure, a broad-spectrum penicillin or cephalosporin may have to be added to cover the *Haemophilus influenzae*. *(Mandell et al, pp. 743–744, 1079)*

26. (A) Tacrine is a cholinesterase inhibitor and therefore can cause nausea, vomiting, and diarrhea at recommended doses. Many patients

must discontinue the drug because of these side effects. Ramipril is an angiotensin-converting enzyme (ACE) inhibitor antihypertensive, and its major side effect is hypotension with headache and dizziness. In addition, all ACE inhibitors may cause a clinically insignificant cough. Dexfenfluramine is an appetite suppressant that causes dry mouth and the potential for pulmonary hypertension if taken for extended periods. Zidovudine is an antiviral and is associated with anemia, asthenia, and headaches primarily. Fluoxymesterone causes amenorrhea and other menstrual irregularities in women and gynecomastia and penile erection in males. *(Isselbacher, pp. 1127, 1730, 1838, 2270)*

27. (D) Pertussis is a bacterial infection that presents with the clinical features of whooping cough. The primary problem associated with the vaccine is central nervous system irritation. The absolute contraindications to the future use of the vaccine are an acute neurological illness within 7 days; a convulsion within 3 days; persistent, severe, and inconsolable crying for over 3 hours; or a high-pitched cry within 48 hours. It is also contraindicated in the presence of a hyporesponsive or hypotonic episode, fever to 40.5°C within 48 hours, or an anaphylactic reaction to the vaccine. *(Hathaway et al, p. 217)*

28. (D) Diphenhydramine elixir, alone or mixed with an equal amount of water, or Kaopectate concentrate held and swished around in the mouth for several minutes often relieves the discomfort of oral ulcerations. Lidocaine viscous is also effective as this is a topical anesthetic. Using warm salt water would irritate the vesicles even more and increase the discomfort, while avoidance of pressure and spicy food would decrease overall irritation. *(Scott et al, pp. 23–26)*

29. (E) Astimazole is a once-a-day antihistamine that has shown good effects in the treatment of allergic rhinitis. It has less sedative side effects than older histamine blockers. *(Hardman et al, pp. 588–592)*

30. **(A)** Fluphenazine (Prolixin) is a phenothiazine that has activity at all levels of the central nervous system, as well as on multiple organ systems. It has been used extensively to manage the manifestations of psychotic disorders. This medication has a side effect of extrapyramidal reactions such as acute dystonia. *(Hardman et al, pp. 417–420)*

31. **(B)** Oxybutynin (Ditropan) exerts a direct antispasmodic effect on smooth muscle and inhibits the muscarinic action of acetylcholine on smooth muscle. As such, it has wide usage in managing patients with voiding difficulties. The anticholinergic effect of Ditropan is minimal. *(Hardman et al, p. 158)*

32. **(D)** Triazolam (Halcion) is a type of benzodiazepine. It is a hypnotic with a short duration of action. It increases the duration of sleep and decreases the frequency of nocturnal awakenings. It is recommended for short-term management of insomnia characterized by difficulty in falling asleep, frequent nocturnal awakenings, and/or early morning awakenings. *(Hardman et al, p. 373)*

33. **(E)** Glyburide is a second-generation oral sulfonylurea. These agents are used in the treatment of type II diabetics, along with dietary restrictions to control the serum glucose levels. The mechanism of action is believed to involve increase in the production of insulin from the pancreatic beta cells and an increase in the sensitivity of peripheral tissues to insulin. *(Hardman et al, pp. 1507–1510)*

34. **(D)** Promethazine (Phenergan) is a phenothiazine derivative that has many uses, some of which include treatment of allergic rhinitis, urticaria, and nausea, and as a preoperative sedative. *(Hardman et al, p. 592)*

35. **(A)** Enalapril (Vasotec) is a newer antihypertensive agent belonging to the category of angiotensin-converting enzyme (ACE) inhibitors and is similar to captopril. It is indicated for the control of mild to moderate hypertension and chronic congestive heart failure. It has the convenience of once-a-day dosing. *(Hardman et al, pp. 743–751)*

36. **(B)** Famotidine (Pepcid) is classified as an H_2-receptor antagonist. It, as well as cimetidine and ranitidine, is useful in the treatment of peptic ulcer disease by inhibiting gastric acid secretion. *(Hardman et al, p. 906)*

37. **(D)** Terfenadine (Seldane) is a relatively new antihistamine that is chemically and pharmacologically distinct from other antihistamines. It is very well tolerated and causes little, if any, sedation because of minimal to no anticholinergic activity. This has been a point in favor of this drug over conventional antihistamines. *(Hardman et al, p. 590)*

38. **(A)** Flurazepam (Dalmane) is a sedative hypnotic of the benzodiazepine group. It has its major use as a sleeping aid; however, the prolonged half-life may create a "hung-over" sensation. Other benzodiazepines, such as triazolam (Halcion), have shorter half-lives and reduce this side effect. *(Hardman et al, pp. 361–370)*

39. **(A)** Methyldopa (Aldomet) is an antihypertensive agent belonging to the centrally acting sympatholytic group of drugs. Its major side effect is drowsiness. Other less common side effects include hemolytic anemia and hepatitis. About 20% of patients on methyldopa for a year will develop a positive Coombs' test. *(Hardman et al, p. 787)*

40. **(A)** Diphenhydramine (Benadryl) is an antihistamine belonging to the ethanolamine group associated with the highest incidence of drowsiness as a side effect. In fact, Benadryl is often used as a hypnotic, especially in hospitalized patients. *(Hardman et al, p. 590)*

41. **(A)** Ipratropium, an anticholinergic agent used in treating asthmatics, especially the subgroup who experience psychogenic exacerbation, produces bronchodilation that develops more slowly and is usually less intense than that produced by adrenergic agonists. *(Hardman et al, p. 665)*

42. (A) Salmeterol is a long-acting beta$_2$-adrenergic agonist that produces bronchodilation. It is not suitable, however, for treatment of acute bronchospasm. It is especially useful in prevention of nighttime asthma attacks. *(Hardman et al, p. 665)*

43. (B) Nitroprusside dilates both arterioles and venules, and its hemodynamic response results from a combination of venous pooling and reduced arterial impedance. *(Hardman et al, pp. 798, 830)*

44. (B) Amrinone causes vasodilation by way of its c-GMP-phosphodiesterase inhibition. It is approved for short-term support of the circulation in advanced heart failure. It causes a fall in systemic vascular resistance and increases the force of contraction of cardiac muscle. *(Hardman et al, pp. 830, 833–834)*

45. (B) Nimodipine has a very high lipid solubility and is therefore useful in relaxing the cerebral vasculature and is effective in inhibiting cerebral vasospasm in patients with neurological defects thought to be caused by vasospasm after subarachnoid hemorrhage. *(Hardman et al, pp. 771–774)*

46. (C) Ondansetron is the prototype of a series of serotonin receptor antagonists being explored for various GI disorders. It is especially effective in treating chemotherapy-induced nausea and vomiting. *(Hardman et al, p. 259)*

47. (E) Fluoxetine and others (sertraline, paroxetine, fluvoxamine, venlafaxine) are a group of selective serotonin reuptake inhibitors shown to be effective in treating depression. *(Hardman et al, p. 259)*

48. (A) Buspirone is a serotonin receptor agonist used clinically as an anxiolytic agent in mildly anxious patients. It lacks beneficial actions in severe anxiety and panic attacks. *(Hardman et al, p. 259)*

49. (D) The effects of cisapride on the motility of the stomach and small bowel resemble those of metoclopramide without the side effects that result from dopamine antagonism. It improves gastric emptying, enhances lower esophageal sphincter tone, and stimulates esophageal peristalsis. *(Hardman et al, p. 933)*

50. (B) Sumatriptan is a serotonin agonist and thus restores blood flow to the brain parenchyma during a migraine attack. Because of this, it is effective in the treatment of an acute migraine attack. *(Hardman et al, p. 259)*

REFERENCES

Hardman IG, Limbird LE, Molinoff PB, Ruddon RW. *Goodman & Gilman's The Pharmacological Basis of Therapeutics*, 9th ed. New York: McGraw-Hill; 1996.

Hathaway WE, Hay WW Jr, Groothius JR, Paisley JW. *Current Pediatric Diagnosis and Treatment*, 11th ed. Norwalk, CT: Appleton & Lange; 1993.

Isselbacher KJ, Braunwald E, Wilson JD, Martin JB, Fauci AS, Kasper DL. *Harrison's Principles of Internal Medicine*, 13th ed. New York: McGraw-Hill; 1996.

Katzung BG. *Basic and Clinical Pharmacology*, 5th ed. Norwalk, CT: Appleton & Lange; 1992.

Mandell GL, Douglas RG Jr, Bennett JE (eds). *Principles and Practice of Infectious Disease*, 3rd ed. New York: Churchill Livingstone; 1990.

Saunders CE, Ho MT. *Current Emergency Diagnosis and Treatment*, 4th ed. Norwalk, CT: Appleton & Lange; 1992.

Tierney LM Jr, McPhee SJ, Papadakis MA, Schroeder SA. *Current Medical Diagnosis and Treatment*, 36th ed. Stamford, CT: Appleton & Lange; 1997.

CHAPTER 7

Psychiatry
Questions

Catherine Judd, PA-C, and Janean R. Schepp, BS, PA-C

DIRECTIONS (Questions 1 through 23): Each of the numbered items or incomplete statements in this section is followed by answers or by completions of the statement. Select the ONE lettered answer or completion that is BEST in each case.

Questions 1 through 23

1. The differential diagnosis of schizophrenia does NOT include

   (A) major depression
   (B) temporal lobe epilepsy
   (C) congestive heart failure
   (D) panic disorder
   (E) alcohol withdrawal

2. An acute manic episode is characterized by a mood that is elevated, expansive, or irritable. Associated symptoms include all EXCEPT

   (A) hyperactivity and reduced need for sleep
   (B) religious preoccupation and spending sprees
   (C) increased self-esteem (grandiosity)
   (D) increased productivity, elevated frustration tolerance, and good humor
   (E) poor concentration and poor social judgment

3. A major depressive episode is MOST associated with which symptom in addition to depressed mood?

   (A) anhedonia
   (B) nausea and vomiting
   (C) panic attacks
   (D) normal sleep and appetite
   (E) psychosis

4. All the following are TRUE about insomnia EXCEPT

   (A) When found, it is always indicative of an underlying disorder.
   (B) Its significance depends on its timing in the usual pattern of sleep.
   (C) It can be associated with bad habits, such as lack of exercise or use of tobacco or caffeine.
   (D) It can be associated with the use of alcohol or other drugs.
   (E) It can be a symptom of depression.

5. Recommended sleep hygiene methods for patients complaining of insomnia include all EXCEPT

   (A) avoiding caffeine, nicotine, and alcohol
   (B) avoiding prolonged naps
   (C) establishing a set wake-up time
   (D) establishing a set time of going to sleep
   (E) exercising regularly

6. Which of the following characteristics is NOT included in the criteria for diagnosing attention deficit hyperactivity disorders (ADHD) in children?

   (A) an inability to remain seated in the classroom
   (B) difficulty following instructions or completing tasks
   (C) intrusiveness and frequent interruptions into conversations or activities of others
   (D) marked distress over minor changes in environment or schedule
   (E) impulsivity and engaging in physically dangerous activities

7. Which of the following are commonly abused prescription drugs?

   (A) methamphetamine (Dexedrine), alprazolam (Xanax)
   (B) imipramine (Tofranil), carbamazepine (Tegretol)
   (C) fluoxetine (Prozac), clozapine (Clozaril)
   (D) bethanechol (Urecholine), buspirone (BuSpar)
   (E) amitriptyline (Elavil), sertraline (Zoloft)

8. Choose the statement that is FALSE concerning alcohol withdrawal syndrome.

   (A) It causes elevated blood pressure with orthostatic drop.
   (B) Patients are in serious danger of seizures.
   (C) It can cause hallucinations and delirium.
   (D) It responds to treatment with antidepressants.
   (E) Nausea or vomiting can be common.

9. Withdrawal from sedative/hypnotic types of drugs

   (A) resembles alcohol withdrawal syndrome
   (B) resembles opiate withdrawal syndrome
   (C) cannot produce seizures
   (D) resembles cocaine withdrawal syndrome
   (E) usually causes somnolence

10. Which of the following is TRUE regarding opiate withdrawal syndrome?

    (A) It carries a risk of status epilepticus.
    (B) Patients have observable piloerection, dilated pupils, and diarrhea.
    (C) It causes auditory hallucinations.
    (D) It is life-threatening.
    (E) It cannot be induced by an opiate antagonist.

11. The DSM-IV criteria for the diagnosis of schizophrenia include all EXCEPT

    (A) characteristic symptoms persisting for at least 1 month
    (B) impairment of social, work, or interpersonal relations
    (C) disturbance not due to effects of a substance
    (D) not due to a general medical condition
    (E) persistence of a mood disorder throughout the illness

12. Psychosis is a symptom of an underlying disorder. When an acutely psychotic patient is encountered, the differential diagnosis should include

    (A) acute drug reaction
    (B) bipolar (manic/depressive) disorder
    (C) major depression
    (D) schizophrenia
    (E) all of the above

13. Specific phobias must be distinguished from panic disorder, in that phobias

    (A) often cause panic attacks in public places
    (B) consist of a persistent fear of a specific object
    (C) are best treated with medication
    (D) are uncommon in the general population
    (E) are seen as reasonable by the patient

14. Somatoform disorders are characterized by all EXCEPT

(A) symptoms that suggest a physical ailment

(B) negative physical and laboratory findings

(C) a concomitant physical ailment

(D) intentional patient malingering

(E) clinically significant distress

15. Reversible causes of dementia in the elderly include

(A) a major depressive episode

(B) vitamin deficiency

(C) prescription medication effects

(D) hydrocephalus

(E) all of the above

16. Common causes of irreversible, chronic, progressive dementia do NOT include

(A) Alzheimer's disease

(B) Parkinson's disease

(C) multiple small strokes

(D) alcoholism

(E) urinary tract infection

17. In addition to a complete history, physical, and neurological examination, a workup of the patient presenting with dementia should include all the following EXCEPT

(A) thyroid function studies

(B) serum B_{12}

(C) CT scan and electroencephalogram (EEG)

(D) lumbar puncture and cerebrospinal fluid examination

(E) folate determination

18. The scope of mental status examination includes

(A) attention

(B) memory

(C) language

(D) executive skills

(E) all of the above

19. Besides lithium carbonate, which of the following can be used to treat bipolar disorder?

(A) fluoxetine (Prozac)

(B) amitriptyline (Elavil)

(C) clozapine (Clozaril)

(D) divalproex sodium (Depakote)

(E) methylphenidate (Ritalin)

20. Caution must be used in prescribing benzodiazepines, such as alprazolam (Xanax), because of all the following EXCEPT

(A) potential for dependence

(B) drowsiness

(C) abnormal motor movements

(D) impaired motor control

(E) risk of withdrawal syndrome

21. Antipsychotic medication, such as haloperidol (Haldol), can cause such neurological side effects as

(A) acute dystonia

(B) abnormal motor movements

(C) motor agitation

(D) parkinsonism

(E) all of the above

22. The borderline personality is characterized by all of the following EXCEPT

(A) manipulative behavior, including suicidal

(B) unstable self-image or sense of self

(C) tempestuous interpersonal relationships

(D) impulsivity and frequent mood shifts

(E) persistent psychotic thinking

23. Personality disorders are

(A) caused exclusively by biological factors

(B) usually not seen in patients with other psychiatric disorders

(C) often associated only with discrete episodes of mental illness

(D) maladaptive traits that cause impairment or emotional distress

(E) easily treated with pyschotropic medications

DIRECTIONS (Questions 24 through 32): Each group of items in this section consists of lettered headings followed by a set of numbered words or phrases. For each numbered word or phrase, select the ONE lettered heading that is most closely associated with it. Each lettered heading may be selected once, more than once, or not at all.

Questions 24 through 27

(A) anxiolytic
(B) selective serotonin reuptake inhibitor (SSRI)
(C) sedative/hypnotic
(D) antipsychotic
(E) monoamine oxidase inhibitor (MAOI)

24. Sertraline (Zoloft)

25. Lorazepam (Ativan)

26. Flurazepam (Dalmane)

27. Clozapine (Clozaril)

Questions 28 through 30

(A) generalized anxiety disorder
(B) panic disorder
(C) both
(D) neither

28. Discrete spontaneous episodes

29. Sustained state of tension and irritability

30. Depression

Questions 31 and 32

(A) preoccupation with body size and weight
(B) binge eating accompanied by some extreme measure to prevent weight gain
(C) both
(D) neither

31. Anorexia nervosa

32. Bulimia nervosa

DIRECTIONS (Questions 33 through 49): Each of the numbered items or incomplete statements in this section is followed by answers or by completions of the statement. Select the ONE lettered answer or completion that is BEST in each case.

Questions 33 through 49

33. What form of psychotherapy would you recommend for a patient with schizophrenia who has required three psychiatric hospitalizations in the last 2 years?

(A) insight-oriented psychotherapy
(B) psychoanalysis
(C) biofeedback
(D) supportive psychotherapy
(E) brief dynamic psychotherapy

34. Alzheimer's disease

(A) can only be definitively diagnosed by a brain biopsy
(B) presents with ataxia, incontinence, and dementia
(C) accounts for 90% of dementias
(D) is characterized by a stepwise, progressive, downhill course
(E) has an inherited familial pattern

35. Memory loss in Alzheimer's disease may be delayed in some cases by

(A) droperidol
(B) ergoloid mesylates
(C) piracetam
(D) thioridazine
(E) tacrine

36. A 60-year-old male patient becomes delirious on hospital day twelve. What is the MOST likely cause of the delirium?

(A) hypoxia
(B) hypoglycemia
(C) hypoperfusion
(D) drug withdrawal
(E) medication side effects

37. Which of the following types of hallucinations tend to be MOST common in demented patients?

    (A) auditory
    (B) tactile
    (C) visual
    (D) olfactory
    (E) gustatory

38. Which of the following antipsychotic medications is associated with agranulocytosis?

    (A) haloperidol (Haldol)
    (B) chlorpromazine (Thorzaine)
    (C) clozapine (Clozaril)
    (D) thioridazine (Mellaril)
    (E) thiothixene (Navane)

39. Akathisia, a side effect of some neuroleptic medications, is characterized by

    (A) numbness and tingling
    (B) muscle stiffness
    (C) psychomotor retardation
    (D) inability to sit still
    (E) diminished spontaneity

40. A 66-year-old woman manifests akinesia, shuffling gait, masked facies, excessive salivation, and a pill-rolling tremor. The MOST likely diagnosis is

    (A) senile tremor
    (B) multiple sclerosis
    (C) Parkinson's disease
    (D) lithium toxicity
    (E) Huntington's disease

41. Anorexia nervosa is commonly associated with all of the following EXCEPT

    (A) distorted body image
    (B) history of truancy
    (C) increased activity level
    (D) endocrine dysfunction
    (E) metabolic alterations

42. Which of the following is MOST characteristic of patients with bulimia nervosa?

    (A) The patient feels in control of eating behavior.
    (B) At least five binge eating episodes occur a week.
    (C) Diuretic abuse is common.
    (D) They have little concern with body shape.
    (E) Major depression and anxiety are common.

43. Panic disorder with agoraphobia is characterized by

    (A) fear of a specific object or situation
    (B) persistent and exaggerated fear of humiliation or embarrassment in social situations
    (C) excessive fear of situations in which escape or obtaining help would be difficult
    (D) discrete attacks of anxiety
    (E) chronic anxiety, apprehension, and somatic symptoms of anxiety

44. A 32-year-old college professor diagnosed with "organic brain dysfunction" is seen for evaluation. The patient was knocked unconscious in a car accident 1 year ago. Since then he has been unable to get into a car and "panics" whenever he is close to an automobile. He continues to function well at work and in his marriage, but insists on walking wherever he goes. Physical, neurological, and mental status exams are normal. The patient is MOST likely suffering from

    (A) agoraphobia
    (B) conversion disorder
    (C) panic disorder
    (D) postconcussion syndrome
    (E) specific phobia

45. A 22-year-old female college graduate was admitted with symptoms of withdrawal, severe psychomotor retardation and waxy flexibility, and inability to take care of herself. She lies in bed all day. Her answers are monosyllabic. Her affect is flat. Two years ago she was admitted with similar symptoms. Which is the MOST likely diagnosis?

(A) dysthymic disorder
(B) schizophrenia, disorganized
(C) major depression, recurrent episode
(D) mental retardation
(E) schizophrenia, catatonic type

46. When lithium is used to treat bipolar affective illness, which lab tests are used in routine monitoring of the patient for side effects?

(A) white blood cell (WBC) count
(B) liver enzymes
(C) glucose
(D) creatinine
(E) electrolytes

47. Narcolepsy is characterized by

(A) daytime "sleep attacks"
(B) cataplexy
(C) sleep paralysis
(D) hypnogogic hallucinations
(E) all of the above

48. Which diagnosis should be strongly suspected in an overweight, hypertensive, middle-aged male who complains of daytime somnolence and whose wife complains that he snores?

(A) coronary artery disease
(B) chronic obstructive pulmonary disease
(C) obstructive sleep apnea syndrome
(D) major depression
(E) narcolepsy

49. Which of the following medications is prescribed for children with attention deficit disorder?

(A) amitriptyline (Elavil)
(B) phenelzine (Nardil)
(C) methylphenidate (Ritalin)
(D) carbamazepine (Tegretol)
(E) lorazepam (Ativan)

DIRECTIONS (Questions 50 through 53): Each group of items in this section consists of lettered headings followed by a set of numbered words or phrases. For each numbered word or phrase, select the ONE lettered heading that is most closely associated with it. Each lettered heading may be selected once, more than once, or not at all.

Questions 50 through 53

Choose the diagnostic category that BEST describes each of the following patients.

(A) affective disorder
(B) bipolar affective disorder
(C) schizophrenia
(D) dementia
(E) none of the above

50. A 59-year-old white male presents to your office with a history of gradual decline in memory for major events, expresses an inappropriate affect oriented only to person, and family reports that the symptoms get worse at night. Which diagnostic category would you initially consider?

51. You are on call to the emergency department when you are asked to evaluate a 42-year-old male who has been brought in by the family in the past for treatment of depression; however, over the last week he has exhibited increased energy, decreased sleep, excessive spending, and increased risk-taking behavior. On mental status exam, you see a black male oriented to person, place, time, and date. He is overactive with elevated mood, pressured speech, is easily distracted and difficult to interrupt. What would you suspect as the likely diagnosis?

52. Your first patient of the day while in a family clinic is an 18-year-old male you have never seen before. He is sitting in the exam room alone. His mental status exam reveals he is fully oriented, but his affect is inappropriate. He indicates a belief that people are trying to harm him, and he has bizarre hand gestures. He also believes that people can read his mind. This could be a presentation of what diagnostic category?

53. A 32-year-old female was referred to your office for evaluation. Upon entering the room you see a tearful, slow-to-react female who describes a gradual worsening in feelings of worthlessness and anhedonia for the last month. She is unkempt. She is fully oriented. What diagnostic category does this scenario fit?

DIRECTIONS (Questions 54 through 60): Each of the numbered items or incomplete statements in this section is followed by answers or by completions of the statement. Select the ONE lettered answer or completion that is BEST in each case.

Questions 54 through 60

54. A prominent feature of cocaine withdrawal is

(A) somnolence
(B) depression
(C) psychosis
(D) muscle cramping
(E) abdominal pain

55. Which of the following antidepressant medications would be the safest in a patient with compromised cardiac status?

(A) Prozac (fluoxetine)
(B) Elavil (amitriptyline)
(C) Tofranil (imipramine)
(D) doxepin
(E) trazodone

56. Clozaril (clozapine) is an antipsychotic used to treat refractory schizophrenia. Routine monitoring is performed for

(A) leukoplasia
(B) eosinophilia
(C) agranulocytosis
(D) thrombocytopenia
(E) leukopenia

57. The Minnesota Multiphasic Personality Inventory (MMPI) is used to

(A) assess the organic component of psychiatric illness
(B) discover unconscious psycodynamic concerns
(C) evaluate cognitive functioning
(D) identify areas of psychopathology
(E) can easily be manipulated by an intelligent patient wishing to present a postive picture

58. Psychiatric conditions associated with HIV infection include which of the following?

(A) depression
(B) acute psychosis
(C) mania
(D) delirium
(E) all of the above

59. The most common neurological problem in AIDS is

(A) AIDS encephalopathy
(B) peripheral neuropathy
(C) cerebrovascular accident
(D) transient ischemic attacks
(E) carpal tunnel syndrome

60. A patient is determined to be "incompetent" if he or she is

(A) psychotic
(B) disoriented
(C) dangerous to himself/herself and others
(D) unable to make decisions in his/her own best interest
(E) unable to determine right from wrong

Answers and Explanations

1. **(C)** The differential diagnosis of schizophrenia includes other psychiatric disorders, some general medical illnesses, and some drug effects. *(Hales et al, p. 416)*

2. **(D)** A manic episode does exhibit elevated mood, increased energy, rapid thought processes, and a reduced need for sleep. However, energy is poorly focused and judgment is impaired, so activities are often disorganized and counterproductive. *(Goodwin and Jamison, p. 92)*

3. **(A)** The DSM-IV criteria for major depressive disorder include markedly diminished interest or pleasure (anhedonia), change in sleep or appetite, depressed mood, and diminished ability to think or concentrate. Psychosis may occasionally occur during a major depression, but it is not a frequent feature. Panic attacks may coexist with major depression. *(Hales et al, p. 469)*

4. **(A)** Insomnia is a symptom. It can indicate a medical illness, bad habits, substance abuse, or psychiatric disorders. *(Hales et al, pp. 837–838)*

5. **(D)** Establishing a set wake-up time and avoiding naps are generally effective at getting sleepy the same time every night. Regular exercise helps to deepen sleep. Use of alcohol, tobacco, and caffeine are to be discouraged. *(Hales et al, p. 838)*

6. **(D)** The child with ADHD demonstrates difficulty in following instructions, completing tasks, and remaining seated in the classroom. Also present are impulsivity and intrusiveness. *(Garfinkel et al, pp. 156–157)*

7. **(A)** Dexedrine is an amphetamine and Xanax is a benzodiazepine, and as such, are subject to abuse. Tofranil, Prozac, Elavil, and Zoloft are antidepressants. Tegretol is a neuroleptic, Clozaril an antipsychotic, and BuSpar is a nonbenzodiazepine anxiolytic. *(Hales et al, pp. 377, 394)*

8. **(D)** Alcohol withdrawal can cause autonomic hyperactivity, including hypertension and vomiting. Seizures can occur because of lowering of the seizure threshold. Delirium and hallucinations can occur suddenly or 2 to 3 days after stopping alcohol ingestion. Benzodiazepines are the treatment of choice for withdrawal. *(Hales et al, pp. 369–371)*

9. **(A)** Withdrawal from benzodiazepines is similar to alcohol withdrawal in that it can cause anxiety, seizures, insomnia, postural hypotension, vomiting, and delirium. *(Galanter and Kleber, p. 182)*

10. **(B)** The withdrawal syndrome consists of profuse diarrhea, piloerection, pupillary dilation, abdominal and muscle cramps, and rhinorrhea. The syndrome can be triggered by administration of a narcotic antagonist. *(Galanter and Kleber, p. 300)*

11. **(E)** Even though continuous signs of the disturbance must be present for 6 months, char-

acteristic symptoms must be present for 1 month, or less if treated. One or more areas of functioning are decreased. The disturbance is not due to the effects of a substance or general medical condition and a mood disorder is brief relative to the duration of the active and residual phases. *(Hales et al, p. 415)*

12. **(E)** Many different causes must be considered for a psychotic episode. These include numerous psychiatric disorders, some general medical illnesses, and drug reactions. *(Hales et al, p. 417)*

13. **(B)** Specific phobias consist of a persistent and unreasonable fear of an object or situation. The patient realizes this fear is unreasonable, but experiences intense anxiety or distress in the situation. Treatment of choice is *exposure* to the object or situation. *(Hales et al, pp. 522, 531)*

14. **(D)** A diagnosis of somatization disorder includes a history of physical complaints before age 30 that occur over a period of several years. Reported symptoms suggest a physical ailment, but are not supported by physical exam and laboratory findings. There may be a concomitant physical ailment. The symptoms cause clinically significant distress, but are not intentionally produced. *(Hales et al, pp. 596–604)*

15. **(E)** Reversible (nondegenerative) causes of dementia can include dementia syndrome of depression, hydrocephalus, toxic disorders, and metabolic disorders, as well as others. *(Coffey and Cummings, p. 371)*

16. **(E)** Urinary tract infections are treatable with antibiotics and therefore are a reversible cause of dementia. All other answers represent irreversible causes. *(Coffey and Cummings, pp. 306, 390, 434, 467)*

17. **(D)** A National Institute on Aging task force recommends numerous tests to diagnose dementia, including complete blood count (CBC), electrolytes, serum B_{12} and folate, thyroid screen, CT scan, and EEG (as well as

other tests as needed). Lumbar puncture will not reveal useful information in most cases of dementia to warrant its use. *(Hales et al, pp. 281–282)*

18. **(E)** The principal congnitive domains of the Mental Status Exam include attention, memory, language, visuospatial skills, calculation, and executive skills. *(Coffey and Cummings, p. 113)*

19. **(D)** Divalproex has been found to be as effective as lithium in treating the core symptoms of elation, grandiosity, and insomnia. It may be more effective than lithium in treating mixed or dysphoric mania, rapid cycling variants, and mania secondary to organic illness. *(Bowden et al, pp. 918–924)*

20. **(B)** Drowsiness may be a benefit or side effect of benzodiazepines. It has been repeatedly shown that driving or operating machinery can be adversely affected by the use of benzodiazepines. When benzodiazepines are used in higher than usual doses, the chances of dependence increase. When they are abruptly discontinued, there is greater incidence of withdrawal. *(Hales et al, p. 958)*

21. **(E)** Neurological side effects from neuroleptics are common. They can occur at any time during treatment and may not be reversible, even after treatment is stopped. Clozaril may cause fewer extrapyramidal side effects, but has a higher incidence of agranulocytosis. *(Hales et al, pp. 444–445)*

22. **(E)** Diagnostic criteria for borderline personality disorder include unstable image of self, difficulty with interpersonal relationships, affective instability, manipulative behavior, and recurrent suicidal behavior. Persistent psychotic thinking is not a common feature. *(Hales et al, p. 714)*

23. **(D)** According to DSM-IV, personality disorders are inflexible and maladaptive personality traits that cause subjective stress, significant impairment in social or occupational functioning, or both. This deviation must be consistently present since adolescence or

early adulthood. Because these traits are pervasive, they are not easily treated, even with psychotherapy. *(Hales et al, pp. 701–704)*

24. **(B)** Sertraline is a selective serotonin reuptake inhibitor (SSRI). It tends to have fewer side effects than the older tricyclic antidepressants. *(Koe, pp. 13–16)*

25. **(A)** Lorazepam is a short-acting benzodiazepine. It is a frequently used treatment for anxiety. *(Hales et al, p. 516)*

26. **(C)** Flurazepam is also a benzodiazepine. It is more commonly used to induce sleep. *(Hales et al, p. 950)*

27. **(D)** Clozapine is an antipsychotic used in treatment-resistant schizophrenia. It may have fewer extrapyramidal side effects than traditional antipsychotics, but carries the risk of angranulocytosis. *(Kane et al, pp. 789–796)*

28. **(B)** Panic disorder is characterized by sudden onset of pounding heart, shortness of breath, dizziness, and extreme anxiety. Patients often feel as though they are about to die. The initial attack often occurs in young adulthood. In severe forms, it can progress to development of phobias associated with situations in which panic attacks have previously occurred. *(Hales et al, p. 498)*

29. **(A)** Generalized anxiety disorder is characterized by the development over time of chronic feelings of tension, anxiety, and restlessness. Discrete episodes of frank panic do not occur. Abuse of alcohol or sedatives often occurs in an attempt to self-medicate. *(Hales et al, p. 500)*

30. **(C)** The difference between major depression disorder, generalized anxiety disorder, and panic disorder can often be quite blurred. In all three disorders, depressed mood and anxiety can coexist. In anxiety and panic disorders, the onset of tension or panic attacks often precedes the onset of depressed mood by a significant period of time. *(Hales et al, pp. 495–500)*

31. **(A)** Anorexia nervosa is a disorder characterized by a refusal to maintain a normal body weight. The person has a distorted body image and sees herself/himself as fat even when severely undernourished. Such persons are preoccupied with body size and shape. *(Hales et al, p. 859)*

32. **(C)** Bulimics have a disorder characterized by binge eating during which they feel a lack of control over their eating behavior. Bulimics, like anorexics, have a preoccupation with their weight and body features. They engage in means to prevent weight gain, such as self-induced vomiting, abuse of laxatives, fasting between binges, or overly strenuous exercise. *(Hales et al, pp. 865–866)*

33. **(D)** Individual psychotherapy alone has not been shown to improve the outcome for schizophrenic patients over the use of medication alone. For many patients recovering from an acute episode, help with living accommodations, food, clothing, income, child care, and medical care are needed immediately. *(Stoudemire, pp. 166–167)*

34. **(A)** Alzheimer's disease presents with memory impairment. At least one of the following may be present: aphasia, apraxia, or agnosia. The course of illness is insidious, progressive and irreversible. *(Stoudemire, pp. 102–107)*

35. **(E)** Multicenter trials using tacrine to treat mildly to moderately demented patients indicate that a subgroup of patients show temporary improvement. Although tacrine causes reversible elevations in liver transaminase levels, the FDA has approved the drug for patients with Alzheimer's disease. *(Kaplan and Sadock, p. 2664)*

36. **(E)** Dementia is the second most common disabling condition of the elderly (arthritis is first). Many geriatric patients have treatable conditions that should be investigated. These include such conditions as hypothyroidism, heart disease, renal disease, and medication side effects. *(Kaplan and Sadock, p. 1159)*

37. **(C)** Hallucinations of all types occur, but visual hallucinations tend to be the most common. Gustatory and olfactory hallucinations occur in psychoses and epilepsy. Auditory hallucinations occur in conjunction with persecutory delusions in delusional disorders. Tactile hallucinations are reported in delirium and withdrawal, particularly from opiates. *(Stoudemire, p. 116)*

38. **(C)** Clozapine is an atypical antipsychotic with demonstrated efficacy for treatment of refractory schizophrenic patients. Although it is not associated with significant extrapyramidal side effects or tardive dyskinesia, there is a 1-2% risk of agranulocytosis. Because of the risk of agranulocytosis, patients are required to have their white blood cell count monitored weekly. Haloperidol, chlorpromazine, thioridazine, and thiothixene do not cause agranulocytosis. *(Stoudemire, p. 165)*

39. **(D)** Akathisia is a common reaction to neuroleptic medications which occurs shortly after initiation of treatment. Akathisia is an extrapyramidal disorder manifested by an unpleasant feeling of restlessness and the inability to sit still. Patients may pace or become agitated in response to the disorder. Numbness and tingling are not side effects of neuroleptic medications. Other extrapyramidal symptoms include drug induced parkinsonism and acute dystonic reactions (muscle stiffness). Psychomotor retardation and diminished spontaneity are not directly attributed to side effects of neuroleptic medication. *(Stoudemire, p. 513)*

40. **(C)** Parkinson's disease is characterized by the triad of akinesia, rigidity, and tremor. Signs and symptoms of lithium toxicity include tremor, weakness, ataxia, drowsiness, dysarthria, nausea and vomiting, and tinnitus that can progress to seizures and coma. Huntington's disease is seen in patients in their thirties and forties. Multiple sclerosis presents with motor and sensory losses, scanning speech, and nystagmus. *(Stoudemire, p. 122)*

41. **(B)** Patients with anorexia experience endocrine dysfunction, such as amenorrhea with decreases in luteinizing (LH) and follicle-stimulating hormone (FSH) secretion, and metabolic alterations that conserve energy. Patients experience distorted body image and extreme fear of being fat. Excessive or compulsive exercise is relatively common. *(Stoudemire, pp. 356–358)*

42. **(E)** Patients with bulimia nervosa have concurrent major depression or anxiety disorders in up to 75% of cases. They engage in eating binges and feel as if their eating is out of control. They do not ordinarily misuse laxatives or diuretics, but engage in at least two binge eating episodes per week for a minimum of 3 months. *(Stoudemire, p. 358)*

43. **(C)** Panic disorder with agoraphobia is characterized by anxiety about being in places or situations from which escape might be difficult (or embarassing) or in which help may not be available in the event an unexpected or situationally predisposed panic attack occurs. *(Stoudemire, p. 236)*

44. **(E)** Specific phobia usually is an excessive and unrealistic circumscribed fear of a focal object or situation. Exposure to the phobic stimulus produces an anxiety response, expectation of exposure may produce anticipatory anxiety, and the object or situation is avoided or endured with considerable discomfort. The phobia is related to situations and results in marked distress or some degree of impairment in activities or relationships. *(Stoudemire, p. 251)*

45. **(E)** Schizophrenia has been classified into subtypes. Catatonic schizophrenia is dominated by motoric abnormalities, such as rigidity, posturing, or waxy flexibility. Other symptoms of schizophrenia are present, such as impairment of social or occupational functioning. *(Stoudemire, pp. 144–145)*

46. **(D)** Lithium is excreted by the kidneys; thus, blood levels are dependent upon renal func-

tion. Lithium can also have long-term effects on renal and thyroid function. Lithium-induced hypothyroidism can be a side effect of lithium treatment and is treated with thyroid replacement. Thus, in addition to routine lithium blood levels, renal and thyroid function should be monitored. *(Stoudemire, pp. 533–537)*

47. **(E)** Narcolepsy is a disorder involving more than just excessive daytime sleepiness. Hypersomnolence is more commonly caused by other disorders or poor habits. The diagnosis of true narcolepsy, which is relatively rare, can be made only in the presence of at least one of the other symptoms. Sleep attacks plus cataplexy is considered pathognomic of narcolepsy. An all-night polysomnograph and daytime sleep latency testing are confirmatory. *(Stoudemire, pp. 640–642)*

48. **(C)** Obstructive sleep apnea is a common cause of excessive daytime somnolence. Snoring is a common observable sign of upper airway obstruction. This is not a benign condition. In addition to sleepiness being quite debilitating and potentially dangerous, lowered pO_2 during sleep and other physiologic changes can lead to hypertension and potentially fatal cardiac arrhythmias. *(Stoudemire, pp. 637–640)*

49. **(C)** Methylphenidate (Ritalin), along with methamphetamine (Dexedrine), and pemoline (Cylert) are stimulants commonly used to treat children with attention-deficit hyperactivity disorders. Amitriptyline and phenelzine are antidepressants. Carbamazepine is an anticonvulsant with several psychiatric uses. *(Stoudemire, pp. 435–439)*

50. **(D)** Dementia has disturbances to both short- and long-term memory, and interferences with social and occupational functioning. Care should be taken to rule out the reversible causes of delirium, such as medication interaction or metabolic derangements. *(Stoudemire, p. 115)*

51. **(B)** Bipolar affective disorder exhibits erratic and disinhibited behavior. Patients are fre-

quently overextended in their activities and responsibilities. They exhibit low frustration tolerance and vegetative symptoms such as diminished need for sleep, as well as changes in diet and weight. *(Kaplan and Sadock, p. 85)*

52. **(C)** In schizophrenia, one can see psychotic symptoms that impair function and affect feelings, thinking, and behavior. These might include hallucinations involving auditory, tactile, visual, or olfactory senses. *(Stoudemire, pp. 147–151)*

53. **(A)** Depression is are characterized by abnormal feelings of dysphoria and anhedonia. Depressive disorders can be divided into unipolar or bipolar. They respond well to mood-stabilizing agents. *(Stoudemire, p. 201)*

54. **(B)** The most common symptom of acute cocaine withdrawal after heavy use is depression. This can also be accompanied by anxiety and irritability. Often, cocaine abusers also abuse sedative medications or alcohol in an attempt to self-medicate these feelings. Cocaine does not produce a physical withdrawal syndrome as do opiates, sedative/hypnotics, or alcohol. *(Stoudemire, pp. 323–324)*

55. **(A)** Prozac is a serotinin reuptake inhibitor, as is Paxil and Zoloft. In general, these agents have no significant cardiac conduction delay and do not produce orthostatic hypotension. No adverse cardiovascular effects have been noted in cases of overdose. *(Kaplan and Sadock, p. 258)*

56. **(C)** A special concern with the use of clozapine is agranulocytosis which occurs in about 1% to 2% of patients. If not detected early this can be fatal. If detected within one to two weeks the medication can be discontinued, and the process usually reverses. Once a patient recovers from the agranulocytosis, he/she cannot be restarted as it will recur. The manufacturer recommends that weekly CBCs be obtained on all patients while on clozapine. *(Stoudemire, p. 165)*

57. **(D)** The MMPI is a well-standardized test that has been used extensively for more than

40 years. It does not take the place of a careful psychiatric examination, but auguments it. It includes sophisticated internal validation factors that point out certain patterns of manipulation on the part of the patient. *(Stoudemire, pp. 86–89)*

58. **(E)** Organic mental disorders are associated with HIV infection and manifest as psychiatric symptoms. Periodic assessment of mental status in HIV-positive patients is important as these symptoms may be managed with appropriate agents. *(Stoudemire, pp. 122–123)*

59. **(A)** AIDS dementia complex is also known as AIDS encephalopathy. The major clinical manifestations are gradual onset of memory deficits, diminished concentration, apathy, social withdrawal, psychomotor retardation, and depression in an HIV-positive patient. Some of these symptoms can be improved with psychotropic medications. *(Stoudemire, pp. 614–616)*

60. **(D)** Competency is a legal term used to define the ability of a person to make decisions based on his/her own best interest. It is further broken down to pertain to the specific task at hand, such as competency to draw up a will, make a contract, or participate in a legal defense. A person may be deemed competent to perform some tasks and not others. *(Stoudemire, pp. 574, 606–607)*

REFERENCES

Bowden CL, Brugger AM, Swann AC, et al. Efficacy of divalproex vs lithium and placebo in the treatment of mania. *JAMA.* 1994; 271(12): 918–924.

Coffey CE, Cummings JL. *Textbook of Geriatric Neuropsychiatry.* Washington, DC: American Psychiatric Press; 1994.

Galanter M, Kleber HD. *Textbook of Substance Abuse Treatment.* Washington, DC: American Psychiatric Press; 1994.

Garfinkel BD, Carlson GA, Wells EB. *Psychiatric Disorders in Children and Adolescents.* Philadelphia: Saunders; 1990.

Goodwin FK, Jamison KR. *Manic-Depressive Illness.* New York: Oxford University Press; 1990.

Hales RE, Yudofsky SC, Talbott JA. *Textbook of Psychiatry,* 2nd ed. Washington, DC: American Psychiatric Press; 1994.

Kane J, Honigfeld G, Singer J, Meltzer H, and the Clozaril Collaborative Study Group. Clozapine for the treatment-resistant schizophrenic. *Arch Gen Psychiatr.* 1988; 45: 789–796.

Kaplan HI, Sadock BJ (eds). *Synopsis of Psychiatry,* 6th ed. Baltimore: Williams & Wilkins; 1991.

Kaplan HI, Sadock BJ (eds). *Synopsis of Psychiatry,* 7th ed. Baltimore: Williams & Wilkins; 1994.

Koe BK. Preclinical pharmacology of setraline: A potent and specific inhibitor of serotonin reuptake. *J Clin Psychiatr.* 1990; 51(12; supp B): 13–17.

Stoudemire A. *Clinical Psychiatry for Medical Students,* 2nd ed. Philadelphia: Lippincott; 1994.

CHAPTER 8

Obstetrics and Gynecology
Questions

Denyse M. Mahoney, PA-C

DIRECTIONS (Questions 1 through 44): Each of the numbered items or incomplete statements in this section is followed by answers or by completions of the statement. Select the ONE lettered answer or completion that is BEST in each case.

Questions 1 through 44

1. Which of the following mother's offspring would require treatment with hepatitis B immune globulin and hepatitis B vaccine at birth?

   (A) mother who has been immunized with hepatitis B vaccine and is surface antibody positive
   (B) mother with active hepatitis A
   (C) mother who is HBsAg positive
   (D) mother with convalescent titers for hepatitis A
   (E) an unregistered mother who has risk factors for hepatitis B

2. A 36-year-old woman gives birth to a child with spina bifida. Which of the following would be correct information when counseling her about future pregnancies?

   (A) The chance of having another child with a neural tube defect is no different from the general population.
   (B) All future pregnancies would be affected, and she should consider permanent sterilization.
   (C) She should be advised to take a vitamin supplement of folic acid prior to her next conception.
   (D) She should be advised to have an alpha-fetoprotein drawn at 10 weeks with her subsequent pregnancies.
   (E) She should be advised to begin folic acid supplements at 12 weeks and continue through the end of pregnancy.

3. A patient was delivered by cesarean section and is presently 2 days postop. She is found to have a swollen, erythematous right leg with a positive Homan's sign. Which of the following did NOT contribute to her present complication?

   (A) decreased blood flow from her lower extremities during the last weeks of pregnancy
   (B) hypercoagulable state of pregnancy
   (C) decreased activity secondary to postoperative state
   (D) use of oxytocin to stimulate labor
   (E) delivery by cesarean section

4. Which of the following would be a sign and/or symptom of postpartum mastitis?

   (A) bloody discharge from the nipple
   (B) engorgement of breast within 48 hours after onset of lactation
   (C) areas of inflammation, redness, and induration of one breast
   (D) green discoloration of breast milk
   (E) increased breast milk production from infected side

5. Which of the following would NOT cause a higher incidence of breech presentation?

    (A) fetal anomalies
    (B) first pregnancy at an early age
    (C) uterine anatomic abnormalities
    (D) premature onset of labor
    (E) grandmultiparity

6. A 28-year-old female presents to the emergency department with a 4-day history of swelling and pain in her vagina. On examination she has a right Bartholin's abscess: the abscess is 4 cm in size, fluctulant, and erythematous. In addition, she has right inguinal adenopathy. Which of the following would be the BEST definitive therapy?

    (A) outpatient surgical correction by marsupialization
    (B) incision and drainage in the emergency department
    (C) PO antibiotics and local treatment with warm soaks
    (D) use of steroids to decrease initial swelling, prior to surgery
    (E) admission to hospital for IV antibiotics and definitive surgery

7. A 25-year-old patient has undergone a rapid, spontaneous vaginal delivery followed by a prolonged third stage of labor, and an eventual manual removal of the placenta. She continues to bleed heavily after placental removal, with an estimated blood loss of greater than 1,000 mL. What would be the initial step to control the hemorrhage?

    (A) rapid infusion of IV pitocin
    (B) administration of SQ terbutaline
    (C) ligation of the uterine artery
    (D) packing of the uterus
    (E) insertion of a Swan–Ganz catheter for more accurate monitoring of cardiovascular status

8. An 18-year-old Gravid 2 Para 0 presents for her first prenatal visit at 16 weeks' gestation. Routine cervical cultures are performed for gonorrhea, and a monoclonal antibody test for chlamydia is obtained. The chlamydia test is positive. Which of the following is the BEST treatment?

    (A) doxycycline 100 mg PO bid for 10 days
    (B) Bactrim DS one tab PO bid for 10 days
    (C) ceftriaxone 250 mg IM
    (D) erythromycin 500 mg PO q6 hours for 7 days
    (E) Keflex 500 mg PO q6 hours for 10 days

9. A 35-year-old patient presents to labor and delivery at 18 weeks' gestation, complaining of fullness in her vagina. On pelvic exam, the cervix is 6 cm with ballooning of the membranes into the vagina. Additional information you might obtain from the patient that would explain her present condition would be

    (A) history of previous septic abortion
    (B) previous second-trimester abortion that was without contractions
    (C) a known, balanced, chromosomal abnormality in the patient
    (D) a history of having an amniocentesis 2 weeks prior to admission
    (E) a history of having an abnormal Pap during the pregnancy that required colposcopy

10. A woman has undergone a suction curettage for a hydatidiform mole. What subsequent steps should be done to ensure she does not develop choriocarcinoma?

    (A) Serial serum beta HCG levels should be obtained every 1 to 2 weeks until negative.
    (B) Prophylatic chemotherapy should be administered.
    (C) The patient should be advised to never conceive again.
    (D) The patient should undergo a radical hysterectomy and bilateral salpingo-oophorectomy.
    (E) Beta HCG levels should be obtained monthly for 1 year.

11. At 34 weeks' gestation, a patient's fundal height measures 40 cm. The sonogram at that time reveals polyhydramnios. What else may be found on ultrasound at this time?

(A) large ovarian cyst
(B) calcification of the placenta
(C) placenta previa
(D) fetal congenital anomalies
(E) an estimated fetal weight that is indicative of intrauterine growth retardation

12. Preterm labor occurs more frequently in twin gestations. Which of the following antenatal complications does NOT occur with greater frequency in a twin gestation?

(A) fetal anomalies
(B) preeclampsia
(C) intrauterine growth retardation
(D) gestational diabetes
(E) maternal anemia

13. Respiratory depression is a known side effect of intravenous magnesium sulfate (a medication commonly used in pregnant women). Which of the following is the BEST means of monitoring the amount of magnesium administered and preventing this complication?

(A) observing changes in the fetal heart rate
(B) checking maternal deep tendon reflexes
(C) serum magnesium
(D) monitoring blood pressure
(E) hourly respiratory rates

14. A 32-year-old patient presents to labor and delivery at 37 weeks' gestation with a complaint of vaginal bleeding. Her history includes two previous cesarean sections. A sonogram performed showed the following (see Figure 8–1). Which of the following procedures should be performed on this patient?

(A) stat dose of subcutaneous terbutaline
(B) bedrest with IV fluids
(C) induced vaginal delivery
(D) bimanual pelvic exam
(E) repeat cesarean section

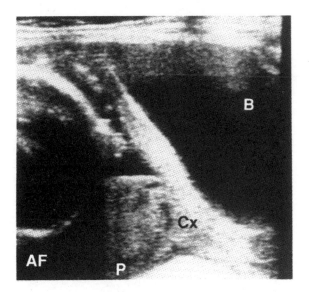

Figure 8–1. A 32-year-old patient at 37 weeks' gestation. AF, amniotic fluid; B, maternal bladder; Cx, cervix; P, placenta.

15. At 36 weeks, a 28-year-old patient presents with a complaint of leaking fluid from her vagina. Which of the following would be a positive test for rupture of membranes?

(A) an L/S ratio of greater than two
(B) the presence of "ferning" on a glass slide made from fluid obtained from the posterior fornix
(C) a low estimate of amniotic fluid volume on ultrasound
(D) testing with nitrazine paper to show that the fluid is acidic
(E) the presence of spinnbarkeit in the cervical mucus

16. A 32-year-old G3P1 presents in labor at 34 weeks' gestation with spontaneous rupture of membranes. She is started on penicillin G, 5 mU IV; the medication is given to treat which organism?

(A) *Chlamydia*
(B) *Listeria monocytogenes*
(C) *Neisseria gonorrhoeae*
(D) group B beta streptococcus
(E) *Escherichia coli*

17. Which of the following medications is NOT used to arrest preterm labor?

    (A) magnesium sulfate
    (B) indomethicin
    (C) ritodrine
    (D) ethanol
    (E) terbutaline

18. Pregnancy complicated by insulin-dependent diabetes prior to gestation has which of the following additional complications?

    (A) increase in fetal congenital anomalies
    (B) increased cesarean section rate
    (C) increased incidence of preeclampsia/eclampsia
    (D) increase in fetal respiratory distress syndrome
    (E) all of the above

19. A 33-year-old gestational diabetic presents for her 34-week prenatal appointment. To begin postnatal counseling at this time; which of the following would be important to stress to this patient?

    (A) She should be counseled to have a bilateral tubal ligation, because further pregnancies might jeopardize her health.
    (B) After delivery she can resume her pre-pregnancy dietary habits as the majority of gestational diabetes become euglycemic after pregnancy.
    (C) She should continue monitoring her serum glucose after delivery to determine whether she is going to be diabetic in the future.
    (D) She should be counseled about diet and weight control after pregnancy.
    (E) She should be advised to avoid use of oral contraceptives because they may predispose her to developing type II diabetes.

20. A 26-year-old female visits a woman's clinic for the first time after the birth of her 3-year-old for a routine pelvic exam and Pap test. The results of the Pap test showed a high-grade squamous intraepithelial lesion. What should the next step in the workup be?

    (A) simple hysterectomy
    (B) repeat the Pap smear in 3 to 6 months
    (C) cryosurgery of the cervix
    (D) LEEP cone biopsy
    (E) colposcopy

21. A 35-year-old woman undergoes a dilation and curettage for irregular menstrual bleeding. The endometrial curettings are consistent with the secretory phase of the menstrual cycle. With this information, which of the following is a correct statement about this patient?

    (A) The patient is entering premature menopause.
    (B) The endometrium is under predominantly estrogen stimulation.
    (C) The patient is taking oral contraceptives.
    (D) The patient has ovulated.
    (E) The patient has Asherman syndrome.

22. When reviewing the events of a patient's labor, what is the MOST predictive factor in determining whether she will develop a post-operative infection after cesarean section?

    (A) history of previous cesarean section
    (B) whether cesarean section was an emergency
    (C) duration of labor prior to cesarean
    (D) presence of medical complications, such as preeclampsia or diabetes
    (E) malpresentation of fetus, such as breech or transverse lie

23. On postop day 5, a patient has persistent spiking temperature despite triple antibiotics for 48 hours. She also is found to be tachypneic and tachycardic. What is the MOST important postop complication to rule out?

    (A) pneumonia
    (B) tubo-ovarian abscess
    (C) endomyometritis
    (D) sepsis
    (E) pulmonary embolus

24. A 36-year-old woman with two previous full-term pregnancies presents for her first prena-

tal visit at 12 weeks' gestation. What tests must she be advised to undergo?

(A) immediate high-resolution ultrasound
(B) genetic amniocentesis
(C) maternal serum alpha-fetoprotein at present visit
(D) amniocentesis for chromosomal abnormalities at 24 weeks
(E) chromosomal analysis of herself and of the father of the baby

25. A 27-year-old Black female with chronic hypertension is being monitored during the active phase of labor. Late decelerations are noted on the monitor. What can be surmised from such a fetal heart rate pattern?

(A) The patient has developed superimposed preeclampsia.
(B) The patient has placenta previa.
(C) The decelerations are secondary to head compression and are of no significance.
(D) There is evidence on the fetal heart tracing of placental insufficiency.
(E) The patient should undergo a pelvic exam to rule out cord prolapse.

26. The tracing shown in Figure 8–2 was obtained on a 23-year-old woman at $41^{1}/_{2}$

weeks during antepartum testing. The tracing can be described as

(A) suspicious for fetal compromise
(B) a reactive nonstress test
(C) a negative oxytocin challenge test
(D) a fetal heart pattern consistent with a cord pattern
(E) an indication that the patient must be incorrect on her date of conception

27. A patient is admitted to labor and delivery with contractions every 4 minutes, lasting 45 seconds. On admission, her pelvic exam revealed a 4-cm dilated cervix. One hour later, her cervix was 5-cm dilated. Which of the following is an accurate statement about her labor pattern?

(A) The fetal presentation should be determined because breech presentation progresses rapidly.
(B) An intrauterine pressure catheter should be placed to determine intensity of uterine contractions.
(C) If this is a first pregnancy, she is making good progress.
(D) This is adequate progress for the latent phase of labor.
(E) She has entered her second stage of labor.

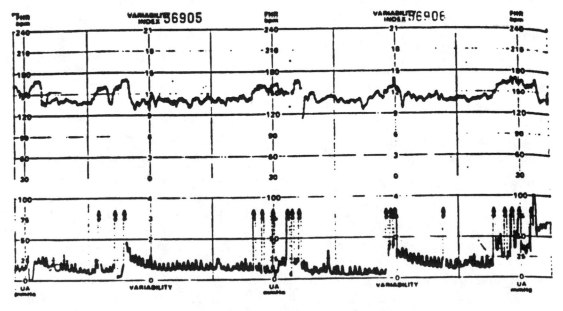

Figure 8–2. A 23-year-old woman at $41^{1}/_{2}$ weeks.

28. A 38-year-old female presents to her family practitioner with complaints of irritability, weight gain, lower abdominal swelling, and difficulty concentrating, which she notes occurs 7 to 10 days before her period begins and resolves on the second or third day of her cycle. She stopped using birth control pills at age 35, and she feels the symptoms have gotten progressively worse since that time. When symptomatic, she is not able to function on her job. Her periods have remained regular every 28 days. What is the MOST likely cause of her symptoms?

    (A) premature ovarian failure
    (B) secondary dysmenorrhea
    (C) polycystic ovary syndrome
    (D) premenstrual syndrome
    (E) depression

29. A 9 pound 8 oz. baby is delivered with mid-forceps to a 32-year-old multiparous patient. The placenta delivered spontaneously without difficulty. The uterus appears to be well contracted with pitocin, but the patient continues to bleed vaginally, presenting bright, red blood. What is the MOST likely cause of this persistent bleeding?

    (A) retained placental products
    (B) lacerations of the cervix or vagina
    (C) previously undiagnosed coagulopathy
    (D) bleeding is from a rectal tear, secondary to the forceps
    (E) uterine atony

30. A 27-year-old woman presents in labor at term with a history of a previous cesarean section for cephalopelvic disproportion. What is the most important item of historical information needed prior to attempting vaginal delivery after a cesarean?

    (A) birth weight of previous baby
    (B) length of labor in previous pregnancy
    (C) strength of contractions in present labor
    (D) uterine incision in previous cesarean section
    (E) indication for primary cesarean section

31. At 11 weeks' gestation, a patient presents to the emergency department with a complaint of vaginal bleeding and lower abdominal cramping. On pelvic exam, there is a large amount of blood in the vagina, and placental tissue is present in the os. This describes which kind of spontaneous abortion?

    (A) inevitable
    (B) septic
    (C) missed
    (D) incomplete
    (E) induced

32. A 17-year-old female presents at the GYN clinic requesting an abortion. She is presently 10 weeks' pregnant. What would be the safest, most efficient means of abortion at this time?

    (A) intra-amniotic saline injection
    (B) suction curettage after cervical dilation with prostaglandin suppository
    (C) hysterotomy
    (D) dilation and curettage
    (E) administration of IV oxytocin

33. At 16 weeks' gestation, a patient presents with a complaint of vaginal bleeding. Her quantitative beta-HCG is higher than expected at 16 weeks' gestation, and her fundal height is approximately a 16- to 18-week size. Although she denies a past history of hypertension, her blood pressure is 140/90. No fetal heart sounds can be heard on doptone, and there is no sign of a fetus on ultrasound. What would be her MOST likely diagnosis?

    (A) threatened abortion
    (B) incomplete abortion
    (C) hydatidiform mole
    (D) fetal demise at 16 weeks
    (E) twin gestation

34. A 28-year-old patient presents to labor and delivery at 38 weeks with a history of sudden onset of sharp pain in her lower abdomen and back, which has since subsided. On evaluation, her blood pressure is 150/100, and there is no detectable fetal heart movement

on ultrasound. She also complains of profuse vaginal bleeding. As observed on the fetal monitor, she is having frequent contractions. What is the MOST likely cause of fetal demise?

(A) placenta previa
(B) gestational diabetes
(C) disseminated intravascular coagulopathy (DIC)
(D) placental abruption
(E) chronic renal failure

35. A woman at 20 weeks' gestation is diagnosed with fetal demise. She has elected to await the onset of spontaneous labor. What blood test should be drawn at this time to avoid a major complication of intrauterine fetal demise?

(A) beta-HCG
(B) PT, PTT, and fibrinogen
(C) liver function test
(D) complete blood count (CBC)
(E) prolactin level

36. At 42 weeks' gestation, a patient's labor is induced. At 5 cm dilated, she undergoes an artificial rupture of membranes with very little fluid present. What other characteristic of a postdate pregnancy might be present at the time of rupture of membranes?

(A) chorioamnionitis
(B) blood-tinged fluid
(C) vernix present in fluid
(D) meconium-stained fluid
(E) hyperstimulation of uterine contractions

37. At a prenatal clinic, a 32-year-old patient presents at 26 weeks' gestation. On history, you find her first child weighed $9^1/_2$ pounds. Her second child was stillborn. What screening test would you order at this time?

(A) alpha-fetoprotein
(B) VDRL
(C) blood type and Rh
(D) 50-g glucose challenge
(E) toxoplasmosis titers

38. A 29-year-old patient presents to the emergency department at 17 weeks' gestation with a complaint of right upper-quadrant and right lower-quadrant pain of 6 hours' duration. The pain is associated with nausea and vomiting. On exam, she has diffuse abdominal tenderness and decreased bowel sounds, and her fundal height is consistent with dates and is nontender. She has no costovertebral angle (CVA) tenderness. Her temperature is 102.4°F and the white blood cell (WBC) count on her complete blood count (CBC) is 18,000. Her urinalysis shows no WBCs or proteinuria. What is the MOST likely diagnosis?

(A) hyperemesis graviderm
(B) acute appendicitis
(C) pylonephritis
(D) unilateral pelvic inflammatory disease (PID)
(E) degenerating myomata

39. Complications secondary to anesthesia are one of the most common causes of maternal mortality. The MOST common life-threatening complication of general anesthesia in the pregnant woman is

(A) hypotension
(B) atelectasis
(C) aspiration
(D) uterine atony
(E) eclampsia

40. A 24-year-old patient presents to a GYN clinic for a routine exam. Her OB/GYN history is significant for having her first child at age 16 and her second at age 18. Since separation from her husband at age 19, she has had several sexual partners. On pelvic exam, she has condylomata acuminata on her labia. What malignancy is this woman at risk for?

(A) ovarian cancer
(B) AIDS
(C) endometrial cancer
(D) cervical cancer
(E) cancer of the labia

41. A 21-year-old patient presents to Planned Parenthood requesting birth control. She states her second pregnancy was unplanned and occurred because she forgot to take her birth control pills for several days in a row. Her OB/GYN history is significant for having two living children, two abortions, and a possible history of pelvic inflammatory disease (PID) approximately 1 year ago. Which of the following would be the BEST means of birth control for this patient?

    (A) contraceptive sponge
    (B) intrauterine device
    (C) bilateral tubal ligation
    (D) DEPO-PROVERA
    (E) condoms

42. A 30-year-old patient complains of progressively worse dysmenorrhea. Her pain begins 2 to 4 days prior to onset of bleeding and is associated with spotting. In addition, she complains of pain on intercourse (dyspareunia). You think the patient may have endometriosis. What is the best way to make the diagnosis?

    (A) a 6-month course of danazol (Danocrine) to see whether the symptoms subside
    (B) pelvic ultrasound
    (C) treatment with prostaglandin synthetase inhibitors to see whether the symptoms abate
    (D) diagnostic laparoscopy
    (E) diagnostic hysteroscopy

43. Which menstrual irregularity would MOST likely occur in a woman suffering from anorexia nervosa or in a woman who is a marathon runner?

    (A) menorrhagia
    (B) amenorrhea
    (C) oligomenorrhea
    (D) polymenorrhea
    (E) metrorrhagia

44. A 25-year-old woman presents with a history of prolonged episodes of amenorrhea followed by prolonged bleeding. She has been sexually active for 6 years and has never conceived. On physical exam, she is obese and somewhat hirsute. On pelvic exam, her ovaries are enlarged bilaterally. The MOST likely diagnosis is

    (A) progesterone-secreting tumor on the ovaries
    (B) hyperprolactinemia syndrome
    (C) congenital adrenal hyperplasia
    (D) polycystic ovary (PCO) syndrome
    (E) hypothyroidism

DIRECTIONS (Questions 45 through 52): Each group of items in this section consists of lettered headings followed by a set of numbered words or phrases. For each numbered word or phrase, select the ONE lettered heading that is most closely associated with it. Each lettered heading may be selected once, more than once, or not at all.

Questions 45 through 48

For the number of weeks of gestation, match the events of pregnancy that occur at the time of pregnancy.

    (A) 6 weeks
    (B) 28 weeks
    (C) 20 weeks
    (D) 16 to 20 weeks
    (E) 14 weeks

45. Fundal height at umbilicus

46. Fetal movements first perceived by mother

47. Fetal heart motion first seen on transvaginal sonogram

48. Optimal time to draw maternal serum alpha-fetoprotein

Questions 49 through 52

The following are a list of drugs. Match the known side effects if the drug is ingested by a pregnant woman.

    (A) alcohol
    (B) nitrofurantoin
    (C) coumadin
    (D) cocaine
    (E) phenytoin

49. Anomalies are caused by the drug's effect on the fetal clotting factors.

50. Higher incidence of stillborns secondary to placental abruptions when this drug is used during second and third trimesters.

51. Taken in large amounts the drug causes definitive syndrome in the fetus, but it is unclear whether occasional use causes fetal harm.

52. The maternal benefits of this drug outweigh the known fetal effects.

DIRECTIONS (Questions 53 through 73): Each of the numbered items or incomplete statements in this section is followed by answers or by completions of the statement. Select the ONE lettered answer or completion that is BEST in each case.

Questions 53 through 73

53. A 62-year-old female who is 12 years postmenopausal complains of urinary urgency, frequency, and occasional incontinence. On pelvic exam, her vaginal mucosa appears atrophic: shiny, pale pink with white patches, and bleeds slightly to touch. Her urinalysis and urine cultures are negative. How would you BEST treat this patient?

    (A) antibiotic by mouth
    (B) testosterone cream to be applied to affected areas
    (C) vaginal suppositories containing sulfa antibiotics
    (D) estrogen-containing cream per vagina

    (E) a surgical procedure that would correct a prolapsed bladder

54. A 26-year-old female who is G2P2 and whose last menstrual period (LMP) was 8 weeks earlier presents to the emergency department with a complaint of lower abdominal pain and vaginal bleeding described as spotting. Her vital signs are stable, and on abdominal exam she has good bowel sounds and no tenderness. On pelvic exam, she has mild cervical motion tenderness and a 6- to 8-week size uterus. Her serum beta-HCG is positive and her hematocrit is 39. You suspect a threatened abortion but want to rule out ectopic pregnancy. What would be the next appropriate step?

    (A) pelvic ultrasound with transvaginal probe
    (B) diagnostic laparoscopy
    (C) serial quantitative beta-HCG every day for a week
    (D) exploratory laparotomy
    (E) culdocentesis

55. A 39-year-old female G2P1Ab1L1 presents to the emergency department with lower abdominal pain, vaginal bleeding, and a 6-week history of amenorrhea. Her GYN history is significant for history of oral contraceptive use in the past and a spontaneous miscarriage. In addition, she has had an episode of pelvic inflammatory disease (PID) and subsequent secondary infertility, for which she has recently undergone diagnostic laparoscopy. On presentation she was orthostatic and a culdocentesis performed in the emergency department was positive for blood. Exploratory laparotomy revealed an ectopic pregnancy. What risk factor did this patient have for developing an ectopic pregnancy?

    (A) a history of spontaneous abortion
    (B) a history of laparoscopy
    (C) a history of oral contraceptive use
    (D) advanced maternal age
    (E) a history of PID

56. A 19-year-old G0P0 female presents to the emergency department with a complaint of lower abdominal pain and fever of 2 days' duration. Her last period was normal and ended 3 days prior to the onset of pain. On physical exam, her temperature was 101°F, and she had decreased bowel sounds and bilateral lower abdominal tenderness with rebound tenderness. On pelvic exam, she had cervical motion tenderness and bilateral adnexal tenderness. The diagnosis of pelvic inflammatory disease (PID) was made and the patient was admitted for IV antibiotic therapy. Which of the following two organisms are MOST likely to cause the infection?

    (A) *Neisseria gonorrhoeae* and *Chlamydia trachomatis*
    (B) *Neisseria gonorrhoeae* and *Bacteroides*
    (C) *Chlamydia trachomatis* and *Mycoplasma hominis*
    (D) *Neisseria gonorrhoeae* and *Clostridium difficile*
    (E) *Chlamydia trachomatis* and *Mycoplasma hominis*

57. A 22-year-old G2P2 presents to the GYN clinic with a history that her boyfriend had a positive culture for gonorrhea. She complains only of a vaginal discharge. On abdominal exam, she has mild bilateral lower abdominal tenderness; and on pelvic exam, a mucopurulent discharge from the cervix and mild cervical motion tenderness. She appears to have mild pelvic inflammatory disease (PID). Because she could tolerate medication by mouth, she is treated on an outpatient basis. Which of the following regimens are adequate treatment for outpatient PID?

    (A) vibramycin 100 mg bid PO
    (B) 2.4 million U procaine penicillin IM with probenicid and erythromycin 25 mg PO for 7 days
    (C) trimethoprim-sulfamethoxazole, 2 tabs PO bid for 7 days
    (D) ceftriaxone 250 mg IM for one dose, and doxycycline 100 mg PO bid for 10 days
    (E) ofloxacin 400 mg PO bid for 14 days

58. A 65-year-old woman comes to your office for a routine gynecological exam. Her last menstrual period was over 15 years ago and she denies any postmenopausal bleeding. On examination she has atrophic changes of the vulva and the vagina, her uterus is of normal size, her left ovary is slightly palpable but her right ovary cannot be felt. What should your next step in the evaluation of her exam be?

    (A) Refer her to a gastroenterologist because left-sided masses in an elderly woman are usually diverticulitis.
    (B) Reassure her that the exam is normal and encourage her to return in 1 year.
    (C) Have her return in 6 weeks to reevaluate the size of her left ovary.
    (D) Order a pelvic/abdominal sonogram and transvaginal sonogram.
    (E) Perform an endometrial biopsy.

59. A 24-year-old female presents with a complaint of labial bumps that are painful when she urinates. On questioning the patient, she reveals she has felt feverish and has had generalized malaise. On pelvic exam, she has several vesicular lesions on the labia and a few ulcerative lesions. The lesions are painful to touch. Which of the following could be the cause of this patient's symptoms?

    (A) condylomata acuminata
    (B) secondary syphilis
    (C) lymphogranuloma venereum
    (D) primary syphilis
    (E) herpes

60. A 49-year-old G2P2 female has a known history of uterine myomata that are approximately 16-week size. Within the past year, her periods have become progressively heavier and longer. A dilation and curettage performed 6 months earlier showed no pathology and failed to decrease the bleeding. Her hematocrit is 25, but the patient is not orthostatic and does not complain of dizziness. Which of the following would be the MOST likely next step in her therapy?

    (A) abdominal myomectomy
    (B) laparoscopic-assisted myomectomy

(C) a 3-month course of leuprolide acetate (lupron depot)

(D) transfusion with two units of packed cells

(E) total abdominal hysterectory

61. Endometrial hyperplasia is a pathology found in women with irregular menstrual bleeding. It is characterized by excessive growth of the endometrium, which is usually a result of a persistently high level of estrogen that is unopposed by progesterone. Which of the following women is likely to have endometrial hyperplasia?

(A) a young woman suffering from anorexia nervosa

(B) a 35-year-old woman with a long history of anovulatory cycles

(C) a woman with a 10-year history of oral contraceptive use

(D) a woman who has just completed her second dose of medroxyprogesterone acetate, DEPO-PROVERA

(E) a 35-year-old woman with adenomyosis

62. On a routine pelvic examination, a 5-cm cystic mass is palpated on the left side of a 22-year-old female. Her last menstrual period was approximately 13 days prior to the exam. It is decided to give her birth control pills in an attempt to suppress ovarian function. Six weeks later, she is reexamined and the cyst is 10 cm in size. Which of the following would be the next step in treating this patient?

(A) Continue birth control pills and reexamine the patient in 8 weeks.

(B) Perform diagnostic laparoscopy to determine whether the cyst is functional versus neoplastic.

(C) Obtain ultrasound to rule out endometrioma.

(D) Perform exploratory laparotomy to remove the cyst.

(E) Administer a GnRH analog to shrink the cyst.

63. A 19-year-old female who is sexually active and uses no form of birth control presents to the emergency department with a complaint of severe abdominal pain. Her last menstrual period (LMP) was approximately 6 weeks before the onset of the pain. She has a history significant for irregular periods. On abdominal exam, she has decreased bowel sounds and rebound tenderness. On pelvic exam, she has a small amount of dark red blood in her vagina and marked tenderness to cervical motion. Prior to bringing the patient to the operating room for an exploratory laparotomy, which test would be helpful in differentiating whether this patient has a ruptured corpus luteal cyst versus ectopic pregnancy?

(A) hemoglobin and hematocrit

(B) urinary pregnancy test sensitive to 25 mIU beta-HCG

(C) white blood cell count on complete blood count

(D) vaginal sonogram to see whether there is free fluid in the cul-de-sac

(E) quantitative beta HCG

64. A 45-year-old woman presents with a complaint of irregular menstrual periods and occasional episodes of hot flashes. On physical exam her external genitalia are slightly pale and the vaginal mucosa is thinned. Her uterus is of normal size, as are her ovaries. Which of the following would BEST describe her clinical and physical findings?

(A) She is peri-menopausal.

(B) She is pregnant.

(C) She is menopausal.

(D) She has premature ovarian failure.

(E) She has polycystic ovaries.

65. A 40-year-old G3P3 woman goes to her gynecologist for a routine GYN exam. Which is/are part of a routine gynecological exam?

(A) bimanual pelvic exam

(B) breast exam

(C) speculum exam of the cervix and vagina

(D) rectovaginal exam

(E) all of the above

66. When performing a pelvic exam, it is important to

    (A) adequately drape the patient to avoid excessive exposure
    (B) insist that family members, including the patient's husband, leave the examining room
    (C) proceed rapidly so the patient has no opportunity to express fear or discomfort
    (D) refrain from informing the patient that a particular part of the exam will be painful
    (E) make sure the patient cannot see you as you perform the exam

67. A 49-year-old female presents with a complaint of hot flashes and amenorrhea of 10 months' duration. Her pelvic exam reveals atrophic external genitala and a normal-size uterus and normal ovaries bilaterally. Her breast exam is within normal limits, and her most recent mammogram was 8 months ago and was negative. You prescribe hormone replacement, a combination of a conjugated estrogen and a progestational agent. Which of the following is NOT an additional advantage of hormone replacement?

    (A) prevention of endometrial cancer
    (B) decreased risk for developing cardiovascular disease
    (C) prevention of osteoporosis
    (D) relief of urogenital symptoms of atrophy
    (E) improvement in sexual satisfaction

68. When obtaining a menstrual history, which of the following is NOT an important question to ask?

    (A) duration and amount of menstrual flow
    (B) color of blood on day 1 of the cycle
    (C) age of onset and frequency of menses
    (D) date of last menstrual period and whether it was normal
    (E) presence of intermenstrual bleeding

69. A 42-year-old female with a known history of uterine myomata presents with a complaint of increased bleeding during menses and spotting 4 to 5 days prior to onset of period. On pelvic exam, she has a 14-week size irregular uterus, consistent with fibroids. On speculum exam, there is a small polyp that can be seen in the endocervical canal. Which of the following would be an appropriate procedure for this patient to undergo next?

    (A) endometrial biopsy with endocervical curettage
    (B) ultrasound of the pelvis
    (C) abdominal hysterectomy
    (D) CAT scan of the pelvis
    (E) colposcopy

70. A 23-year-old crack abuser presents to the emergency department with a complaint of vaginal spotting and no period for 6 weeks. A pregnancy test is positive and her pelvis is consistent with a 6-week gestation. She is discharged with the diagnosis of threatened abortion. Two days later, she returns and miscarries. A VDRL drawn at the time of the initial visit is found to be positive. Upon questioning, the patient then remembers having a bump on her vulva approximately 4 weeks earlier. If the patient failed to get treatment at this time, which of the following symptoms would she most likely develop?

    (A) condylomata acuminata on the vulva
    (B) maculopapular skin rash, often on the palms of the hands and soles of the feet
    (C) mucopurulent discharge from the cervix
    (D) vesicular lesions on the vulva that are painful to touch
    (E) signs of pelvic inflammatory disease (PID)

71. A 27-year-old G2P1Ab1 at 32 weeks' gestation presents to her obstetrician with a complaint of not feeling the baby move for 24 hours. On ultrasound, intrauterine fetal demise is confirmed; there is no sign of fetal movement and there is no fetal cardiac motion. The patient is induced and delivers spontaneously approximately 12 hours later. Which of the following is an appropriate means of helping parents deal with the loss of the child?

(A) Allow the parents to hold and examine the stillborn child, if they choose.

(B) Heavily medicate the mother during labor and particularly the delivery, so she will have no recollection of the delivery.

(C) The patient should be reassured that she is young and can easily conceive again.

(D) Discourage the father (or other support person) from being present during labor and delivery to spare him the pain.

(E) The patient and husband should be encouraged not to name the child or to take pictures, so as not to have bad memories of the pregnancy.

72. A 32-year-old G3P2Ab1 female at 40 weeks' gestation is being monitored in labor and develops the fetal heart rate depicted in Figure 8–3. Which of the following is TRUE about this patient's tracing?

(A) These are late decelerations.

(B) This pattern is an indication for a stat cesarean section.

(C) This fetal heart rate pattern indicates that the patient is in the second stage of labor.

(D) These are variable decelerations.

(E) The patient needs pitocin to increase the frequency of contractions.

73. A 16-year-old female is seen in the emergency department as a rape victim. She undergoes a physical and pelvic exam. Prior to being discharged from the emergency department, she should be offered which of the following?

(A) follow-up visit in order to be tested for pregnancy and obtain a repeat VDRL

(B) information on how to contact a rape crisis counselor

(C) treatment for gonorrhea and chlamydia

(D) medication to prevent pregnancy

(E) all of the above

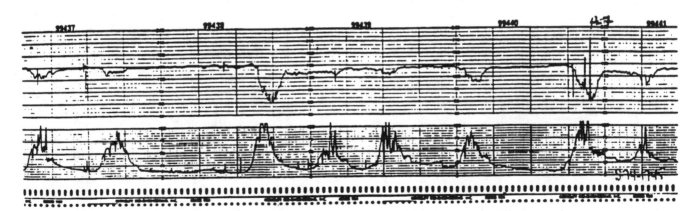

Figure 8–3. A 32-year-old G3P2Ab1 female at 40 weeks' gestation.

Answers and Explanations

1. **(C)** The Centers for Disease Control and Prevention recommend that babies born to mothers who are hepatitis B surface antigen positive should be treated to prevent mother-to-newborn transmission. Treatment has been found to prevent transmission by 90%. Neonates born to mothers who are hepatitis B surface antigen positive have a high incidence of developing acute and chronic hepatitis, hepatoma, and cirrhosis. Treatment consists of hyperimmune serum globulin (HBIG) and the hepatitis B vaccine (HBvac). These are both given at birth, and the HBvac is given in two more doses, beginning at 1 month of age. Mothers who have been immunized with the hepatitis B vaccine and are hepatitis B antibody positive are protected against hepatitis B and therefore cannot transmit the virus to their children. There is no risk of transmission of hepatitis A to the neonate. One study showed that mothers who have not registered for prenatal care were at greater risk of being hepatitis B surface antigen positive, and therefore the neonatal was at greater risk of transmission. But there is no indication for prophylaxis, until tests for hepatitis B surface antigen are positive. *(Burrow and Ferris, p. 332; Sammuels and Cohen, pp.753–757)*

2. **(C)** Neural tube defects (NTD) occur because of failed closure of the neural tube between the third and fourth week of embryologic development. The most common malformations that occur because of this failed closure are anencephaly, encephalocele, and spina bifida. Neural tube defects are the second most common birth defect in the United States. It has been shown that in women who have had a previous child affected with an NTD, preconceptual and use in the first 3 months of pregnancy of a folic acid supplement will decrease the incidence of having another child with an NTD. Although not yet proven, this regimen could prevent the occurrence of NTDs in women with no previous history. At this time, the American College of OB/GYN recommends that women who have had a child or aborted a fetus with an NTD should take 4 mg of folic acid a day, beginning 1 month prior to attempting conception and for the first 3 months of pregnancy. Women who have had a child with an NTD should be counseled that they have a 10 times greater risk of having another child with an NTD. But, particularly with the possibility of decreasing this risk with the use of folic acid, these women do not need to be counseled to have permanent sterility. Screening for NTDs is offered to all pregnant women and is done by obtaining a maternal serum alpha-fetoprotein at $15^1/_2$ weeks to $20^1/_2$ weeks of gestation, not 10 weeks. But in a woman with a history of a child with an NTD, early screening in the second trimester (after 12 weeks) by obtaining an amniotic fluid alpha-fetoprotein and acetylcholinesterase should be offered. Because normal closure of the neural tube occurs by day 26 of fetal development, beginning supplementation in the 12th week would be too late. *(Rose and Mennuti, pp. 605–618)*

3. **(D)** The patient's symptoms are describing a deep vein thrombosis (DVT), a known complication in the pregnant and postpartum/postoperative patient. The factors that· increase the risk of DVT in a pregnant or recently pregnant woman are the hypercoagulable state of pregnancy. A number of blood coagulation factors rise during pregnancy. These include fibrinogen, factor VIII, factor VII, and other vitamin K–dependent clotting factors. During pregnancy, depression of the systemic fibrinolytic activity occurs, which returns to normal after delivery. In the puerperium, however, there are secondary rises of fibrinogen and circulatory platelets. Answers A and C are anatomical/mechanical reasons for increased chance of DVT. Decreased blood flow from the lower extremities occurs secondary to the enlarged uterus and, because of decreased patient mobility, can be secondary to an operative delivery, such as forceps or cesarean section. DVT is 3 to 16 times more common after a cesarean section than after a spontaneous vaginal delivery. *(Creasy and Resnick, p. 792; Cunningham et al, p. 478; Hacker and Moore, p. 201)*

4. **(C)** Chills and fever occur with mastitis, as do the localization of an area of redness, hardening, and induration on the breast. Mastitis typically occurs during the third and fourth week postpartum. Postpartum breasts do become engorged within 24 to 48 hours, but bilaterally and without localized induration or erythema. Postpartum engorgement resolves spontaneously with support and application of ice packs. Mastitis does not cause breast milk to change color, but the offending organism, *Staphylococcus aureus,* can be cultured from the breast milk. Treatment consists of an oral (or if necessary, parenteral) penicillinase-resistant antibiotic for 10 days. If an abscess has formed, incision and drainage may be necessary. Increased milk production does not occur, but often mastitis occurs after the mother has attempted to wean the baby and is producing less milk. *(Creasy and Resnick, p. 652; Cunningham et al, p. 485; Hacker and Moore, pp. 132–133)*

5. **(B)** As term approaches, the fetus assumes the longitudinal lie in the vertex presentation. The reason for vertex predominance is the piriform shape of the uterus. Although the fetal head is larger at term than the podalic pole, the breech and flexed extremities are bulkier and, therefore, adapt to the fundus better. Congenital anomalies, particularly anencephalic and hydrocephalic babies, will present more commonly as breech. Presumably, this is because the piriform-shaped uterus accommodates these anomalies more efficiently. Uterine anomalies, such as bicornate and septate uterus, predispose to breech presentation. Prior to 32 weeks, the amniotic cavity is larger and the amount of amniotic fluid is greater; therefore, more fetuses are in the breech presentation. Breech presentation is more common in grandmultiparous women because of relaxed uterine musculature. Age and first pregnancy are not risk factors for breech presentation. *(Cunningham et al, pp. 178–180, 349)*

6. **(A)** Bartholin's glands are bilateral vulvovaginal glands that open into the posterolateral aspect of the vagina. When infected, often unilaterally, the causative agent frequently is *Gonococcus.* After the initial infection, the duct to the gland becomes scarred, and subsequently asymptomatic mucoid-filled cysts will recur or the duct will become reinfected. When a patient presents to the emergency department with acute swelling and severe pain, incision and drainage can be performed to relieve the patient's discomfort. If the patient is not excessively uncomfortable, local treatment with warm soaks or ice can be attempted, with PO antibiotics. Definitive treatment is marsupialization of the gland, which is a means of creating a fistulous tract between the cyst and the skin. This will prevent the development of the chronic mucoid-filled cysts or possible reinfection. Marsupialization can be performed as an outpatient procedure in an operating room and is usually done after the acute episode has subsided, either due to I & D or local therapy. In-hospital IV antibiotics are never needed for Bartholin's abscess and steroids

would not be helpful. *(Hacker and Moore, pp. 4, 343; Jones et al, pp. 589–590)*

7. **(A)** There are several things the practitioner should do once it appears that the patient is bleeding heavily postdelivery. Initially, the practitioner should simultaneously attempt to contract the uterus manually and to administer medications that will cause uterine contractions. Oxytocin is usually given first, and if the uterus does not respond, ergonovine or methylergonovine should be administered. The ergotrates cause sustained uterine contractions and are, therefore, more efficacious but can cause hypertension and hence are contraindicated in some cases. When oxytocin and methylergonovine fail to work or when methylergonovine is contraindicated, a prostaglandin derivative, 15-methyl-prostaglandin F2 alpha, should be administrated. The 15-M prostaglandin can be given intramuscularly (or intrauterine) and has been found to be efficacious once oxytocin and ergotrates have failed. The uterus and vagina should be explored for retained products and lacerations at the same time as the above medications are administered. Packing of the uterus had been used as a means of controlling postpartum hemorrhage but is not an initial step. It is most commonly used in cases of placenta accreta and persistent lower-segment bleeding. When packing is used and is effective, the patient's vital signs should be carefully monitored, as packing can initially conceal continued hemorrhage. Terbutaline should not be given in any instance of postpartum bleeding because it causes uterine relaxation and would subsequently cause more bleeding. As with any situation when there is the potential for shock to develop, the patient's cardiovascular status should be monitored. At least one, if not two, large-gauge IV catheters should be placed, and specimens for blood crossmatch should be obtained. Invasive, central monitoring would not be necessary in the initial treatment of postpartum hemorrhage, but would be indicated if the patient required extensive fluid, blood and blood product, replacement, or if the patient developed dis-

seminated intravascular coagulation (DIC). *(Creasy and Resnick, pp. 533–534; Cunningham et al, pp. 417–419; Hacker and Moore, pp. 292–293).*

8. **(D)** *Chlamydia trachomatis* is an obligate intracelluar bacterium. It is very difficult to culture; therefore, monoclonal antibody tests are performed and are felt to be almost as accurate as cultures. Cervical infection at the time of delivery will often result in neonatal chlamydial conjunctivitis or neonatal pneumonia. Chlamydial infection in the mother also has been implicated in the development of preterm birth and preterm premature rupture of membranes. It is, therefore, important to test every patient on her first prenatal visit and to treat positive results. Chlamydia is very sensitive to tetracycline and doxycycline, but these medications are never used during pregnancy because they are teratogenic. Erythromycin is the drug of choice; it is safe to use in pregnancy, and the organism is sensitive to it. Bactrim has some effect on chlamydia but is not used as a first-line medication in pregnancy. Ceftriaxone is not very effective against chlamydia, nor is Keflex. Women at greater risk for having chlamydia are young women under the age of 20, those of lower socioeconomic status, patients with several sexual partners, and patients who have or have had other sexually transmitted diseases. *(Creasy and Resnick, pp. 683–685; Cunningham et al, pp. 853–854; Hacker and Moore, p. 185)*

9. **(B)** The patient's condition is describing an incompetent cervix. Patients with an incompetent cervix typically present in the second trimester with the complaint of spotting and a bulging feeling in their vagina. They do not complain of painful contractions. On pelvic exam, there is cervical dilation with the membranes bulging through the os in an hourglass configuration. Although the exact cause of incompetent cervix is not known, it has been associated with previous cervical trauma, including dilation and curettage, conization, and cautery of the cervix, but colposcopy alone is not a risk factor. Abnormal cervical development has been noted as one of the genital tract abnormalities that occur in

women whose mothers were exposed to diethylstilbestrol (DES). Incompetent cervix is known to occur in these women. A previous first-trimester abortion is not associated with a higher incidence of incompetent cervix. Babies born to women with incompetent cervix do not have a chromosomal abnormality. Spontaneous abortion can occur after amniocentesis, but it is typically associated with painful contractions and spontaneous rupture of membranes. (*Cunningham et al, pp. 498–499*)

10. **(A)** Gestational trophoblastic neoplasia (GTN) consists of benign GTN, most often hydatidiform mole, and malignant GTN, which includes nonmetastatic and metastatic GTN. Approximately 20% of women who have a hydatidiform mole will go on to develop some form of malignant GTN, one of which is choriocarcinoma. To best detect these patients, serum beta-HCG tests are drawn every 1 to 2 weeks until they are negative. In addition, a woman who has had a mole should not become pregnant for 1 year, as pregnancy would interfere with the means of following the trophoblastic disease. Once beta-HCG levels are negative, the patient needs to be followed monthly for 6 months and then every 2 months for 1 year. Should the level of HCG plateau or begin to rise, the patient should undergo further workup and eventually receive chemotherapy. In nonmetastatic GTN, single-agent chemotherapy is effective with either methotrexate or actinomycin D. Prophylactic chemotherapy was considered a possibility in some centers, but morbidity and mortality associated with therapy did not outweigh the benefits. A radical hysterectomy is not indicated for any stage of GTN, but hysterectomy at the time of diagnosis of a hydatidiform mole is acceptable for a woman who has finished childbearing. It is not necessary to remove the adnexa, but it is still necessary to follow beta-HCG levels to detect possible metastatic trophoblastic tissue. (*Creasy and Resnick, pp. 1120–1123; Cunningham et al, pp. 540–553*)

11. **(D)** Polyhydramnios or hydramnios is excessive amniotic fluid. In most cases of mild polyhydramnios, there is no etiology, but moderate to severe hydramnios is usually associated with fetal anomalies. The anomalies are primarily those of the central nervous system, which includes anencephaly, and gastrointestinal anomalies, such as esophogeal atresia. These anomalies are easily diagnosed on ultrasound. Other conditions in which hydramnios occurs are diabetes, immune and nonimmune hydrops, and in one twin of a twin gestation. A large ovarian cyst may be found in a woman with a greater than expected fundal height, but would not be found concurrently with polyhydramnios. Calcification of the placenta occurs with postdate pregnancy or in intrauterine growth retardation, both of which are usually associated with oligohydramnios. (*Creasy and Resnick, pp. 622–623, 946–997; Cunningham et al, pp. 554–556*)

12. **(D)** It is more likely that preeclampsia will develop in twin gestations; it usually occurs earlier in gestation and is more severe. Congenital anomalies of one or both twins is more common in multiple than in single gestations. Frequently, hydramnios accompanies the anomalous twin. Intrauterine growth retardation occurs secondary to intrauterine crowding and subsequent placental insufficiency. The growth retardation can be in both twins or one alone. Other complications of twin gestation are a higher incidence of cesarean section secondary to malpresentation, postpartum hemorrhage secondary to uterine atony, maternal anemia, and a higher incidence of spontaneous abortion. (*Cunningham et al, pp. 629–647; Hacker and Moore, pp. 244–249*).

13. **(C)** Magnesium plasma levels of 4 to 7 mEq/L are known to prevent eclamptic seizures. When the levels are above 10 mEq/L, respiratory depression develops. It is, therefore, advantageous to follow plasma levels periodically, approximately every 8 hours, to prevent toxicity. A clinical means of monitoring magnesium levels is to follow the intensity of patellar deep tendon reflexes. Preeclampsia tends to be a hyperstimulatory state; thus, the deep tendon reflexes tend to be hyperreflexic. Magnesium sulfate has a

depressive effect on this hyperreflexia; it, therefore, becomes a good bedside means of monitoring magnesium levels and therefore its affect on the respiratory system. If patellar reflexes return to normal, it can be presumed that the magnesium levels are within the therapeutic, but not toxic, level. But loss of patellar reflexes is associated with plasma levels greater than 10 mEq/L and impending respiratory depression. Therefore, this is not an exact means of monitoring magnesium levels. Although administration of $MgSO_4$ will cause decreased fetal heart rate variability, this is not an adequate or consistent means of monitoring plasma levels. Because $MgSO_4$ has only a minimal effect on lowering blood pressure, it is not a good means of monitoring levels. Even though monitoring respiratory rate frequently is necessary when a patient is on magnesium, once the respiratory rate is significantly affected, the level could be in the toxic range. *(Creasy and Resnick, pp.829–831; Cunningham et al, pp. 681–682)*

14. **(E)** The figure (8–1) in the sonogram is showing a complete placenta previa. The sonogram is the most definitive means of diagnosing a placenta previa. A bimanual exam would be completely contraindicated, as it would result in severe hemorrhage secondary to digital disruption of the placental site. A sterile speculum exam can be performed if done in an environment where emergency cesarean section is readily available. Because the patient is 37 weeks, there would be no reason to treat the patient conservatively with IV fluids and bedrest. If the patient is preterm and active bleeding has subsided, it is possible to treat conservatively. The patient would then remain on strict bedrest, avoid use of tampons and douching, and refrain from sexual intercourse. If the previa is partial or low-lying and the patient is preterm, conservative treatment may result in avoiding cesarean section; as gestation progresses, the placenta may move away from the cervical os. A vaginal delivery would be completely contraindicated in the instance presented in the question because it is a complete previa at 37 weeks and there is no chance that the placenta would migrate upward. A repeat ce-

sarean section would be the only reasonable course of action in this case. The patient's history of previous cesarean is the probable etiology of the placenta previa. Previas are more common in women who have undergone previous cesarean sections, multiparous patients, and patients of advanced maternal age. Terbutaline is used to cause uterine relaxation and in preterm labor. *(Creasy and Resnick, pp. 602–608; Cunningham et al, pp. 712–714)*

15. **(B)** The accurate diagnosis of spontaneous rupture of membranes is important to ascertain whether the patient has begun labor (premature rupture of membranes) or if the patient is in premature gestation, prior to 37 weeks (preterm premature rupture of membranes). To evaluate for spontaneous rupture of membranes a sterile speculum examination is performed with the patient in the dorsal lithotomy position. Evidence of rupture of membranes would be clear or blood-tinged fluid in the posterior fornix of the vagina, or pooling, and escape of clear fluid from the cervical os when the patient coughs. The fluid is then checked with nitrazine paper. Because amniotic fluid is basic with a pH of approximately 7.0 to 7.5 and vaginal secretions are 4.5 to 5.5, it can be surmised that, if the fluid obtained from the vagina turns nitrazine paper blue (indicative of a higher pH), it is amniotic fluid. Ferning also is a phenomenon of the basic amniotic fluid in the acidic vagina. A ferning pattern is seen on the glass slide when placed under the light microscope. Spinnbarkeit is the long thin, profuse mucus obtained from the cervix after ovulation; it is not found in a pregnant woman. Although in preterm rupture of membranes, it is important to obtain amniotic fluid from the vaginal fornix for lecithin/sphingomyelin (L/S) ratio, the L/S ratio is an indication of fetal lung maturity, not a test for the presence or absence of ruptured membranes. Ultrasound determination of amniotic fluid volume is an important means of evaluating premature and preterm rupture of membranes, but it is not a means of diagnosing rupture of membranes. (For instance, in postdate pregnancies, intrauterine growth retardation, and fetal congenital

anomalies, amniotic fluid is decreased but is not secondary to rupture of membranes.) (*Cunningham et al, pp. 309, 557–558; Gregg, pp. 241–247; Hacker and Moore, pp. 462, 557*)

16. **(D)** Group B beta streptococcus (GBS) is normal lower genitourinary tract flora in many adult women and men and is generally asymtomatic. It is responsible for two different neonatal infections. Early-onset disease occurs within the first 7 days of life and is characterized by the development of respiratory distress, pneumonia, septicemia, and death. Late-onset disease is characterized most commonly by meningitis and occurs usually after the first week of life. Colonization of the genital or anorectal area is associated with preterm rupture of membranes and preterm labor. Within the past year, the Centers for Disease Control and Prevention and the American College of Obstetrics and Gynecology have published guidelines for treatment. The guidelines offer two possible treatment paths, which differ on a "risk" versus "culture-positive" basis. The risk factor treatment plan is to treat with penicillin G 5 mU IV as a loading dose followed by 2.5 mU IV every 4 hours until delivery if the mother has the following risk factors: previously delivered an infant who had GBS-invasive disease; GBS bacteruria during pregnancy; delivery at less than 37 weeks' gestation; duration of ruptured membranes greater than or equal to 18 hours or an intrapartum temperature of greater than or equal to 100.4°F (38°C). The alternative guidelines include all of the risk factors above *and* women who are culture positive at 35 to 37 weeks' gestation. The treatment choice is the same for both pathways. Chlamydia also is associated with a higher incidence of preterm labor, premature rupture of membranes, and neonatal disease, which includes conjunctivitis, pneumonitis, and otitis media. But chlamydia is very sensitive to erythromycin, and if the patient and her sexual partner are compliant with treatment, it is generally eradicated prior to the onset of labor. Patients are usually tested for chlamydia at their first prenatal visit and treated immediately. *Listeria monocytogenes* also causes neonatal infection, which includes pneumonitis, meningitis, and conjuctivitis, but it is very rare and most commonly occurs after the mother ingests contaminated foods. (The *Listeria* can be found in unpasteurized milk and milk products.) Gonococcal infection also has been implicated in the development of preterm labor and preterm rupture of membranes; if not treated at the time of birth it can cause opthalmia, arthritis, or sepsis, but women with the above risk factors are much more likely to have GBS than gonorrhea. *Escherichia coli* is the most common bacteria isolated from positive urine cultures in pregnant women; once it is treated, with the correct antibiotics, cultures should be repeated. If repeat cultures are negative, then further treatment is not necessary at the time of labor. (*Hacker and Moore, pp. 182–185; Keene, pp. 16–28; Schuchat et al, pp. 1–20*)

17. **(D)** Magnesium sulfate and ritodrine are two of the more commonly used tocolytic agents. The presumed effect of magnesium is that it works as an antagonist to calcium at the myometrial level. $MgSO_4$ is given in the same dose for preterm labor as in preeclampsia: a 4-g loading dose followed by 2 g/hour. Ritodrine is a beta-adrenergic agonist. Its effect is on the adrenergic receptors of the smooth muscle of the myometrium to decrease its contractile potential. Ritodrine also has some $beta_1$-activity; it therefore can cause maternal tachycardia and subsequent chest pain, and ECG changes consistent with ischemia. It also can cause pulmonary edema and hyperglycemia. Terbutaline, another beta-adrenergic agonist, is also very commonly used as a first-line drug for tocolysis; it has similar side effects as ritodrine, but these side effects tend to be clinically less severe. Because a significant number (approximately 20%) of patients with preterm contractions respond to bedrest and hydration, these measures should be instituted prior to the use of medications. The ability to actually stop preterm labor with these tocolytic agents has been questioned. Some studies have shown no significant difference in preterm delivery when use of tocolytic agents is compared to conservative therapy of bedrest and hydration. Because prostaglandins are involved in the initiation

of myometrial contractions and, therefore, of labor, the use of prostaglandin synthetase inhibitor drugs (such as indomethacin) can be used to arrest preterm labor. These medications have significant fetal effects and are, therefore, never used as initial means of tocolysis. The side effects are premature closure of the fetal ductus arteriosus and the development of oligohydramnios. Such medications are used only for short periods of time and only after other medications have been tried and failed. Ethanol was once used intravenously to arrest labor, but its effect of intoxication, lethargy, and respiratory depression in the mother and fetus have since discouraged its use. *(Cunningham et al, pp. 756–758; Hacker and Moore, pp. 270–275).*

18. **(E)** Congenital anomalies are increased threefold in fetuses born to women who are diabetic prior to pregnancy. Clinicians feel that this rate is greatly decreased if the mother is in excellent diabetic control prior to conception. Congenital heart defects are the most common anomalies, followed by neural tube defects. Women with diabetes have a higher incidence of cesarean section delivery. A primary reason is the higher incidence of macrosomia and subsequent cephalopelvic disproportion, as well as the possibility of shoulder dystocia. There is general disagreement about the timing of delivery of a diabetic woman. Many centers feel that women should be delivered prior to 40 weeks because of the higher incidence of intrauterine fetal demise after 36 weeks. Elective induction, especially with an unfavorable cervix, often leads to cesarean section. The cesarean section rate for diabetic women (gestational and pregestational) is approximately 50%. There is a fourfold increase in preeclampsia/eclampsia in women with overt diabetes and gestational diabetics with fasting hyperglycemia. Because the lungs of babies born to diabetic mothers mature at a later gestational age, they have an approximately five times greater chance of having respiratory distress syndrome. This makes elective delivery prior to 38 weeks a very difficult decision. Amniocentesis for lung maturity often is performed prior to elective delivery. A lecithin/sphin-

gomyelin (L/S) ratio greater than 2 has been found to be inaccurate in predicting fetal lung maturity in diabetic mothers. If present, phosphatidylglycerol (PG) is the best indicator of fetal lung maturity. *(Cunningham et al, pp. 816–822)*

19. **(D)** Women who are gestational diabetics are at greater risk for developing glucose intolerance in the future. This risk is significantly decreased if the patient maintains her ideal body weight, therefore women who are gestational diabetics should be counseled to continue weight control and diet after the pregnancy is over. Most women who are gestational diabetics do not remain glucose intolerant immediately after pregnancy. Therefore monitoring serum glucose after delivery will not be indicative of future predisposition for diabetes. But approximately one half of gestational diabetics will become glucose intolerant within 10 years of the pregnancy; this risk is decreased if the patient can maintain a good weight control. Women who are gestational diabetics are at increased risk for developing gestational diabetes in future pregnancies but this will have no long-term effects on their health. Only women who have pregestational diabetes with vascular involvement and any patient requesting permanent sterilization should be counseled to have a bilateral tubal ligation. There is no increased risk to developing type II diabetes when women who are gestational diabetics use oral contraceptives. *(Walsh and Hoody, pp. 25–27)*

20. **(E)** High-grade squamous intraepithelial lesion is part of the nomenclature used for describing abnormal Pap tests. It was developed in 1988 at a meeting of experts and cytopathologists in Bethesda, MD, and is refered to as the Bethesda System; it is the accepted means of reporting results of Pap smears. High-grade squamous intraepithelial lesion (SIL) is equivalent to moderate dysplasia/CIN II, severe dysplasia/CIN III, and carcinoma in situ/CIN III. High-grade SIL on a Pap smear is an indication for further evaluation by colposcopy. Low-grade SIL is equivalent to mild dysplasia/CIN I and hu-

man papilloma virus (HPV) effects. The treatment of low-grade SIL is controversial. Since only 2% to 30% of these lesions progress to a higher-grade lesion, some practitioners feel the treatment for SIL is to repeat the Pap smear every 3 months for 1 year. If one of the repeat Paps comes back showing atypical squamous cells of undetermined significance/premalignant change or SIL the patient should be referred for colposcopy. Because low-grade lesions on cytology often are not reliable, others feel that all women with low grade SIL should be referred for colposcopic evaluation. Certainly, women who are suspects for poor compliance and have low-grade SIL for the first time on Pap should be referred for colposcopy, as they may not return for the suggested repeated smears every 3 months. If the Pap smear is normal after three intervals, the patient can be referred for routine screening. Routine screening varies according to past history of abnormal Pap, the patient's risk factors for SIL, and sexual history; but in general the American Cancer Society and American College of Obstetrics and Gynecology recommend that sexually active teenagers and all woman 18 years or older should have a pelvic exam and Pap test yearly. After a woman has had three consecutive normal Pap tests and she has no risk factors for cervical cancer or SIL, then the practitioner may use his or her discretion to determine the interval of routine testing. A LEEP cone biopsy is done after colposcopy, when indicated; cyrosurgery is seldom used for the treatment of abnormal findings on a Pap test. Simple hysterectomy is not a procedure done for a SIL of any grade. (Gries-Griffin, pp. 17–20; Scott, pp. 71–76)

21. **(D)** In the normal menstrual cycle, the endometrium undergoes hormonal stimulation in preparation for implantation of the fertilized ovum. During the first half of the cycle, the endometrium is under the influence of estrogen, which is secreted from the developing follicle. This estrogen causes cellular proliferation of the endometrium, termed the *proliferative phase.* After ovulation, progesterone is secreted from the corpus luteum, and the effect of this hormone on the en-

dometrium is to cause secretion of glycogen and mucus from the glandular cells. This phase is termed the *secretory phase* and depends upon the occurrence of ovulation with the subsequent development of a corpus luteum. This patient could not be going through premature menopause because she has ovulated. Because a secretory endometrium is secondary to progesterone stimulation, this patient's endometrium could not be predominantly under estrogen stimulation. The second choice is therefore incorrect. The third choice also is incorrect because oral contraceptives prevent ovulation and therefore the development of the corpus luteum and secretion of progesterone. Asherman syndrome is intrauterine adhesions, which is characterized by amenorrhea and can only diagnosed on hysteroscopy. (Cunningham et al, p. 495; Hacker and Moore, pp. 454–456; Jones et al, pp. 68–78)

22. **(C)** Duration of labor prior to cesarean section is the most predictive factor in whether a patient develops a postoperative infection. It was previously believed that the number of pelvic exams while in labor and duration of rupture of membranes were equally predictive, but controlled studies showed that it was the length of labor that determined the number of pelvic exams and the possibility of ascending infection secondary to rupture of membranes. Although diabetes and other medical complications do affect the incidence of postoperative infection, they are not the most causative. (Burrow and Ferris, p. 350)

23. **(E)** The diagnosis of pulmonary embolus (PE) is very difficult to make. The most common sign present is tachypnea. Pulmonary embolus is the most dangerous complication of deep vein thrombosis (DVT). It occurs approximately five to seven times more frequently in women who have undergone cesarean section. A ventilation–perfusion scan often is the means of diagnosing a PE and is accurate, except in cases of obstructive or constrictive lung disease, heart failure, and pulmonary infiltrate. The definitive diagnosis can be made best on pulmonary angiography. An arterial blood gas is helpful in mak-

ing the diagnosis. (A) would be a good possibility except that the patient with pneumonia should be responding to triple antibiotics. Tubo-ovarian abscess is infrequent as a complication of cesarean section. It is more commonly seen in pelvic inflammatory disease (PID) that failed to respond to triple antibiotics after 48 hours. A patient with sepsis should respond to triple antibiotics. *(Cunningham et al, pp. 479–480; Hacker and Moore, pp. 201–202)*

24. **(B)** Age 35 has been arbitrarily designated as the age at which a mother must be advised to undergo genetic amniocentesis to rule out Down syndrome. The risk of an offspring with Down syndrome at age 30 is 1 in 885, whereas at age 35, it is 1 in 365; at age 40, it is 1 in 100, and at age 45, it is 1 in 35. Although a woman may decide against amniocentesis, it is the practitioner's responsibility to advise her of the incidence of Down syndrome in her age group and to refer her to available genetic counseling. Additional indications for genetic counseling and possible amniocentesis are previous history of a child born with a chromosomal abnormality; family history of a chromosomal abnormality or Down syndrome; high risk for neural-tube defect; previous child or family member with neural tube defect (NTD), elevated maternal serum alpha-fetoprotein, and family history of serious X-linked hereditary disorder. Chorionic villus sampling (CVS) can also be used for prenatal genetic diagnosis. It is performed between 9 and 12 weeks' gestation, thus allowing for earlier diagnosis, but it cannot be used to diagnose NTDs. *(Cunningham et al, pp. 570–587; Hacker and Moore, pp. 94–101)*

25. **(D)** Late decelerations are a result of uteroplacental insufficiency. A late deceleration occurs when the fetal heart rate begins to slow after the onset of the contraction and returns to baseline after the contraction is completed. Late decelerations by definition must be repetitive and are often the consequence of fetal hypoxia and subsequent acidosis. Many maternal factors cause uteroplacental insufficiency and subsequent intrauterine growth retardation. Some of these factors are

severe preeclampsia, chronic hypertension, chronic renal disease, severe diabetes with vascular involvement, and heavy maternal smoking. Although it is very likely that a patient with chronic hypertension with superimposed preeclampsia might develop late decelerations, the diagnosis of superimposed preeclampsia cannot be made solely on a fetal heart rate pattern. The diagnosis would instead be made if the patient developed hyperflexia, proteinuria, and generalized edema, in addition to her chronic hypertension. A patient with placenta previa would more than likely develop vaginal bleeding and fetal bradycardia. Decelerations secondary to head compression are early decelerations, and if they are not severe, are of no consequence. A prolapsed cord would typically show a cord pattern (variable deceleration) or bradycardia on fetal monitoring. *(Cunningham et al, pp. 291, 298, 764–765)*

26. **(B)** A nonstress test (NST) is called reactive if there are two fetal heart rate accelerations accompanying a fetal movement within a 20-minute period. The fetal heart rate accelerations should be 15 beats per minute above the baseline, lasting for 15 seconds. A reactive NST is a means of ensuring fetal well-being in the antepartum period in a high-risk pregnancy. Indications for conducting antepartum testing are gestational or insulin-dependent diabetes, postdate pregnancy (starting between $40^1/_2$ weeks and 41 weeks), intrauterine growth retardation, preeclampsia, chronic hypertension, history of previous preterm delivery or stillbirth, and multiple gestations (ie, twins, triplets). Because this pattern is reactive, it is, therefore, not suspicious for fetal compromise. An oxytocin challenge test (OCT) entails administration of oxytocin to cause contractions. There are no contractions on this tracing. A positive OCT is one in which late decelerations occur consistently with contractions and is indicative of some degree of fetal compromise. A negative OCT is one in which late decelerations do not occur consistently. OCTs are performed when the NST is nonreactive or if on NST there are spontaneous contractions with late or suspicious decelerations. There is no

way on fetal heart rate tracings to determine fetal age. A cord pattern would show variable decelerations, which do not appear on the above tracing. *(Cunningham et al, pp. 291–292, 1291–1292)*

27. **(C)** A woman in labor with her first pregnancy should dilate 1.2 cm per hour once she has entered the active phase of labor. The active phase of labor is defined as the onset of rapid change in cervical dilation and usually occurs after reaching 4 cm dilation. A multiparous patient usually dilates 1.5 cm in the active phase. The latent phase precedes the active phase and is defined as the onset of regular uterine contractions, but with slow dilation of the cervix. In a nulliparous patient, the latent phase should last no longer than 20 hours; in multiparous women, approximately 14 hours. (A) is incorrect because it implies the situation is describing more rapid progress than normal, which is not true. (B) implies that progress is inadequate and therefore necessitating an intrauterine pressure catheter. (D) is also incorrect because the question does not describe the latent phase. (E) is incorrect because the second stage of labor is determined from full dilation until delivery of the baby. *(Burke, p. 31)*

28. **(D)** Premenstrual syndrome is made up of many different symptoms that are both physical and psychological. The most common symptoms are feeling bloated, weight gain, loss of efficiency, irritability, difficulty concentrating, tiredness, mood swings, and depression. A woman will experience the symptoms cyclically, in a repetitive relationship to her menses; they will also subside at the same time in her cycle. Symptoms can begin as early as the day of ovulation and end by at least the fourth day of menstrual flow. Women at risk for developing the syndrome are those with a family history, ages 35 to 45, and a history that the symptoms subsided during pregnancy or while taking ovulatory inhibiting medications such as birth control pills. Premenstrual syndrome is associated with ovulation; therefore, it would not occur in premature ovarian failure or polycystic

ovary syndrome, both of which are anovulatory cycles. Secondary dysmenorrhea is pain that occurs with menses, but not exclusively. It often occurs in women in their thirties and forties and is associated with clinical entities such as endometriosis, chronic pelvic inflammatory disease (PID), and adenomyosis. It does not have the behavioral and psychological features as PMS. Clinical depression can be misdiagnosed as PMS. The primary means of differentiating the two is the association of PMS symptoms to the menstrual cycle. Women with a primary diagnosis of depression will have their symptoms throughout the cycle but these can get worse just prior to menstruation. *(Hacker and Moore, pp. 334–337; Johnson, pp. 637–643)*

29. **(B)** The information in the question gives numerous reasons for postpartum bleeding. They are uterine overdistention secondary to a large baby; midforceps delivery and therefore the possibility of cervical tears; and multiparity, which predisposes to a less contractive uterus. The information given states, however, that the uterus is well contracted; thus uterine atony would be an incorrect answer, as would retained products, because the placenta delivered spontaneously. Midforceps delivery is associated with a higher incidence of cervical and vaginal lacerations; therefore, careful inspection of the cervix and vagina should follow such a delivery. In the above incident, lacerations would be the most likely answer. Causes of excessive postpartum bleeding (postpartum hemorrhage) are overdistention of the uterus secondary to a large infant; polyhydramnios or multiple gestation; midforceps and rotation forcep delivery; delivery through an incompletely dilated cervix; the use of halothane anesthetics, which cause uterine relaxation, and finally, women who had very rapid or very slow dilation. Retained placenta and abnormally adherent placenta, such as placenta accreta, increta, or percreta are also causes of postpartum hemorrhage. Because the question states that the placenta delivered spontaneously, accreta could not be a likely cause. Previously undiagnosed coagulopathy might be a cause for postpartum hemorrhage, but in the

above case is not the most likely cause. Rectal tears or fourth-degree lacerations are more common with forceps delivery but are usually easily repairable and, therefore, do not cause much bleeding. *(Cunningham et al, pp. 405–406, 415–418, 436)*

30. **(D)** Knowledge of the uterine scar is the most important factor in determining whether a patient is a candidate for vaginal delivery after a cesarean section (VDAC). The safest and most commonly used incision is the lower segment transverse incision. A classical incision on the uterus is known to easily rupture during labor. The low transverse incision ruptures less than 2% of the time. Therefore, VDAC is contraindicated in patients who have a classical incision. It is questionable whether patients with a low vertical incision on the uterus should undergo a trial of labor. The incidence of spontaneous rupture is minimal, but greater than low transverse. The indication for the primary cesarean section should not be a deterrent because the success rate of VDAC in patients with a recurrent indication, such as cephalopelvic disproportion or failure to progress, is approximately 60%. Length of labor and intensity of present contractions have no effect on the decision to allow a patient a trial of labor. *(Cunningham et al, pp. 408, 446)*

31. **(D)** Incomplete abortions are characterized by heavy vaginal bleeding and placental tissue present in a dilated cervical os. The bleeding is heavy because there has been incomplete separation of the placenta and, therefore, inadequate myometrial contraction of the blood vessels. Bleeding from an incomplete abortion can be severe enough to cause marked hypovolemia and shock. Inevitable abortion occurs when a patient has crampy abdominal pain and bleeding, and upon pelvic exam, the cervical os is partially open. Leaking membranes may be seen from the cervical os or the vaginal vault. Septic abortion occurs when the signs and symptoms of spontaneous abortion are accompanied by a temperature elevation greater than 38°C. This diagnosis is made only after other sources of

fever have been excluded, such as urinary tract infection (UTI). A missed abortion is one in which the fetus dies but the products of conception are retained. A patient typically notes loss of pregnancy signs, such as nausea, vomiting, and breast tenderness. On sequential pelvic exams, the uterus fails to enlarge and, in fact, will decrease in size. On ultrasound, there is no evidence of fetal viability, and it is often used to verify the diagnosis. Induced abortion is one in which the mother elects to terminate the pregnancy. *(Cunningham et al, p. 497; Hacker and Moore, pp. 416–421)*

32. **(B)** Suction curettage is the safest means of elective abortion in the first trimester. It is more efficient if preceded by a preliminary means of dilating the cervix. This can be accomplished with prostaglandin suppository in the vagina or with laminaria tents inserted into the cervix. Intra-amniotic saline injection is infrequently used and only during the second-trimester. Hysterotomy, dilation and extraction, and the use of oxytocin are reserved for second-trimester abortions. The use of prostaglandin-induced labor for second trimester terminations has increased in frequency; the prostaglandins used are either E_2 or F_2 alpha and are used intra-amniotic or intravaginally. This method does entail that the patient go through labor and is associated with a high rate of retained placenta requiring manual removal. *(Cunningham et al, pp. 502–505; Hacker and Moore, pp. 421–424)*

33. **(C)** Hydatidiform mole is one component of gestational trophoblastic neoplasm (GTN). Moles occur in a gestation in which there is a proliferation of trophoblastic tissue. It can be a complete mole, in which there is no sign of a fetus, or a partial mole, in which the fetus may be viable, or there are findings consistent with a nonviable fetus. The most common symptom of hydatidiform mole is several episodes of vaginal bleeding. A size-to-dates discrepancy also is common. Approximately one half of the patients are larger than dates, and one fourth are smaller. The trophoblast is responsible for production of human chorionic gonadotropin (HCG);

therefore, the levels of beta-HCG in the serum are often greater than expected for the weeks of gestation. The occurrence of preeclampsia prior to 20 weeks is highly suggestive of hydatidiform mole. On ultrasound, there are very characteristic findings, and it is the best means of diagnosing a mole. (A) is incorrect because with a threatened abortion at 18 weeks, there should be fetal heart tones. An incomplete abortion usually occurs prior to 12 to 14 weeks and would more than likely be characterized by a decreasing beta-HCG level. A fetal demise at 16 weeks would also have decreasing beta-HCG levels and would not be associated with hypertension. In twin gestation, there would be a higher level of beta-HCG and a larger fundal height, but at 16 weeks, fetal heart tones should be heard. (*Cunningham et al, pp. 541–545; Hacker and Moore, p. 15*)

34. **(D)** Placental abruption is the separation of the placenta before delivery of the fetus. Separation can occur in various degrees, and it can be partial or complete. Abruption can be associated with vaginal bleeding or the bleeding may remain hidden within the uterus. If the separation is of a significant degree, the blood loss will be extensive because the uterus cannot contract down upon the torn vessels that supply the placenta. The fetus's blood supply is subsequently disrupted and fetal death occurs. The mother also is severely affected. She will develop shock secondary to blood loss and also has a high chance of developing a consumptive coagulopathy. The coagulopathy is most often hypofibrinogenemia with elevation of fibrinogen-fibrin degradation products. Pregnancy-induced and chronic hypertension often are associated with placental abruption. It also is seen in trauma, short umbilical cord, sudden decompensation of the uterus, and uterine anomaly. Placenta previa does present at term with vaginal bleeding, but infrequently with fetal demise, and is not typically associated with hypertension. Gestational and nongestational diabetes is associated with a higher incidence of fetal demise at term, but the patient's presentation is more consistent with an abruption. Disseminated intravascular coagulopathy (DIC) is a known complication of preeclampsia and abruption, but would probably not cause fetal demise without some other precipitating event, such as abruption. Chronic renal failure is associated with a higher incidence of fetal wastage, but the case presented is more consistent with an acute occurrence. (*Cunningham et al, pp. 701–712*)

35. **(B)** A consumptive coagulopathy, primarily hypofibrinogenemia, occurs within 4 to 6 weeks of intrauterine fetal demise. It is felt to be secondary to the release of thromboplastin from the dead fetus. Because the products of conception tend to shrink postdemise and labor is more effective if initiated on its own, a woman is allowed to await spontaneous labor if she so chooses. She must be monitored for the possibility of coagulopathy with weekly PT and PTT, plus fibrinogen and platelet counts. The use of prostaglandin E_2 and F_2 alpha has increased the number of women who have elected immediate termination, because it has greatly increased the success of induction of labor. The release of thromboplastin affects only the coagulation factors, and, therefore, there should be no change in liver function tests. The hemoglobin and hematocrit levels would fall if the patient went into DIC, but that would occur significantly after the change in coagulation factors. Prolactin levels would have no effect on the incidence of DIC postfetal demise. (*Cunningham et al, pp. 716–719*)

36. **(D)** A pregnancy that progresses past 42 weeks is associated with increased fetal morbidity and mortality. One reason for the increased fetal risk is decreased amniotic fluid with subsequent cord compression. Cord compression may result in fetal distress, which in turn causes fetal defecation in utero and subsequently meconium-stained fluid. Because postdate pregnancies are associated with these complications and an increased risk of intrauterine demise, patients are monitored from $40^1/_2$ weeks. This monitoring can be in one or more of the following ways: nonstress testing, biophysical profile, or oxytocin challenge test. These tests have all been associated with high false-positive and false-

negative results. In many cases, induction is performed at 42 weeks regardless of antepartum test results. Babies born after 42 weeks' gestation can either be large for dates, which increases the risk for failed induction, cephalopelvic disproportion, and shoulder dystocia, or these babies can be growth-retarded. A growth-retarded fetus has a greater chance for stress during labor and, when born, appears as if it has lost weight, particularly muscle mass and subcutaneous fat. Chorioamnionitis does not occur more commonly with postdate pregnancy. In fact, it is more common with preterm delivery. Blood-tinged fluid is sometimes associated with partial placental abruption but is not a common finding in postdate pregnancy. The presence of vernix would indicate a preterm or term fetus. Rupture of membranes, either spontaneously or artificially, is usually followed by a greater intensity of contractions, but usually not hyperstimulation. (Cunningham et al, pp. 759–763)

37. **(D)** The optimal time to screen for gestational diabetes is between 24 and 28 weeks. In some patients, pregnancy is a diabetogenic state. Human placental lactogen is a hormone secreted by the placenta, with levels increasing during the latter half of pregnancy. This hormone has an anti-insulin effect in the mother and, in predisposed patients, will cause glucose intolerance. The glucose challenge test (also called the 50-g glucola, or O'Sullivan) is the most commonly employed screening test. It consists of taking 50 g of glucola in a nonfasting state and having a plasma glucose drawn 1 hour later. If the plasma glucose is 135 to 140 mg/dL, the patient then must undergo a 3-hour glucose tolerance test. All pregnant women should undergo routine screening for gestational diabetes by 28 weeks. Women with a significant obstetric or family history should be screened at their first prenatal visit, even if it is before 28 weeks. Criteria for this screening are maternal age greater than 30, a family history of diabetes, a prior macrosomic baby, a baby with a congenital anomaly, or a stillborn. Women who are hypertensive or obese also have a higher incidence of gestational di-

abetes. Alpha-fetoprotein screening is accurate only between 15 to 20 weeks. Although women infected with syphilis have a high incidence of stillborns, they should undergo treatment after the first obstetric loss. Babies infected with syphilis are usually growth-retarded, not macrosomic. Rh-negative women should receive RhoGAM at 28 weeks, but their blood type and Rh should be drawn at the first prenatal visit. Babies that have congenital toxoplasmosis are generally smaller for gestational age and are microcephalic or hydrocephalic. (Cunningham et al, pp. 617–619, 812–816)

38. **(B)** Acute appendicitis is the most important surgical diagnosis to rule out during pregnancy. It is also one of the most difficult diagnoses because the enlarging uterus displaces the appendix and, therefore, the location of pain. Moreover, many of the presenting complaints of appendicitis are common complaints of pregnancy, such as nausea, anorexia, and vomiting. A mild leukocytosis also is common in pregnancy, particularly during the third trimester. If the diagnosis of appendicitis is a serious consideration, the patient should undergo exploratory laparotomy. To delay would increase the occurrence of severe peritonitis, gangrene, spontaneous abortion, preterm labor, and increased maternal morbidity. Another possible surgical complication of pregnancy that could be present in the above patient is acute cholecystitis. Hyperemesis gravidarum would be an unlikely diagnosis because it is primarily a first-trimester phenomenon and is not associated with a fever or markedly elevated WBC count. If this patient had pyelonephritis, she would probably have costal vertebral angle (CVA) tenderness and WBCs in the urine. If pelvic inflammatory disease (PID) occurs at all during pregnancy, it is extremely rare and only before 12 weeks. Degeneration of uterine myomata does cause pain, mild leukocytosis, and slightly elevated temperature. Usually, however, it is not associated with decreased bowel sounds, nausea, and vomiting, and ordinarily there is some uterine tenderness and a palpable myomata. (Cunningham et al, pp. 831–832)

39. **(C)** The aspiration of acidic gastric contents or undigested food particles will cause severe respiratory distress and possibly death. To prevent this complication, the mother should be fasting for 6 to 12 hours prior to general anesthesia, and medication to reverse gastric acidity should be administered immediately prior to intubation. In addition, intubation should be performed with pressure on the cricoid cartilage to occlude the esophogus, and extubation should be performed with the mother awake and on her side. A true fasting state with minimal gastric contents is extremely difficult to achieve in obstetric patients. A woman seldom knows when she will begin labor and, more important, gastric emptying and peristalsis are delayed or inhibited at the onset of labor. Subsequently, all pregnant women should be treated as if they have a full stomach. In the fasting state, the stomach continues to secrete gastric juices that have a very low pH. To neutralize this pH, antacids are administered within 45 minutes of intubation. Maternal hypotension does not accompany general anesthesia, but is the major side effect of spinal and epidural anesthesia. Atelectasis frequently occurs within the first 24 hours after general anesthesia but is not life-threatening. If left untreated, in some instances atelectasis will progress to pneumonia. Three of the inhalation anesthetics used in obstetrics do cause uterine relaxation and in some cases uterine atony. These agents are halothane, enflurane, and isoflurane. They are used in conjunction with nitrous oxide and given in the smallest possible amounts to avoid this complication. Although uterine atony is associated with lower hematocrit postdelivery and greater chance of blood transfusion, these complications are not as life-threatening as aspiration. Eclampsia probably does not occur more often with general anesthesia, and, in fact, in severe preeclampsia/eclampsia, general anesthesia is the preferred means of anesthesia. (*Cunningham et al, pp. 329–339*)

40. **(D)** Cervical cancer and its precursors, low-and-high grade squamous intraepithelial lesions, SIL (previously known as dyplasia or cervical intraepithelial neoplasia), occur more often in women who are sexually active at an early age (before age 20) and who have multiple sexual partners. Originally, women who were married young and had children at a young age were considered at risk, but it is now felt that cervical cancer is due to sexual intercourse at an early age *and* multiple sexual partners. Women who smoke also are at a higher risk of developing cervical cancer. Infection has been considered a possible etiology of SIL. The most commonly implicated agent is the human papillomavirus (HPV), the same virus that causes condylomata accumulata. HPV types 6 through 11 are usually associated with benign lesions such as condylomata and low-grade SIL and are not felt to be related to a high degree of malignancy. Types 16, 18, 31, 33, 35 and additional types are more commonly found in high-grade lesions and cervical cancer and adenocarcinomas. Although strong evidence suggests HPV has either a causative or exacerbative effect on neoplastic changes in the cervix, many women with high-grade SIL or invasive carcinoma have no evidence of the virus. Early sexual relationships and multiple partners have not been a historical finding in women who develop ovarian or endometrial cancer. Endometrial cancer is more common in nulliparous women. Labial cancer occurs at a much later age than the above gynecological neoplasms. AIDS is not considered a cancer, but a woman with SIL should be counseled for AIDS, as some of the risk factors for developing AIDS and SIL are the same. (*Hacker and Moore, p. 177; Jones et al, pp. 58–64, 643–654; Gries-Griffin, pp. 16–20*)

41. **(D)** This patient would be a very good candidate for depomedroxyprogesterone acetate or DEPO-PROVERA. Depomedroxyprogesterone acetate is a synthetic long-acting progestational agent that provides contraception by preventing ovulation. It is given by IM injection, in a 150 mg dosage every 3 months. The patient has indicated in her history that she is not a good candidate for oral contraceptives, because she could not take them regularly. The advantages of depomedroxyprogesterone acetate for this patient is that its every 3-month administration will enhance

compliance and it is effective and reversible. The failure rate for depomedroxyproges-terone acetate is .03%, which is comparable to surgical sterilization at .04% (the rates for oral contraceptives and intrauterine devices are 3% and 12% for condoms.) The patient gave a history of a possible episode of PID: intrauterine devices have been associated with a higher risk of exacerbating PID in a patient with a previous history. This risk is particularly high in a patient with multiple sexual partners, a recent episode of PID, and women under the age of 25. The contracep-tive sponge has been associated with a slightly higher risk of developing toxic shock syndrome and has been taken off the market. Condoms are a good means of preventing the spread of sexually transmitted diseases, are readily available, and are without significant medical contraindications. But this patient is probably looking for a more reliable means of birth control. Bilateral tubal ligation (BTL) would not be the optimal form of birth con-trol for this patient. She is relatively young and BTLs are nonreversible. Recent literature also has shown that the failure rate may actu-ally be closer to 1.9% and that those patients who do conceive are at greater risk for ec-topic pregnancy. The risk for failure and ec-topic pregnancy increases with the years du-ration after the procedure; therefore, women sterilized at a younger age are at greater risk for failure. Moreover, younger women who have undergone surgical sterilization are more likely to regret having the procedure than older women. (*Grimes, pp. 4–13; Hacker and Moore, pp. 453–467; Jones et al, pp. 225–231; Schroder, pp. 18–34*)

42. **(D)** Endometriosis is endometrial-like tissues found outside the uterus that responds to cyclic hormonal stimulation. Because this ec-topic tissue can be found in various locations, most commonly on the ovaries, tubes, uterosacral ligaments, and posterior cul de sac, symptoms of the disease vary greatly. Progressively worse dysmenorrhea, unre-sponsive to prostaglandin (PG) synthetase in-hibitors is a common presenting complaint. Infertility occurs in approximately 20% to 40% of women with endometriosis and is of-ten the reason a woman undergoes a workup. Frequently, women with en-dometriosis also complain of dyspareunia. This is considered to be secondary to en-dometrial implants in the uterosacral liga-ment. Because of the various ways in which endometriosis presents, laparoscopic visual-ization is the only means of definitively for-mulating the diagnosis. Endometrial im-plants are not visualized on ultrasound. However, endometriomas, cysts formed on the ovary secondary to excessive bleeding from endometrial tissue, can be seen on sonography. There is, however, no way of differentiating an endometrioma from a sim-ple ovarian cyst, a dermoid, or other pelvic pathology. Laparoscopic diagnosis should be made prior to the administration of any med-ical therapy, such as danazol. The absence of response to PG synthetase inhibitors may be a means of making the preliminary diagnosis of endometriosis but not the conclusive diag-nosis. Hysteroscopy would be of no help in making the diagnosis, as endometriosis is ex-trauterine. (*Jones et al, pp. 303–326; Szarzynski, pp. 37–47*)

43. **(B)** Women who lose 25% of their ideal body weight secondary to anorexia nervosa and women who engage in vigorous or stressful exercise often have secondary amenorrhea, probably because of hypothalamic dysfunc-tion. These women typically have low go-nadotropin levels and low estrogen levels. Because of their lack of estrogen, findings on physical exam may include decreased breast size, an atrophic vaginal mucosa, and possi-bly absent cervical mucus. In general, these patients are anovulatory. Weight gain and decreased exercise often restore normal hy-pothalamic functioning. Oligomenorrhea, or episodic menstrual bleeding occurring at in-tervals longer than 35 days, is due to anovu-latory cycles. It is seen in women who engage in moderate exercise, but not in anorexia, in which complete cessation of menses is more common. Menorrhagia is cyclic menstrual bleeding that is excessive in amount or dura-tion. Polymenorrhagia, which also is often due to anovulatory cycles, is episodic bleed-ing occurring in cycles shorter than 21 days.

Metrorrhagia is uterine bleeding between periods and is usually due to uterine polyps or carcinoma but can be due to estrogen withdrawal or anovulation. *(Hacker and Moore, pp. 525–527, 532–534; Jones et al, pp. 351–375)*

44. **(D)** The signs and symptoms of polycystic ovarian syndrome (PCO) are due to hyperandrogenism, which is a result of overproduction of androgen by both the ovaries and adrenal gland. Clinically, patients with the syndrome are hirsute, have menstrual irregularity, and are infertile. Approximately 50% of these women are obese, most have acne, and 15% are virilized. The ovaries have multiple follicular cysts, which are arrested in development. The ovarian stroma consists of luteinized thecal cells that produce androgens. This excess androgen plus that produced by the adrenal gland results in increased LH secretions from the pituitary, which in turn continues stimulation of the ovaries and more androgen secretion. The excess androgen is converted peripherally into estrogen. Because women with PCO are anovulatory, this estrogen is unopposed by progesterone. The unopposed estrogen effect on the endometrium places these women at greater risk for developing adenomatous hyperplasia and possibly endometrial carcinoma. The high levels of estrogen also cause the amenorrhea and at other times, excessive bleeding. Congenital adrenal hyperplasia also presents with hirsutism and virilism, but these patients usually have a male body type and do not have enlarged ovaries. Excess androgen production prevents the secretion of progesterone; therefore, this patient's symptoms would not be due to a progesterone-secreting tumor. Patients with hyperprolactinemia usually are amenorrheic but have galactorrhea and are not hirsute. Hypothyroidism also causes amenorrhea, but not hirsutism. *(Hacker and Moore, pp. 535–539; Jones et al, pp. 169–174, 351–375)*

45. **(C)** A fundal height at the umbilicus roughly corresponds to 20 weeks' gestation. On physical examination, there are several ways of determining fundal height and, therefore, gestational age. A fundus palpable to the pubic symphysis is 12 weeks; at the umbilicus, 20 weeks. Those weeks between these two landmarks are approximated. After 20 weeks and before 32 weeks, fundal height is measured with a tape measure in centimeters. Weeks' gestation correspond (±1 cm) to the measured centimeters from the top of the symphysis to the top of the fundus. *(Cunningham et al, p. 1260)*

46. **(D)** Women who have previously been pregnant will first feel fetal movement between 16 and 18 weeks. With a first pregnancy, women will usually feel movement between 18 and 20 weeks. Gestational age can be approximated to when fetal movement is first perceived. *(Cunningham et al, p. 218)*

47. **(A)** At $5^1/_2$ to 6 weeks' gestation, fetal heart motion can be seen on transvaginal sonogram, the gestational sac can be seen at 4 weeks from the last menstrual period. The yolk sac, which appears as a rounded symmetrical circular structure within the gestational sac, can be seen at $5^1/_2$ weeks' gestation and is the first indication of a healthy gestation. *(Howe, pp. 189–193)*

48. **(D)** Maternal serum alpha-fetoprotein is a screening test to detect the presence of numerous fetal abnormalities, the most common of which are neural tube defects. The major protein secreted by the early fetus is alpha-fetoprotein. This protein is secreted into the amniotic fluid and crosses the fetal membranes into the maternal circulation. The level of alpha-fetoprotein is elevated in the amniotic fluid of an abnormal fetus and, therefore, in the maternal serum. This elevation is best detected between 16 and 20 weeks. In addition to open neural tube defects, other abnormalities detected include congenital nephrosis, esophageal and duodenal atresia, exophalos, Turner and Potter's syndromes, fetal death, or fetal blood in amniotic fluid. *(Cunningham et al, p. 277)*

49. **(C)** Coumadin is a small molecule that easily crosses the placenta and is taken up by the fetus. The anomalies it causes are a result of hemorrhage secondary to its anticoagulant ef-

fect. Exposure during the first trimester causes anomalies that are collectively termed *fetal warfarin syndrome*. Use of coumadin during the second and third trimesters causes optic atrophy, cataracts, microcephaly, microphthalmia, blindness, and mental retardation. Heparin is a large molecule that does not cross the placenta and is, therefore, the drug of choice for anticoagulation. *(Cunningham et al, pp. 565–566)*

50. **(D)** The use of cocaine during pregnancy causes an increased chance of placental abruption that is most likely secondary to its vasoconstrictive effects. Because of the placental abruption, there is a higher incidence of stillborn fetuses. Use of cocaine also is felt to cause an increase in preterm delivery and intrauterine growth retardation. *(Cunningham et al, p. 568)*

51. **(A)** Women who are considered alcoholics often produce a child with fetal alcohol syndrome (FAS). Children born with the syndrome have characteristic cardiovascular, limb, and craniofacial defects. In addition, they are found to be growth-retarded, have impaired fine and gross motor function, and lower IQs. The effects on a fetus of a small amount of alcohol ingested during pregnancy is still uncertain. It is best to abstain entirely. *(Cunningham et al, pp. 567–568)*

52. **(E)** Phenytoin (Dilantin) is one of the most commonly used anticonvulsant medications. It is considered a cause of minor craniofacial and digital anomalies but is not definitive if these are secondary to drug versus a genetic disposition found in women who have a seizure disorder. Nonetheless, the adverse effects of terminating the medication, consequent seizures, and potentially causing maternal and fetal hypoxia outweigh the chance of developing the anomalies. If a patient is already pregnant and is well controlled by Dilantin, she should remain on the medication. *(Cunningham et al, p. 566)*

53. **(D)** The patient's symptoms are describing postmenopausal atrophic changes affecting the vagina, bladder, and urethra. The patient may also complain of vaginal discharge, itching, burning, and dyspareunia. These symptoms are all due to estrogen depletion and, therefore, are best treated with estrogen replacement. Replacement can be either in the form of systemic estrogen or local application in the form of vaginal creams or suppositories. Estrogen is well absorbed through the vaginal mucosa; thus, a relatively small dose can be used with minimal systemic effects. Because some estrogen is systemically absorbed, local therapy is still associated with the known complications of estrogen replacement. Oral estrogen with progesterone is effective treatment for atrophic vaginitis/cystitis and has the advantage of also treating osteoporosis. Estrogen administered transdermally via a patch can also be used for atrophic vaginitis and symptoms associated with atrophic changes. It is recommended that women who still have their uterus should also take progesterone, which can be taken by pill or a combined transdermal route. Antibiotics, orally or locally, would not be indicated in the patient, as the urine culture was negative. Testosterone is not indicated to treat atrophic vaginitis. A bladder procedure would not be indicated because the patient did not describe urinary stress incontinence and there was no evidence of a cystocele on examination. *(Baker, pp. 285–287; Hacker and Moore, pp. 544–550; Wehrle, p .18)*

54. **(A)** If on ultrasound an intrauterine pregnancy can be identified, then an ectopic can be reasonably ruled out. On transvaginal sonogram, a fetus with a beating fetal heart can first be visualized at $5^1/_2$ to 6 weeks' gestation; at 4.0 weeks, a gestational sac can be identified. Sonographic findings in the presence of an ectopic pregnancy are generally nonspecific. There may be a sonolucency in the endometrial cavity suggestive of a gestational sac called a *pseudogestational sac*. The adnexa may contain a mass with a mixed echogenic pattern, and there may be fluid in the posterior cul de sac. Serious diagnostic errors have occurred when the pseudogestational sac has been mistaken for a real gestational sac. In the instances when a fetus is not identifiable, it would be advisable to follow

quantitative beta-HCG levels and to closely monitor the patient for changes in her physicial exam and symptoms that would suggest an ectopic pregnancy. Quantitative levels of beta-human chorionic gonadotrophin (beta-HCG) are known to double within 48 hours in a viable pregnancy. In an ectopic pregnancy, the trophoblastic tissue that produces beta-HCG does not function as adequately as in a normal pregnancy and, therefore, this doubling time will not occur. Instead it will either maintain a plateau or rise only a small degree. Obtaining quantitative beta-HCG levels more frequently than every 48 hours will not provide the necessary information and will confuse the situation. Although an ectopic pregnancy must always be suspected when a pregnant woman presents with abdominal pain and bleeding, the above patient's physical findings are not significant enough to subject the patient to either laparotomy or laparoscopy. If the patient had rebound tenderness or more severe tenderness on pelvic exam, a culdocentesis would be an appropriate diagnostic procedure, but would not be the next step, prior to vaginal sonogram. (*Cunningham, pp. 520–522; Emerson and McCord, pp. 199–203, Hacker and Moore, pp. 417–419, 425–435*)

55. **(E)** Ectopic pregnancy is responsible for the greatest number of maternal deaths in the first trimester and second most common in all three trimesters. The incidence of ectopic pregnancy is increasing in the United States. The increase in sexually transmitted diseases and subsequent tubal damage and pelvic adhesions are primarily responsible for the rise in ectopic pregnancy. A woman who has had PID has a sevenfold increase in her chance of developing a tubal pregnancy. A history of spontaneous abortion is not a risk factor for ectopic pregnancy, but there is a possibility that a history of induced abortion is a risk factor. A recent history of having undergone laparoscopy is not a risk factor for ectopic pregnancy, but a recent study suggested that previous abdominal/pelvic surgery may be a risk factor. Several studies have shown that the majority of the time the ectopic implantation occurs on the right side. Advanced ma-

ternal age does not place a patient at increased risk. Birth control pills change the cervical mucosa and make it less permeable to the gonorrhea bacteria. Women on the pill are, therefore, somewhat protected against the development of PID. Additional factors that have been implicated in the increased incidence of ectopic pregnancy, but remain unproven, are tubal surgery secondary to tubal reanastomsis; tubal ligation, and conservative surgery at the time of ectopic pregnancy. (*Hacker and Moore, pp. 425–428; Ramirez et al, pp. 733–739*)

56. **(A)** The patient in the question has many of the classic presenting signs and symptoms of acute PID. Because of her age, the severity of her presenting symptoms, and most important, her parity, she is a good candidate for in-hospital treatment. Gonorrhea and chlamydia are the most commonly implicated organisms in PID. Gonococcal PID typically presents with symptoms of fever, lower abdominal pain, and tenderness. Chlamydial PID, on the other hand, is more indolent; symptoms are usually mild tenderness and low-grade temperature. Unfortunately, chlamydia causes as much, if not more, tubal damage as gonorrhea, and is, therefore, as likely to cause infertility. Anaerobic bacteria are typically the etiologic agents in a second episode of PID and would not be the most common cause of an initial episode. Two strains of mycoplasma have also been implicated in the etiology of PID: *Mycoplasma hominis* and *Ureaplasma urealyticum*, but are not the most common etiologic causes of PID. *Clostridium difficile* is the organism responsible for pseudomembranous enterocolitis, a side effect of antibiotic administration, usually with ampicillin and clindamycin. (*Hacker and Moore, pp. 387–389, Hinman, pp. 75–80*)

57. **(D)** Forty-five percent of women who culture positive for gonorrhea have concurrent chlamydia. Antibiotic therapy must, therefore, treat both these organisms. Because of the increasing prevalence of penicillin-resistant strains of *Neisseria gonorrhoeae*, ceftriaxone, which is highly effective against even resistant strains, is presently the drug of

choice for gonorrhea. Doxycycline or any of the tetracyclines is the drug of choice for chlamydia, but some strains of gonococcus are resistant to tetracycline. Combined therapy with ceftriaxone and doxycycline is, therefore, the best outpatient treatment for PID. Cefoxitin 2 g IM with probenecid 1 g PO can replace ceftriaxone. Trimethoprim-sulfamethoxazole is effective against both gonorrhea and chlamydia, but resistant strains of both organisms have developed against the drug. Ofloxacin 400 mg PO bid for 14 days plus either clindamycin 450 mg PO qid for 14 days or Flagyl 500 mg PO bid for 14 days is the alternative choice in penicillin-allergic patients. If a patient fails to improve within 48 hours on an outpatient basis, she should be admitted for IV therapy. In-hospital therapy should include coverage for gonorrhea, chlamydia, and anaerobic bacteria. No single drug is adequate; the following combinations are all possible choices: cefoxitin or cefotetan with doxycycline; gentamycin and clindamycin (clindamycin does cover some strains of chlamydia). The patient should be reexamined 7 to 10 days after completing therapy, and repeat cultures for gonorrhea and chlamydia should be sent at that time. In addition, at the time of diagnosis, the practitioner should make sure the patient's sexual partner is being adequately treated and followed up. (*Hacker and Moore, pp. 392–393; Hinman, pp. 75–80*)

58. **(D)** Any palpable mass on pelvic exam in a woman more than 2 years menopausal is abnormal and requires immediate evaluation. A third of pelvic masses detected in women older than 50 are malignant; in a postmenopausal woman the ovaries are atrophic and should not be palpable. Therefore, this mass is considered malignant until otherwise proven. Ovarian cancer is the leading cause of death from gynecological cancers; primarily because of the difficulty in making the diagnosis at an early stage. The initial evaluation should be expedient and usually includes a pelvic/adominal sonogram and transvaginal sonogram, to further evaluate the ovary. If in fact there is an ovarian mass on sonogram, then the patient should be re-

ferred to a gynecological oncologist for futher evaluation and surgery. Although diverticulitis does occur in older women, a palpable adenexal mass should always be worked up by the gynecologist. Performing an endometrial biopsy might be the next appropriate step if the patient had postmenopausal bleeding, but in this case it would not be helpful in the immediate evaluation of this patient's palpable ovary because the patient did not have any bleeding. (*Dumesic, pp. 40–41; Hacker and Moore, pp. 602–604*)

59. **(E)** Herpes genitalis is a venereal disease caused by the herpes simplex virus. Ninety percent of the time it is caused by the herpes simplex type II virus, and 10% of the time by the herpes simplex type I virus. The initial episode is usually the most severe, although some patients are asymptomatic. The virus can migrate up the nerve fiber and remain dormant, which can cause recurrent episodes. The first episode can be associated with a generalized viremia, and the patient may present with generalized malaise and low-grade fever. Recurrent episodes are usually precipitated by stress, menstruation, and upper respiratory infection. The principal way in which to differentiate the herpetic lesion from other labial lesions is that it is painful to touch. The definitive diagnosis is made on culture. Primary syphilis is characterized by a chancre, usually a singular lesion, that has a punched-out base with rolled edges. Secondary syphilitic lesions are condyloma latum, that are raised, round, plateau-like lesions of various sizes that often occur in clusters. The lesions are extremely infectious and occur on the labia, vulva, the surrounding perineum, and inner thigh and buttocks. Like the chancre lesion characteristic of primary syphilis, these lesions are not painful to touch. Condylomata acuminata is caused by the human papillomavirus (HPV) and is a sexually transmitted disease. These lesions can occur on the vulva, vagina, perineum, or cervix. They are white, verrucous growths that, when large and multiple, are described as cauliflower-like. The lesion of lymphogranuloma venerum is a painless vulvovaginal ulcer progressing to adenitis, usually to the nodes of

the anus and rectum. Chlamydia is the causative agent. *(Hacker and Moore, pp. 380–384)*

60. **(C)** Fibroids, or more correctly, leiomyomata, are benign growths of the myometrium. Their growth is stimulated by estrogen, and once a woman reaches menopause they will generally decrease in size. The woman in the question is 49 years old. As the average age of menopause in American women is 51, it can be assumed that this woman will have less estrogen within approximately 1 to 5 years, with subsequent decrease in the size and bleeding of her leiomyomata. The next therapeutic step should therefore take this information into strong consideration; a 3 month course of leuprolide acetate (lupron depot) a GnRH analog, would be the best choice. GnRH analogs produce a sustained and continuous release of GnRH on the pituitary that eventually results in a decrease in the release of pituitary gonadotrophins and a subsequent decreased production of estrogen from the ovaries. With less estrogen, leiomyomata will decrease in size and bleeding will decrease; this will allow for correction of anemia with iron therapy prior to surgery and often less blood loss at the time of surgery. GnRH analogs are generally given only for a 3-month period because this produces the maximum decrease in the size of the myomata and because of the strong effect the analogs have on bone demineralization. In a woman who is close to menopause, surgery can sometimes be completely avoided following therapy with GnRH analogs, as the patient may become menopausal during or around the time of the treatment. Myomectomy, either laparascopically or abdominally, would seldom be the procedure of choice in a 49-year-old woman because myomectomy is done primarily to preserve fertility and is generally a more complicated procedure. Transfusion would be required only if the patient were symptomatic or if a surgical procedure were immediately contemplated. Because the patient was stable and the use of leuprolide acetate would correct her anemia and make the surgery easier, total abdominal hysterectomy at this time would not be the next therapeutic choice. *(Hacker and Moore, pp. 38–39, 348–352)*

61. **(B)** Endometrial hyperplasia is found on pathological specimen usually on dilation and curettage or on an endometrial biopsy performed in the office. It is considered a premalignant lesion and in some instances will progress to endometrial cancer. It is found in women who experience abnormal uterine bleeding secondary to overstimulation of the endometrium by estrogen unopposed by progesterone. Premenopausally, endometrial hyperplasia occurs in women who are anovulatory; women who fail to ovulate do not form a corpus luteum and, therefore, do not produce progesterone. These women usually have a less severe form of hyperplasia called *simple hyperplasia* or *cystic glandular hyperplasia.* Postmenopausal women with endometrial hyperplasia also have excessive estrogen stimulation of the endometrium without the protective effect of progesterone. This is often seen in women receiving estrogen replacement without progesterone added to the regimen and in women who are not taking exogenous estrogen. The source of estrogen in these women appears to be the peripheral conversion of androsteredione (from the adrenal gland) to estrone. This conversion takes place in adipose tissue and occurs at a greater rate in obese women. Adenomatous hyperplasia is a more severe form of endometrial hyperplasia and is more often found in postmenopausal women. It is more likely to progress to endometrial carcinoma than hyperplasia. In its most severe form, it is called carcinoma in situ. Anorexic women have low levels of both estrogen and progesterone secondary to minimal secretion of FSH and LH. Women on oral contraceptives are anovulatory, but the progesterone component and relatively low levels of estrogen prevent hyperplasia. A patient being treated with medroxyprogesterone acetate also has low levels of FSH and LH and therefore low levels of estrogen. Adenomyosis occurs when there is extension of the endometrial glands and stroma into the uterine musculature. It is characterized clinically by dysmenorrhea and menorrhagia but has no effect on the proliferative and secretory cycles of the ovary. *(Hacker and Moore, pp. 352–354, 374, 543–546, 576–577)*

62. **(D)** If a patient is less than 40 years of age and an adnexal/ovarian cyst is less than 6 cm in size, the patient can be placed on birth control pills and observed for 6 weeks. A large percentage of patients, 60% to 70%, will respond to such a regimen and no adnexal mass will be palpable at the next examination. If the cyst is between 6 and 8 cm and is unilocular on sonography, it also can be observed. Multilocular or solid cysts between 6 and 8 cm should be explored. In the case presented, the cyst not only did not respond to hormonal treatment, but also grew larger. Exploratory laparotomy is the preferred means of treatment for both diagnostic and therapeutic reasons. Although a simple or uniloculated cyst can be differentiated on ultrasound from a multiloculated cyst, differentiating a benign multilocular cyst from a malignant one is impossible on ultrasound. To adequately diagnose the etiology of an adnexal mass, removal and pathological diagnosis are necessary. Laparoscopy again is not adequate in distinguishing whether an adnexal mass is a functional cyst or malignant lesion; looking at the cyst through the laparoscope is therefore not an accepted diagnostic procedure. If the surgeon is skilled at surgical removal of the cyst laparoscopically, with a specimen that could be evaluated pathologically, then this would be acceptable therapy. Functional cysts, such as corpus luteal or follicular greater than 8 cm in size, should be removed to prevent torsion or rupture that can present as a surgical emergency. A GnRH analog would prevent further hormonal stimulation of the cyst, but at this time there is no evidence that their use would shrink the cyst. *(Hacker and Moore, pp. 356–358)*

63. **(B)** This patient requires exploratory laparotomy for either ruptured ectopic pregnancy or ruptured hemorrhagic corpus luteum. Because hemoperitoneum causes an elevation of the WBC count, this test would not help in deciding the origin of the peritoneal irritation. A low hemoglobin and hematocrit (Hbg and Hct) would also be expected in both cases. As the presence of a corpus luteal cyst frequently causes prolonged amenorrhea with irregular or nominal bleeding, the only way to determine whether this patient's amenorrhea is secondary to pregnancy is to obtain a pregnancy test. Urinary pregnancy tests that are sensitive to 25 mIU/mL of urinary human chorionic gonadotropin are positive in more than 95% of ectopic pregnancies. Free fluid on vaginal sonogram would occur with either a ruptured hemorrhagic corpus luteum or a ruptured ectopic and would not be helpful in differentiating between the two. A quantitative beta-HCG would not be necessary, because a positive urine pregnancy test would be sufficient to determine that the patient was pregnant. *(Hacker and Moore, p. 428)*

64. **(A)** This woman's symptoms and physical findings are characteristic of the perimenopausal period: a time when ovarian functioning is decreasing and levels of estrogen and progesterone levels are decreasing. Menstrual irregularities often are the first indication of decreased hormonal levels. Vasomotor symptoms, often described as hot flashes, also are common during this period. These symptoms generally start as feelings of intense heat beginning in the chest and progressing upward to the neck and head. They typically occur at night, are accompanied by profuse diaphoresis, and can cause sleep irregularities. Women also may complain of decreased sexual desire during this period, due to the loss of estrogen effects on the vaginal mucosa resulting in atrophic changes, decreased lubrication, and subsequent dyspareunia. Although this patient could conceive, because some cycles can be associated with ovulation, it would be unlikely given that the patient has a normal-size uterus, and pregnancy is a hyperestrogen state, inconsistent with the patient's findings on pelvic exam. Because the patient is still menstruating, menopause is not a possible explanation: menopause is defined as the cesssation of menses for at least 12 months. The patient is 45 years old, so premature ovarian failure is not a possiblity. In addition, most patients with this syndrome are amenorrheic. A patient with polycystic ovaries often is amenorrheic but can have irregular menses. Unlike perimenopausal women, these patients tend

to have excessive estrogen. (*Hacker and Moore, pp. 526–527; Wehrle, pp. 16–21*)

65. (E) A large percentage of women see only their gynecologist routinely. The general health care of women then falls into the hands of the practitioner who does routine GYN exams. Obviously, a bimanual exam of the pelvic organs (uterus, ovaries, tubes, and bladder) is part of the gynecological exam, as is inspection of the cervix and vagina on speculum exam. A breast exam and an explanation of self-examination are important. Breast cancer is the most common malignant neoplasm in women. Early detection via routine exam, self-exam, and screening mammography allows for greater cure rates. Screening mammograms should be done first at age 35 to 40 for a baseline and then repeated at physician-determined intervals (usually 1- to 2-year intervals) between ages 40 to 50. After age 50, it is suggested that women undergo annual mammography. Women at increased risk for breast cancer should have their baseline mammogram at age 35 and their subsequent mammograms at closer intervals. Performing a recto-vaginal exam is uncomfortable for many patients, but it allows the examiner to better asses the posterior cul-de-sac, the position of the uterus, particularly retroverted uteri and to further assess adenexal masses. Moreover, as colon cancer is the fourth most common cancer in women it can alert the practitioner to the possibility of a rectosigmoid mass. (*Dumesic, p. 39–46; Hacker and Moore, pp. 443–445*)

66. (A) The ability of a practitioner to perform a pelvic exam adequately depends on the patient's preparation for the examination. Communication prior to and throughout the exam is extremely important. Patients tolerate such exams much better when they are informed of what the practitioner is doing or about to do and can see the practitioner's face as the exam is performed. Preparation by adequately draping the patient is a good means of keeping the patient comfortable and somewhat lessens the sense of self-consciousness and loss of control many women experience during a pelvic examination. The exam should be gradual, again to allow the patient to express discomfort with any part of the exam. Although it may make the examiner uncomfortable, allowing one family member to remain in the examination room may help the patient tolerate the procedure better. When the patient is an adolescent, allowing a mother or sister in the room may greatly decrease her anxieties. Some patients will actually feel more uncomfortable with the husband or a family member remaining in the room. Again, good communication with the patient will alert the practitioner to this possibility. The patient should be informed when a part of the exam may be painful. To avoid doing so may prevent the completion of the exam secondary to the patient's mistrust of the examiner and general discomfort. When informing the patient of impending pain, stress that the discomfort will be far lower if the patient can relax and not tighten up in response to the anticipated pain. (*Dumesic, pp. 39–46*)

67. (A) Hormone replacement therapy will not prevent the development of endometrial cancer, and administering estrogen alone will actually increase the incidence of endometrial cancer. Women who still have their uterus should therefore always be given a progestational agent along with estrogen. Estrogen replacement in a menopausal or perimenopausal woman will decrease the risk for cardiovascular disease. The increased risk for developing cardiovascular disease in the menopausal woman is related to lipid metabolism: low-density lipoproteins and cholesterol increase and high-density lipoproteins decrease. Estrogen appears to have a reverse affect on these levels: increasing high-density lipoproteins and decreasing low-density lipoproteins. Adding progesterone to the hormone replacement regimen has a somewhat negative effect on the benefits of estrogen. There is an overall positive effect on the lipid profile. Bone density begins to decrease in a woman's early twenties, but is significantly accelerated by estrogen depletion, and in many women will lead to osteoporosis. A significant degree of bone loss occurs within the first several years of menopause; the recently menopausal and peri-menopausal woman is therefore the most likely to benefit from hormone replacement. Women of Northern European descent, smokers, drinkers, and women who have been sedentary are at greater risk of developing osteoporosis. Urinary urgency, dysuria, incontinence, and increased incidence of bladder infections occur with estrogen depletion and improve with hormone replacement. Because lack of estrogen will cause loss of vaginal secretions and elasticity, resulting in dyspareunia; many menopausal and perimenopausal women will have decreased sexual drive and satisfaction. These symptoms are relieved with hormone replacement. *(Baran, pp. 321–324; Wehrle, pp. 16–21.)*

68. **(B)** Whether a patient is being interviewed during a routine exam or being seen for a gynecological emergency, a thorough menstrual history is important. First, the date of the last menstrual period (LMP) should be obtained and whether the LMP was normal in amount, duration, and interval. The patient should also be asked about her two previous periods and whether they were normal. Next the patient should be asked about her menstrual cycle: is it regular in interval, and what is the interval? A normal menstrual cycle is 28 to 30 days. A history of irregular cycles is indicative of anovulatory cycles or other endocrine abnormalities. Duration of menstrual flow, presence of clots, and amount of bleeding and associated pain are additional information that should be obtained. The color of the blood is generally not information needed as it is not suggestive of any pathology. Age of menarche and onset of menopause and perimenopausal symptoms are also important in menstrual history. Intermenstrual bleeding can be spotting just prior to menses or at time of ovulation. It can also be indicative of uterine cancer and should always be investigated. Finally, a history of premenstrual syndrome should be elicited. The symptoms are extremely variable and include bloating, painful breast swelling, fatigue, depression, anxiety, irritability, and hostility. *(Hacker and Moore, pp. 15–16, 334–336; Jones et al, pp. 5–6)*

69. **(A)** An endometrial biopsy can be performed in an office or clinic with either local anesthesia in the form of paracervical block or just premedication with analgesics. The endometrium is sampled with an extremely small suction-type curette in 4 to 6 different sites. In the case of this patient, as in any woman suspected of having cancer, an endocervical curetting should be performed prior to obtaining endometrial samples. In the case where polyps are visualized in the endocervical canal, they can be of either endocervical or endometrial origin. The polyps can often be removed in the office if they are small, but if they are of considerable size, they should be removed in an operating room. Endometrial polyps are seldom malignant in premenopausal women, but in menopausal or postmenopausal women they should be removed in the operating room to allow adequate dilation of the cervix to remove all the polyps for pathological diagnosis. The patient's increased menstrual bleeding is probably secondary to her known myomata. Submucosal myomata will often cause excessive bleeding. Curettage will decrease this bleeding; it thus becomes not only a diagnostic but also a therapeutic procedure. Endometrial sampling, whether by dilation and curettage (D&C) or endometrial biopsy, is indicated in any woman 40 years of age or older who has intermenstrual bleeding or a marked change in her bleeding pattern. It should be performed prior to performing a hysterectomy, as the need for additional surgery and nodal sampling would change if the patient had a malignancy. A sonogram would adequately identify myomata but would not be helpful in determining whether there have been malignant endometrial changes. A CAT scan provides greater imaging than ultrasound, particularly if pelvic or periaortic nodes are suspected, but it still does not provide the necessary pathological diagnosis for this patient. Colposcopy would not be the procedure of choice, as no endometrial sampling is routinely performed with this procedure. *(Hacker and Moore, p. 350; Jones et al, pp. 19–25, 723–726)*

70. **(B)** Syphilis, particularly in people who use IV drugs and crack or cocaine, is greatly increasing in frequency. It is theorized that many women are exchanging sex for drugs and that is why it is increasing in this population. Primary syphilis is characterized by a chancre that is a nontender, ulcerative lesion usually found on the vulva, but it can be also found in the vagina or on the cervix. It will appear between 10 and 60 days from the time of inoculation and spontaneously regress after 4 to 6 weeks. It usually is associated with nontender, inguinal lymphadenopathy. Because serologic tests are usually negative at this time, the primary means of making the diagnosis is by obtaining a specimen from the lesion. The spirochete can be seen on darkfield microscopy. Secondary syphilis occurs anywhere from 3 to 6 weeks after the appearance of the chancre. It is characterized by a macular papular skin rash, often on the palms of the hands and soles of the feet; generalized malaise and anorexia; and condylomata lata lesions. These lesions are broad exophytic excrescences that are found on the vulva, thighs, and buttocks and are extremely infectious. Sampling from these lesions again reveals the spirochete under the darkfield microscope. The VDRL is positive at this time, and inguinal adenopathy is also present. Benzathine penicillin G, 2.4 million U in a one-time dose is the treatment for primary, secondary, or latent syphilis (less than 1 year's duration). Tertiary syphilis, which may affect any organ system of the body, particularly the central nervous system, is treated with three doses of benzathine penicillin G at weekly intervals. When it is not possible to document the duration of infection, the treatment of choice is the three doses at weekly intervals. For patients allergic to penicillin, tetracycline, 500 mg orally for 15 days, is given for primary, secondary, and latent syphilis; 500 mg orally for 30 days for tertiary syphilis. There are no signs of PID with syphilis; and a mucopurulent cervical discharge is characteristically found in cervicitis or PID. Condylomata acuminata is not a lesion found in syphilis; painful vesicular lesions are more characteristic of herpes. (*Hacker and Moore, pp. 186–187, 383–384; Jones et al, pp. 577–579*)

71. **(A)** One of the best means of antepartum fetal surveillance is the mother's perception of fetal movement. Whenever a woman complains of decreased fetal movement, she should immediately undergo fetal monitoring to obtain a reactive tracing and ultrasound to document fetal well-being. Intrauterine demise or neonatal death is not only a medical problem, but also a psychosocial problem. The practitioner who deals with pregnant women must learn how to deal with women who have suffered a stillborn or neonatal loss. Couples should be allowed to see their child and hold or examine the baby. Often the child has undergone maceration or has a disfiguring anomaly. Wrapping the child to conceal or lessen these changes will help reduce the parents' shock. Although mothers and fathers often will opt not to view their dead child, it has been shown that to do so will help the parents accept the death and grieve appropriately. Taking pictures has also been found to help the parents in accepting the child's death. In addition, many parents who originally could not deal with the demise can later return to view the pictures. Mothers should be appropriately medicated for pain and should not be "snowed." Being knocked out with good amounts of amnesiacs and analgesics will take away the realization that the child was actually born dead. Often, these women will not accept that their babies were stillborn but in fact believe that something was done to kill the child. Again, an awareness of the stillbirth enhances the mother's ability to appropriately grieve. Allowing the father to remain with the mother during the labor and delivery will allow him to better accept the reality of the child's death. It also will allow the couple to provide each other with support and encouragement. Often in an attempt to help the mother with the pain of labor and delivery of a stillborn, the practioner forgets that the father too has lost a child. Reminding the mother that she can conceive again actually

minimizes the death of her child and does not contribute to the mourning process. *(Capitulo and Maffia, pp. 81–86)*

72. **(D)** Variable deceleration is caused by umbilical cord compression. The onset of the decelerations varies according to its relationship to the contraction and the shape of the deceleration varies when compared to the other decelerations. Variable decelerations occur when the cord is around the baby's neck or a limb and when there is oligohydramnios. Changing the mother's position from the right side to left side, or placing her in Trendelenburg or knee-chest position may relieve the pressure on the cord and subsequently resolve the variable decelerations. Severe variable decelerations, those lasting greater than 60 seconds, often occur during the second stage of labor, as the patient starts to push, but do not exclusively occur in the second stage, and therefore, it cannot be assumed that the patient is in this stage of labor. Late decelerations begin after the onset of the contractions and occur consistently at the same time of each contraction and appear similar in form. Late decelerations usually are indicative of some kind of uteroplacental insufficiency such as chronic hypertension, pregnancy-induced hypertension, sudden and severe maternal hypotension. Placing the patient on her left side will cause maximum blood flow to the placenta and often alleviates the late decelerations. Variable decelerations by themselves are not an indication for an emergency cesarean section; if they are associated with decreased fetal heart rate variability, are persistent, deeper, prolonged (variables with a late component), or more frequent, then a cesearean may be the best course. The contractions depicted on the tracing are every 2 to 4 minutes and would not need to be increased in frequency with pitocin stimulation. *(Hacker and Moore, pp. 252–257; Freeman and Garite, p. 75)*

73. **(E)** Rape makes up about 7% of all violent crime in this country. Approximately 3 to 10 times as many rapes are committed than are reported. Practitioners who care for women at some time in their career must deal with women who have been raped. Practitioners are called upon to obtain evidence and treat the patient, both medically and psychologically. The patient should be treated for both gonorrhea and chlamydia at the time she is initially seen. A baseline VDRL and pregnancy test should also be drawn, and the patient should be seen again in 6 weeks to repeat these tests and to repeat GC and chlamydial cultures. The patient must be informed about the possibility of pregnancy. A certain percentage of women are protected against pregnancy with a preexisting form of birth control such as birth control pills, IUD, bilateral tubal ligation, or hysterectomy. In women unprotected by preexisting means of birth control, postcoital contraception should be offered. This is usually in the form of the birth control pill Ovral (ethinyl estradiol 50 mg/dL and norgestrel 0.5 mg) given as two tabs PO immediately and then two tabs in 12 hours. The patients should be instructed that this dose can cause nausea and vomiting. In addition, the patient should be offered HIV counseling and testing. *(Hacker and Moore, pp. 486–489; Jones et al, pp. 525–533)*

REFERENCES

Baker VL. Alternatives to oral estrogen replacement. *Prim Care Mature Woman, Obstet Gynecol Clin North Am.* 1994; 21(2).

Baran DT. Osteoporosis: Monitoring techniques and alternative therapies. *Prim Care Mature Woman, Obstet Gynecol Clin North Am.* 1994; 21(2).

Burke L. The use of the Friedman curve in labor management. *Cincinnatti J Med.* 1975; 56: 29–36.

Burrow GB, Ferris TF. *Medical Complications during Pregnancy.* Philadelphia: Saunders; 1988.

Capitulo KL, Maffia A. *The Perinatal Bereavement Team: Development and Function, Women and Loss.* New York: Praeger; 1985.

Creasy RK, Resnick R. *Maternal Fetal Medicine, Principals and Practices,* 3rd ed. Philadelphia: Saunders; 1994.

Cunningham FG, MacDonald PC, Gant NF. *Williams Obstetrics,* 18th ed. Norwalk, CT: Appleton & Lange; 1989.

Dumesic DA. Pelvic examination: What to focus on in menopausal women. *Consultant: Consul Prim Care.* 1996; 36(1).

Emerson DS, McCord ML. Clinician's approach to ectopic pregnancy. *Clin Obstet Gynecol.* 1996; 39(1).

Freeman RK, Garite TJ. *Fetal Heart Rate Monitoring.* Baltimore: Williams & Wilkins; 1981.

Gregg AR. Introduction to premature rupture of membranes. *OB/GYN Clin North Am.* 1992; 19(2).

Gries-Griffin J. Abnormal Pap test results. *Adv Phys Assist.* 1995; 3(7).

Grimes DA (ed). The Contraceptive Report. *Update Female Steril. 1996; VII(3).*

Hacker NF, Moore JG. *Essentials of Obstetrics and Gynecology,* 2nd ed. Philadelphia: Saunders; 1992.

Hinman AR (ed). Sexually transmitted diseases treatment guidelines. *MMWR.* 1996; 42(rr-14).

Howe RS. Early pregnancy: Normal and abnormal. *Clin Obstet Gynecol. 1996; 39(1).*

Johnson SR. Clinician's approach to the diagnosis and management of premenstrual syndrome. *Clin Obstet Gynecol.* 1992; 35(3).

Jones HW, Wentz AC, Burnett LS. *Novak's Textbook of Gynecology,* 11th ed. Baltimore: Williams & Wilkins; 1988.

Keene GF. Group B strep colonization and infection in pregnancy. J *Am Acad Phys Assist.* 1995; 8(6).

Ramirez NC, Lawrence WD, Ginsburg KA. Ectopic pregnancy, a recent five-year study and review of the last 50 years' literature. *J Reprod Med. 1996; 41(10).*

Rose CR, Mennuti MT. Preconceptional folate supplementation and neural tube defects. *Clin Obstet Gynecol.* 1994; 37(3).

Sammuels P, Cohen A. Pregnancies complicated by liver disease and liver dysfunction. *Obstet Gynecol Clin North Am.* 1992; 19(4).

Schroder RK. With the first injectable contraceptive, birth control becomes a seasonal issue. *Adv Phys Assist.* 1995; 3(3).

Scott PM. Abnormal Pap smears: When is colposcopy needed? J *Am Acad Phys Assist.* 1996; 9(1).

Szarzynski JE. Endometriosis, a diagnostic and therapeutic challenge. *Phys Assist.* 1993; 17(5).

Walsh HJ, Hoody DL. Gestational diabetes: Screening and diagnosis. *Adv Phys Assist.* 1995; 3(6).

Wehrle KE. The in between time: A guide to perimenopause. *Adv Phys Assist. 1996; 4(1).*

CHAPTER 9

Practice Test
Questions

DIRECTIONS (Questions 1 through 64): Each of the numbered items or incomplete statements in this section is followed by answers or by completions of the statement. Select the ONE lettered answer or completion that is BEST in each case.

Questions 1 through 64

1. Which congenital defect is MOST often recognized at birth or on the first day of life and is lethal if not corrected?

   (A) tetralogy of Fallot
   (B) transposition of the great vessels
   (C) patent ductus arteriosus
   (D) atrial septal defect
   (E) ventricular septal defect

2. Which of the following tests is best for monitoring adequate blood sugar control in the diabetic?

   (A) 12 midnight blood sugar
   (B) glycohemoglobin level (HbAlc)
   (C) 24-hour urine for glucose
   (D) 6 PM blood sugar
   (E) 8 AM insulin level

3. Clozaril (clozapine) is an antipsychotic used to treat refractory schizophrenia. Routine monitoring is performed for

   (A) leukoplasia
   (B) eosinophilia
   (C) agranulocytosis
   (D) thrombocytopenia
   (E) leukopenia

4. Which nervous structure is at greater risk during anterior cervical microdiscectomy?

   (A) superior laryngeal nerve
   (B) recurrent laryngeal nerve
   (C) cervical sympathetic chain
   (D) vagus nerve
   (E) inferior laryngeal nerve

5. The MOST reliable physical finding in acute appendicitis is

   (A) hyperesthesia of the skin overlying the right lower quadrant
   (B) localized right lower-quadrant tenderness
   (C) tenderness on rectal examination
   (D) psoas sign
   (E) observation of bilious vomiting

6. A 15-year-old patient presents with a complaint of severe menstrual cramps that prevent her from attending school and maintaining her normal daily activity. The pain usually occurs on the first day of her menses and has gotten progressively worse since the onset of menarche at age 13. A pelvic exam is without significant findings. You make the diagnosis of primary dysmenorrhea. The MOST appropriate treatment is

   (A) Tylenol with codeine
   (B) oral contraceptives
   (C) prostaglandin synthetase inhibitors
   (D) diagnostic laparoscopy
   (E) tocolytic agents

7. Clinical features of Cushing's syndrome include

   (A) thick skin
   (B) hirsutism
   (C) improved strength
   (D) hair loss
   (E) abdominal pain

8. Hepatitis B vaccine is recommended to all the following EXCEPT

   (A) infants born to a hepatitis B surface antigen (HBsAg)–positive mother
   (B) established hepatitis B–infected individuals
   (C) promiscuous heterosexuals
   (D) persons receiving an accidental needle-stick from HBsAg–positive blood or body fluids
   (E) health care professionals exposed regularly to blood

9. The primary means by which oral contraceptives prevent pregnancy is

   (A) inhibition of endometrial implantation of the embryo
   (B) inhibition of the release of prolactin and, therefore, prevention of ovulation
   (C) inhibition of the release of estrogen from the follicle and, therefore, ovulation
   (D) inhibition of spermatozoa by pill-induced changes in the cervical mucus
   (E) inhibition of the midcycle gonadotropin surge and, therefore, ovulation

10. The mechanism of action of calcium-channel blockers in the treatment of angina pectoris is

    (A) reduction of the excitation–contraction–coupling mechanism responsible for myocardial and smooth-muscle contraction
    (B) inhibition of the binding of circulating catecholamines to beta-adrenergic receptors
    (C) increase in calcium extrusion from myocardial cells

    (D) increase of diastolic filling of the left ventricle
    (E) increase in the oxygen-binding capacity of hemoglobin

11. Psychiatric conditions associated with HIV infection include

    (A) depression
    (B) acute psychosis
    (C) mania
    (D) delirium
    (E) all of the above

12. Human breast milk offers which of the following advantage(s) to neonates?

    (A) secretory IgA
    (B) will meet all infant nutrition requirements till age 4 to 6 months
    (C) epidermal growth factor
    (D) infant has higher absorption of iron from breast milk
    (E) all of the above

13. An S3 gallop sound in an adult is usually associated with

    (A) hypertension
    (B) pericarditis
    (C) myocardial infarction
    (D) congestive heart failure
    (E) aortic stenosis

14. "Apple core" lesions on barium enema strongly suggest

    (A) diverticulitis
    (B) sigmoid volvulus
    (C) Gardner's syndrome
    (D) carcinoma of the colon
    (E) villous adenoma

15. After delivery of an Rh-positive baby to an Rh-negative mother, the mother is given RhoGAM. When is RhoGAM also indicated in an Rh-negative mother?

    (A) after an ectopic pregnancy
    (B) following amniocentesis

(C) routinely at 28 weeks

(D) following spontaneous or induced abortion

(E) all of the above

16. The most common primary malignancy of the skin is

(A) squamous cell carcinoma

(B) melanoma

(C) neurofibroma

(D) keratoacanthoma

(E) basal cell carcinoma

17. AIDS-associated Kaposi's sarcoma

(A) may present in the lung as nodular infiltrates

(B) is seen primarily in IV-drug users

(C) rarely responds to alpha-interferon administration

(D) when treated with radiotherapy is associated with a high response rate and an improved prognosis

(E) presents with relatively indolent cutaneous lesions

18. Approximately 60% of body weight is composed of water. Which of the following is correct?

(A) two-thirds intracellular

(B) one-third extracellular

(C) plasma fluid is extracellular

(D) interstitial fluid is extracellular

(E) all of the above

19. When performing a Pap smear you are attempting to obtain cells from the area that undergoes dysplastic changes. This area is called the

(A) endocervix

(B) squamocolumnar junction

(C) posterior vaginal fornix

(D) exocervix

(E) internal os

20. Bilateral nonpitting edema is associated with

(A) cardiac disease

(B) lymphedema

(C) renal disease

(D) cirrhosis

(E) venous disease

21. Atrial fibrillation is characterized by

(A) an irregularly irregular rhythm

(B) progressively increasing P-R intervals

(C) varying P-R intervals

(D) a prolonged Q-T interval

(E) a narrowed QRS complex

22. A 78-year-old male presents with a "classic triad" of dementia, incontinence of urine, and difficulty with gait. What would you expect to see on a CT scan of the head?

(A) large ventricles

(B) brain tumor

(C) cerebral atrophy

(D) multiple infarcts

(E) single infarct

23. NPH insulin usually has its peak activity at

(A) 4 to 6 hours

(B) 18 to 24 hours

(C) 10 hours

(D) 6 to 14 hours

(E) 16 hours

24. A toddler presents with a 3-day history of conjunctivitis, coryza, nasal discharge, and a hacking cough. On examination, you notice small, irregular, grayish-white lesions on the upper buccal mucosa. The most likely diagnosis is

(A) rubeola

(B) rubella

(C) roseola

(D) rosacea

(E) rotavirus

25. Which of the following medications is pre-scribed for children with attention deficit dis-order?

    (A) amitriptyline (Elavil)
    (B) phenelzine (Nardil)
    (C) methylphenidate (Ritalin)
    (D) carbamazepine (Tegretol)
    (E) lorazepam (Ativan)

26. A ventricular wall aneurysm may be caused by

    (A) diabetes
    (B) myocardial infarction
    (C) congenital malformation
    (D) high-fat diet
    (E) recurring ventricular tachycardia

27. Which atherosclerotic aneurysm is MOST common?

    (A) abdominal aortic aneurysm
    (B) carotid artery aneurysm
    (C) popliteal aneurysm
    (D) femoral aneurysm
    (E) subclavian artery aneurysm

28. Multiple plantar verrucae (warts) are BEST managed with

    (A) antiviral therapy
    (B) conventional surgical excision
    (C) cryosurgery
    (D) laser surgery
    (E) salicylic acid therapy

29. HIV-infected patients are at increased risk for all the following central nervous system (CNS) diseases EXCEPT

    (A) progressive multifocal leukoen-cephalopathy (PML)
    (B) primary CNS lymphoma
    (C) cryptococcoma
    (D) bacterial meningitis
    (E) TB meningitis

30. A 25-year-old woman requests birth control pills. Before prescribing a combination estro-gen/progesterone pill, you must obtain a negative history of

    (A) previous deep vein thrombosis
    (B) smoking
    (C) type I diabetes
    (D) migraine headache
    (E) hepatitis B

31. Chvostek's and Trousseau's signs can be seen in patients with

    (A) hypercalcemia
    (B) hypomagnesemia
    (C) hypocalcemia
    (D) hypermagnesemia
    (E) hypophosphatemia

32. Hypercalcemia should be suspected if a pa-tient has a serum calcium level of

    (A) 8.0 mg/dL with albumin of 3.0 g/dL
    (B) 9.0 mg/dL with albumin of 3.0 g/dL
    (C) 10.0 mg/dL with albumin of 4.0 g/dL
    (D) 10.0 mg/dL with albumin of 2.0 g/dL
    (E) 9.5 mg/dL with albumin of 3.8 g/dL

33. Which of the following is NOT associated with pancreatitis?

    (A) alcohol
    (B) gallstones
    (C) hyperlipidemia
    (D) carcinoma
    (E) hyperparathyroidism

34. Which study is MOST accurate in confirming the diagnosis of venous thrombosis and the extent of involvement?

    (A) impedance plethysmography
    (B) ultrasound
    (C) ultrasound and real-time B-mode imag-ing
    (D) radiolabeled fibrinogen
    (E) venography

35. Which of the following drugs can cause a maculopapular rash in a patient with infec-tious mononucleosis?

(A) tetracycline

(B) erythromycin

(C) ampicillin

(D) sulfa

(E) cephalosporin

36. The immediate treatment of sustained ventricular tachycardia without a pulse is

(A) bretylium 5 mg/kg IV push

(B) lidocaine 5 mg/kg IV push

(C) procainamide 30 mg/kg IV push

(D) defibrillate up to 3 times

(E) epinephrine 1 mg/kg IV push

37. Studies determining the incidence rate of otitis media show that all of the following statements are true EXCEPT

(A) The peak incidence occurs in the second 6 months of life.

(B) By the first birthday, 62% of all children will have had at least one episode of otitis media.

(C) Administration of the HIB vaccine has been shown to decrease the incidence of otitis media.

(D) The occurrence rate declines after age 6 years.

(E) Age at first episode of acute otitis media has shown to be the most powerful predictive factor concerning future infections.

38. Treatment of an avulsed secondary tooth includes which one of the following?

(A) cleaning the tooth thoroughly by scrubbing all dirt and foreign matter from the tooth

(B) inserting the tooth into the open socket or placing the tooth under the patient's tongue

(C) wrapping the tooth in gauze

(D) referral to a dentist in 7 to 10 days

(E) soaking the tooth in peroxide

39. The standard endocarditis prophylaxis recommendation for dental and surgical procedures is

(A) penicillin G 1 million U IV during the procedure

(B) amoxicillin 500 mg orally 1 hour before the procedure and 2 g 2 hours later

(C) penicillin V 1 g orally 6 hours before the procedure and 2 g 1 hour later

(D) amoxicillin 3 g orally 1 hour before the procedure and 1.5 g 6 hours later

(E) vancomycin 500 mg orally 1 hour before the procedure and 2 g 6 hours later

40. Regarding bilirubin, which of the following is correct?

(A) Bilirubin is formed mostly from the buildup of hemoglobin.

(B) Once formed, bilirubin joins with albumin to form prostaglandins.

(C) Conjugated bilirubin is acted upon by bacteria in the intestine to produce urobilinogen and urobilin.

(D) The hepatic parenchymal cell is a site of bilirubin conjugation with hydrochloric acid.

(E) All bilirubin found in the body is unconjugated.

41. A 34-year-old female has a low-grade squamous intraepithelial lesion on Pap smear and undergoes colposcopy. Which of the following would NOT be an indication for either a LEEP conization or cold knife cone biopsy?

(A) positive endocervical curettage

(B) a higher-grade lesion on biopsy at the time of the colposcopy

(C) inability of the colposcopist to visualize the transition zone

(D) lesions suspicious for carcinoma

(E) cervical intraepithelial neoplasia grade II (CIN II) on colposcopic biopsy

42. The human papillomavirus (HPV) is the causative organism for the common wart as well as genital warts. Regarding genital warts, the following are true EXCEPT

   (A) In the United States, HPV infections have been occurring at five times the rate of genital herpes since the mid-1980s.
   (B) No single treatment is effective in eradicating the virus and preventing recurrence.
   (C) The treatment of choice is cryotherapy.
   (D) The lesions can be confused with condylomata lata of secondary syphilis.
   (E) Of women with cervical dysplasia, more than 50% of male sexual contacts will have HPV.

43. Purple, polygonal papules and plaques are MOST characteristic of

   (A) guttate psoriasis
   (B) granuloma annulare
   (C) lichen planus
   (D) nummular eczema
   (E) vitiligo

44. What is the most common cause of large-bowel obstruction in an adult?

   (A) carcinoma
   (B) volvulus
   (C) diverticulitis
   (D) ulcerative colitis
   (E) Hirschsprung's disease

45. A child is brought to your office with high fever, difficulty swallowing, and drooling over the past several hours. On exam you notice an ill-appearing child with inspiratory stridor, breath sounds that are equal bilaterally, and symmetrical chest movement. The most likely diagnosis is

   (A) epiglottitis
   (B) bacterial pharyngitis
   (C) viral croup
   (D) foreign-body aspiration
   (E) pneumonia

46. Of the following, the BEST and safest way to approach the child described in Question 45 would be

   (A) direct visualization of the pharynx with a tongue blade
   (B) obtaining a lateral soft tissue x-ray prior to exam
   (C) direct visualization with the aid of a laryngoscope
   (D) obtaining a bronchoscopy as soon as possible
   (E) obtaining a rapid strep screen by swabbing the oropharynx

47. Target lesions are pathognomonic of

   (A) erythema marginatum
   (B) erythema multiforme
   (C) erythema annulare
   (D) erythema nodosum
   (E) erythema infectiosum

48. Medications acceptable for prophylaxis of *Pneumocystis carinii* pneumonia (PCP) include trimethoprim-sulfamethoxazole, aerosolized pentamidine, and

   (A) dapsone
   (B) ciprofloxacin
   (C) ethambutol
   (D) clarithromycin
   (E) Cefaclor

49. Which of the following abnormal findings produced by arterial injury is most important?

   (A) pain
   (B) pallor
   (C) pulselessness
   (D) paralysis and paresthesia
   (E) poikilothermia

50. A 50-year-old male presents with abrupt onset of hypertension, headache, palpitations, sweating, weight loss, and anxiety attacks.

Which of the following lab tests would be MOST useful in making the diagnosis?

(A) captopril-induced renal scan

(B) 24-hour urine catecholamines, metanephrines, VMA

(C) 24-hour urine protein and creatinine clearance

(D) renal vein renin levels

(E) serum creatinine

51. Headaches associated with a brain tumor have all of the following characteristics EXCEPT

(A) wakes patient at night

(B) worse in AM, improves throughout the day

(C) worse with coughing

(D) worse with defecation

(E) has an aura

52. Which of the following is the MOST important first step in treating a child who is unresponsive after suspected cardiopulmonary arrest?

(A) applying cardiac monitor

(B) initiating closed chest cardiac massage

(C) determining if patient is having respiratory difficulty and establishing a patent airway

(D) assessing whether circulatory problems exist by checking brachial, femoral, or carotid pulses

(E) establishing an IV line

53. Which of the following is the correct treatment for a positive urine culture in a 14-week-pregnant patient with no urinary tract infection (UTI) symptoms?

(A) repeat the culture and sensitivity, because without symptoms the culture could be false-positive

(B) a 10-day course of antibiotic therapy as an outpatient

(C) admission to the hospital for intravenous therapy

(D) chronic suppressive therapy

(E) repeating the culture and sensitivity within 2 days of initiating therapy in order to test for a cure

54. Varicella

(A) has an average incubation period of about 14 days

(B) causes scarring if not treated aggressively

(C) is associated with subsequent herpes simplex

(D) can be transmitted to adults as shingles

(E) can be confirmed by serological testing at the time of presentation

55. What hormone plays a vital role in urine osmolality?

(A) aldosterone

(B) antidiuretic hormone (ADH)

(C) renin

(D) angiotensin

(E) erythropoietin

56. What substance is secreted by the chief cells of the stomach?

(A) gastrin

(B) pepsin

(C) pepsinogen

(D) gastric acid

(E) glucagon

57. The pathophysiology of respiratory distress syndrome (RDS) involves atelectasis resulting from

(A) decreased lung perfusion

(B) aspiration of meconium

(C) failed pulmonary capillary development

(D) surfactant deficiency

(E) fluid overload

58. On physical exam, hypercalcemia can be detected by

    (A) a positive Chvostek's sign
    (B) carpal pedal spasm
    (C) tetany
    (D) stupor
    (E) none of the above

59. What diagnosis should be strongly suspected in an overweight, hypertensive, middle-aged male who complains of daytime somnolence and whose wife complains that he snores?

    (A) coronary artery disease
    (B) chronic obstructive pulmonary disease
    (C) obstructive sleep apnea syndrome
    (D) major depression
    (E) narcolepsy

60. Prinzmetal's angina (variant angina) is due to

    (A) abnormal coronary anatomy
    (B) coronary artery spasm
    (C) coronary steal syndrome
    (D) abnormal levels of circulating thyroid-stimulating hormone (TSH)
    (E) high serum magnesium levels

61. A 55-year-old white female presents with nonspecific complaints of anorexia, fatigue, hair loss, and dry skin. Physical exam reveals a pale, fair-skinned woman with dry skin, mild vertigo, and a beefy red tongue. Laboratory values reveal hypothyroidism and macrocytic anemia. Which of the anemias listed is MOST commonly associated with the findings?

    (A) anemia of chronic disease
    (B) thalassemia minor
    (C) folate deficiency
    (D) pernicious anemia
    (E) iron deficiency

62. All of the following might normally be found on the neurological exam of a patient with a herniated lumbar disk EXCEPT

    (A) diminished ankle or knee reflexes
    (B) areas of numbness on the leg or foot
    (C) positive Babinski sign on affected side
    (D) weakness of foot inversion or eversion
    (E) weakness of big toe dorsiflexion

63. Which of the following medications is appropriate initial therapy for uncomplicated erysipelas?

    (A) tetracycline
    (B) sulfamethoxazole
    (C) vancomycin
    (D) dicloxacillin
    (E) streptomycin

64. Tardive dyskinesia is seen with large doses of

    (A) paraldehyde
    (B) buspirone
    (C) ethylene glycol
    (D) phencyclidine
    (E) phenothiazides

DIRECTIONS (Questions 65 through 68): Each group of items in this section consists of a set of lettered headings followed by several numbered words or phrases. For each numbered word or phrase, select the ONE lettered heading that is most closely associated with it. Each lettered heading may be selected once, more than once, or not at all.

Questions 65 through 68

Choose the diagnostic category that BEST describes each of the following patients.

    (A) depression
    (B) bipolar affective disorder
    (C) schizophrenia
    (D) dementia
    (E) none of the above

65. A 59-year-old white male presents to your office with a history of gradual decline in memory for major events, expresses an inappropriate affect oriented only to person, and family reports that the symptoms get worse at night. Which diagnostic category would you initially consider?

66. You are on call to the ER when you are asked to evaluate a 42-year-old male who has been brought in by the family in the past for treatment of depression. However, over the last week he has had increased energy, decreased sleep, excessive spending, and increased risk-taking behavior. On mental status exam, you see a Black male oriented to person, place, time, and date. He is overactive with elevated mood, pressured speech, is easily distracted, and difficult to interrupt. What would you suspect as the likely diagnosis?

67. Your first patient of the day while in a family clinic is an 18-year-old male you have never seen before. He is sitting in the exam room alone. His mental status exam reveals he is fully oriented, but his affect is inappropriate. He indicates a belief that people are trying to harm him, and he has bizarre hand gestures. He also believes that people can read his mind. This could be a presentation of what diagnostic category?

68. A 32-year-old female was referred to your office for evaluation. Upon entering the room you see a tearful, slow-to-react female who describes a gradual worsening in feelings of worthlessness and anhedonia for the last month. She is unkempt. She is fully oriented. What diagnostic category does this scenario fit?

DIRECTIONS (Questions 69 through 85): Each of the numbered items or incomplete statements in this section is followed by answers or by completions of the statement. Select the ONE lettered answer or completion that is BEST in each case.

Questions 69 through 85

69. All of the following statements about intermittent claudication are correct EXCEPT

   (A) It is the most common complaint produced by limb ischemia.
   (B) The onset of pain occurs at rest.
   (C) The onset of pain occurs while stretching the affected limb.
   (D) The cessation of pain occurs after rest.
   (E) The symptoms may remain stable for years or improve.

70. A patient has a type III epiphyseal fracture (Salter fracture). This type of fracture is described as

   (A) the epiphyseal plate has slipped from its origin and there is a fracture through the metaphysis producing a triangular metaphyseal fragment
   (B) a crushing injury damaging the epiphyseal plate usually producing growth arrest
   (C) the epiphyseal plate has slipped with a fracture involving the epiphysis
   (D) an intra-articular fracture extending through the epiphysis, epiphyseal plate, and metaphysis
   (E) the epiphyseal plate separates from the metaphysis without displacement or injury to the growth plate

71. Characteristics of a full-thickness burn include which of the following?

   (A) blister formation
   (B) charred appearance
   (C) sensitive to pin prick
   (D) usually heals well spontaneously
   (E) erythema only

72. Which of the following plays a primary role in the development of diverticulosis?

   (A) gender
   (B) geographic region
   (C) familial history
   (D) age
   (E) Northern European ancenstry

73. Adverse reactions to the DPT (diptheria, pertussis, and tetanus) vaccine that occur in more than 5% of the recipients include all of the following EXCEPT

   (A) pain or swelling at the site of injection
   (B) fever higher than 38.0°C
   (C) anorexia or vomiting
   (D) febrile convulsion
   (E) drowsiness following injection

74. All the health problems listed are commonly associated with homozygous sickle cell anemia EXCEPT

    (A) cholelithiasis
    (B) congestive heart failure (CHF)
    (C) aseptic necrosis of the femoral head
    (D) gout
    (E) hypoxemia

75. Narcolepsy is characterized by

    (A) daytime "sleep attacks"
    (B) cataplexy
    (C) sleep paralysis
    (D) hypnagogic hallucinations
    (E) all of the above

76. A hemorrhage complicating duodenal ulcer

    (A) usually is massive secondary to penetration into the gastroduodenal artery
    (B) is a more frequent complication than either obstruction or perforation
    (C) requires gastric resection for its control
    (D) can be controlled by endoscopic techniques with decreased mortality
    (E) can be controlled with simple ligation without the risk of recurrent hemorrhage

77. Ulcerative colitis most frequently involves the

    (A) cecum
    (B) ileum
    (C) left colon
    (D) right colon
    (E) rectum

78. Replacement hormones for adrenal insufficiency have different glucocorticoid strengths. When compared to cortisol, prednisone has how many more times the anti-inflammatory glucocorticoid effect?

    (A) 4.0 × the strength
    (B) 2.0 × the strength
    (C) 10 × the strength

    (D) 30 × the strength
    (E) 40 × the strength

79. Psoriatic arthritis, Reiter's syndrome, ankylosing spondylitis, and the arthritis associated with inflammatory bowel disease are all examples of

    (A) septic arthritis
    (B) seronegative arthritis, or spondyloarthropathies
    (C) classic inflammatory arthritis
    (D) necrotizing vasculitis syndromes
    (E) noninflammatory arthritis

80. A prominent feature of cocaine withdrawal is

    (A) somnolence
    (B) depression
    (C) psychosis
    (D) muscle cramping
    (E) abdominal pain

81. When closing lacerations in the ER setting, it is important to relieve tension on the wound edges to achieve an optimal result. Which is the best technique to reduce wound tension?

    (A) undermining soft tissues
    (B) splinting the affected part
    (C) closing only the top layer of the wound
    (D) application of adhesive strips
    (E) using continuous mattress sutures

82. Principles of fluid resuscitation in the acute management of hypovolemic shock include all of the following EXCEPT

    (A) immediate insertion of central venous catheters
    (B) insertion of large-bore peripheral IVs
    (C) rapid infusion of 2 L of lactated Ringer's solution
    (D) replacement with type-specific blood for life-threatening shock
    (E) close monitoring of vital signs

83. Which of the following operations for duodenal ulcer has the lowest morbidity and mortality?

    (A) proximal gastric vagotomy
    (B) partial gastrectomy
    (C) truncal vagotomy and pyloroplasty
    (D) truncal vagotomy and antrectomy
    (E) truncal vagotomy and gastrojejunostomy

84. Factors that increase the suspicion that a physical injury to a child has a nonaccidental etiology include all of the following EXCEPT

    (A) a history that does not explain the extent or characteristics of the injury
    (B) an explanation of the child's involvement in the traumatic incident that is not compatible with the child's developmental level
    (C) an abnormal delay in seeking medical help
    (D) parents who seem overly anxious and distraught
    (E) a history that varies and continues to change through the course of questioning

85. A patient presents with acute onset of a highly inflammatory monarthritis. His synovial fluid results show a cloudy fluid with decreased viscosity, a markedly elevated number of white blood cells (WBCs), presence of urate crystals, and a negative Gram stain. The patient's MOST likely diagnosis is

    (A) pseudogout
    (B) rheumatoid arthritis (RA)
    (C) gout
    (D) septic arthritis
    (E) systemic lupus erythematosus (SLE)

DIRECTIONS (Questions 86 through 89): Each group of items in this section consists of a list of lettered headings followed by a set of numbered words or phrases. For each numbered word or phrase, select the ONE lettered heading that is most closely associated with it. Each lettered heading may be selected once, more than once, or not at all.

Questions 86 through 89
Match the following vaginal infections with the appropriate description.

    (A) *Trichomonas vaginalis*
    (B) atrophic vaginitis
    (C) gonorrhea
    (D) candidiasis
    (E) bacterial vaginosis

86. Thick, white discharge with vaginal itching and burning; marked erythema of vulvovaginal mucous membranes

87. Vaginal itching and burning; thin, blood-tinged discharge; thin, friable vulvar and vaginal epithelium

88. Soreness with vaginal itching and burning; frothy, yellow-green discharge; diffusely reddened mucous membranes

89. Musty, malodorous discharge, thin, grayish in color

DIRECTIONS (Questions 90 and 91): Each of the numbered items or incomplete statements in this section is followed by answers or by completions of the statement. Select the ONE lettered answer or completion that is BEST in each case.

Questions 90 and 91

90. The most common type of childhood maltreatment seen by health care practitioners is

    (A) failure to thrive (nonorganic)
    (B) physical abuse
    (C) sexual abuse
    (D) emotional/verbal abuse
    (E) neglect

91. At 10 weeks' gestation, a 23-year-old Gravida 1, Para 0 breaks out in a rash that begins first on her face and then spreads downward. One week earlier, she suffered fever, malaise, and myalgias. Which test should be obtained immediately to determine whether her fetus will be affected by an infection resulting in severe congenital abnormalities?

    (A) VDRL
    (B) cervical cultures for gonorrhea
    (C) chlamydial cultures
    (D) rubella titers
    (E) group B beta-strep cultures

DIRECTIONS (Questions 92 through 95): Each group of items in this section consists of a list of lettered headings followed by a set of numbered words or phrases. For each numbered word or phrase, select the ONE lettered heading that is most closely associated with it. Each lettered heading may be selected once, more than once, or not at all.

Questions 92 through 95
For each description of a skin lesion, select the disease with which it is associated.

    (A) contact dermatitis
    (B) herpes zoster
    (C) pityriasis rosea
    (D) rubeola
    (E) scabies

92. Herald patch preceding eruption

93. Vesicular eruption confined to a unilateral dermatome

94. Highly pruritic serpentine burrows

95. Koplik spots

DIRECTIONS (Questions 96 through 136): Each of the numbered items or incomplete statements in this section is followed by answers or by completions of the statement. Select the ONE lettered answer or completion that is BEST in each case.

Questions 96 through 136

96. Asthmatic children

    (A) rarely present before age 5 years
    (B) have a generally poor prognosis
    (C) rarely require pharmacological therapy
    (D) present with hyperreactivity of the airways to a variety of stimuli
    (E) demonstrate rales as the diagnostic feature on physical exam

97. In examining a patient suspected of sustaining vascular injury, which of the following factors yields the LEAST diagnostic information?

    (A) shock
    (B) type of trauma
    (C) fracture
    (D) gender
    (E) color of blood

98. The cardiac murmur commonly heard in an infant with persistent ductus arteriosus is

    (A) late in diastole
    (B) crescendo–decrescendo
    (C) a late systolic continuous machinery sound
    (D) early in systole
    (E) heard only within 24 hours of birth

99. An 8-year-old child presents with onset of periorbital and leg edema following a recent viral upper respiratory tract illness. Urinalysis shows microscopic hematuria, no casts, and heavy proteinuria. What is the BEST initial approach in this child?

    (A) cyclosporine
    (B) cyclophosphamide
    (C) corticosteroids
    (D) no treatment necessary
    (E) renal biopsy

100. The Denver Developmental Screening Test (DDST)

(A) is a screening instrument designed to determine whether a particular child's development falls within the normal range

(B) consists of a progressive sequence of developmental tasks that test personal, social, fine motor/adaptive, language, and gross motor skills

(C) when administered in the office should allow children to demonstrate their best effort and ability

(D) all of the above

(E) none of the above

101. A 28-year-old female presents with sudden onset of shortness of breath, circumoral and carpopedal dysesthesia (tingling sensation), and carpopedal spasm. She complains of vague chest pain. Review of systems is unremarkable except for recent increase in stress at work. Vital signs are respiration 32, pulse 82, blood pressure 110/70, and temperature 98.6°F. ECG is normal. Exam reveals tachypnea, although the patient's breath sounds are normal, and the exam is otherwise normal. The most likely diagnosis is

(A) pneumonia

(B) primary pulmonary hypertension

(C) asthma

(D) hyperventilation

(E) myocardial infarction

102. The following statements concerning the Apgar scoring system are true EXCEPT

(A) A score is given at 1 and 5 minutes.

(B) The 1-minute score is an index of infant asphyxia.

(C) Signs including heart rate, muscle tone, and color are given a score.

(D) A total score of 5 indicates an infant in the best possible condition.

(E) Apgar scoring should continue every 5 minutes until a score of 7 is reached.

103. Which of the following clinical findings is seen with mandibular fractures?

(A) rhinorrhea

(B) malocclusion

(C) raccoon's eyes

(D) Battle sign

(E) Macewen's sign

104. A 40-year-old male presents with a complaint of severe anterior chest pain. His examination demonstrates a blood pressure of 122/80, a loud friction rub, and diffuse ST segment elevation in all leads except for aVR and V1. The most likely diagnosis is

(A) acute myocardial infarction

(B) rupture of the thoracic aorta

(C) acute pericarditis

(D) cardiac tamponade

(E) aortic dissection

105. A 28-year-old white male presents with a 24-hour complaint of sore throat. Upon examination, the tonsils are not markedly enlarged. The supratonsillar fossa is markedly edematous and swollen with the uvula deviated away from the affected side. Which of the following would be the most likely diagnosis?

(A) tonsillar abscess

(B) Ludwig's angina

(C) peritonsillar abscess

(D) retropharyngeal abscess

(E) epiglottitis

106. The evaluation of new-onset seizures in an adult should include all the following EXCEPT

(A) CT scan

(B) chest radiograph

(C) HIV testing

(D) blood urea nitrogen (BUN), electrolytes, and creatinine

(E) fasting blood sugar

107. What is the site of the MOST common form of extracranial vascular disease?

(A) external carotid artery

(B) common carotid artery

(C) internal carotid artery

(D) subclavian artery

(E) vertebral artery

108. Which of the following would indicate a superficial frostbite injury?

    (A) icy, hard, and wooden skin
    (B) intense hyperemia and marked edema
    (C) nonblanchable, waxy-appearing skin
    (D) hemorrhagic blisters and skin necrosis
    (E) purplish blebs on skin surface

109. All of the following are true regarding hepatitis A EXCEPT

    (A) Household contacts should be given immunoglobulin prophylaxis.
    (B) Routine immunoprophylaxis is not necessary for contacts of an office worker.
    (C) An inactivated hepatitis vaccine has been developed and has been shown to be safe and effective in preventing hepatitis A.
    (D) During the clinical phase of hepatitis A, by the time jaundice appears, shedding of the virus has usually decreased substantially.
    (E) The incubation period for hepatitis A ranges from 4 weeks to 6 months.

110. Clinical manifestations of primary syphilis infection include which of the following?

    (A) diffuse macular rash
    (B) generalized lymphadenopathy
    (C) low-grade fever
    (D) painless genital ulcer
    (E) arthralgias and myalgias

111. A 21-year-old thin male presents to your office with a sudden onset of vague chest pain radiating to the left shoulder, dyspnea, and cough. He states that his past medical history is unremarkable except for smoking. The onset of the above symptoms occurred while he was playing basketball. Vital signs are unremarkable except for a pulse of 110 and a respiratory rate of 28. You note decreased breath sounds, hyperresonance, and decreased vocal fremitus on the left thorax. At this time the MOST likely diagnosis is

    (A) mycoplasmal pneumonia
    (B) work-induced asthma

    (C) spontaneous pneumothorax
    (D) bronchial carcinoma
    (E) aortic stenosis with angina

112. During your examination of the patient in Question 111, the x-ray returns to reveal air in the pleural space with visible retracted lung border; there is no pleural effusion. Treatment should consist of

    (A) nitroglycerin IV
    (B) epinephrine subcutaneously
    (C) further investigation with a CT scan of the chest
    (D) aspiration of the air with a large needle or chest tube
    (E) endotracheal intubation

113. A 19-year-old G0P0 sexually active woman presents with a complaint of not menstruating for 6 months. Her past history is significant for an onset of menarche at age 15, with menses occuring only four to six times per year. She is presently using no form of birth control. Initial labs are a negative beta HCG, normal thyroid-stimulating hormone (TSH) test, and normal prolactin level. She is given progesterone, 10 mg PO qd for 10 days and has withdrawal bleeding 7 days later. Her diagnosis is MOST likely

    (A) hyperprolactinemia
    (B) secondary amenorrhea
    (C) secondary infertility
    (D) premature ovarian failure
    (E) primary amenorrhea

114. A young male patient with low back pain, an inflammatory sacroiliitis, and a positive HLA-B27 test would MOST likely have

    (A) psoriatic arthritis
    (B) Reiter's syndrome
    (C) ankylosing spondylitis
    (D) juvenile rheumatoid arthritis
    (E) arthritis of inflammatory bowel disease

115. A positive Lachman's test is indicative of

    (A) medial collateral ligament tear
    (B) lateral collateral ligament tear

(C) anterior cruciate ligament tear

(D) medial meniscus tear

(E) lateral meniscus tear

116. Common clinical and laboratory abnormalities seen in rheumatoid arthritis (RA) include all of the following EXCEPT

(A) normochromic, normocytic anemia

(B) elevated erythrocyte sedimentation rate (ESR)

(C) crystals in the synovial fluid

(D) high titers of rheumatoid factor

(E) subcutaneous nodules

117. A patient is considering permanent sterilization by tubal ligation. What important aspects of the procedure and complications should be explained during presurgical counseling?

(A) that the procedure can easily be reversed

(B) the possibility of development of pelvic inflammatory disease (PID) secondary to the procedure

(C) the possibility of pregnancy after the procedure with a higher incidence of ectopic pregnancy

(D) the possibility that menstrual irregularities may occur after the procedure

(E) that the procedure is associated with an increase in dysmenorrhea

118. All of the following are indicative of a prerenal state EXCEPT

(A) urinary sodium concentration less than 20 mEq/L

(B) high urine osmolality

(C) urine protein excretion greater than 3.5 gm/day

(D) ratio of blood urea nitrogen (BUN) to serum creatinine greater than 20:1

(E) decreased urine volume

119. Which of the following physical findings is/are commonly found with bowel obstruction?

(A) abdominal distention and tympany

(B) localized tenderness

(C) auscultatory "rushes"

(D) rigidity of the abdominal wall

(E) all of the above

120. The most common bacterial pathogen for otitis media at all ages is

(A) Group A beta hemolytic strep

(B) *Escherichia coli*

(C) *Streptococcus pneumoniae*

(D) *Staphylococcus aureus*

(E) *Moraxella catarrhalis*

121. Following a myocardial infarction

(A) aspartate aminotransferase (AST or SGOT) peaks after 72 hours

(B) lactic dehydrogenase (LDH) peaks within 6 hours

(C) the CK-MM isoenzyme is elevated as a result of myocardial necrosis

(D) hypoglycemia is common

(E) the serum creatine kinase (CK) peaks within 24 hours

122. A flat, nonelevated primary skin lesion is referred to as a

(A) papule

(B) macule

(C) wheal

(D) pustule

(E) bulla

123. All of the following physical findings may be associated with mitral stenosis EXCEPT

(A) a diastolic apical rumble

(B) a systolic crescendo–decrescendo murmur

(C) an opening snap

(D) an S3 gallop

(E) a loud S1

124. A 14-year-old anemic patient has the following findings: gallstones, mild icterus, splenomegaly, elevated reticulocyte count, and decreased serum haptoglobin; yet he feels reasonably well. These findings MOST strongly suggest

    (A) autoimmune hemolytic anemia
    (B) von Willebrand's disease
    (C) idiopathic hemochromatosis
    (D) vitamin B_{12} deficiency
    (E) hereditary spherocytosis

125. A 22-year-old female presents to the emergency department with extreme shortness of breath after jogging. No past medical history is immediately available. Vital signs are pulse 120, respiration 32, temperature 98.7°F, and blood pressure 130/84. Exam reveals a lethargic and confused patient; there are diffuse expiratory wheezes and a prolonged expiratory phase. Hyperresonance to percussion is noted. The most likely diagnosis is

    (A) pneumothorax
    (B) bronchial asthma
    (C) bronchiolitis
    (D) pulmonary edema
    (E) pneumonia

126. The most common chronic gastrointestinal bacterial infection to affect humans is

    (A) *Proteus*
    (B) *Bacillus cereus*
    (C) *Helicobacter pylori*
    (D) *Staphylococcus aureus*
    (E) *Escherichia coli*

127. Which of the following clinical and laboratory findings is included in the major manifestations of the revised Jones criteria for the diagnosis of acute rheumatic fever?

    (A) arthralgia
    (B) fever
    (C) elevated erythrocyte sedimentation rate (ESR)
    (D) subcutaneous nodules
    (E) elevated streptococcal antibody titers

128. The MOST common type of burn seen in children is

    (A) spill/scald burn
    (B) immersion/scald burn
    (C) contact thermal burn
    (D) flame burn
    (E) electrical flash burn

129. A couple comes to your office with a complaint that the woman is unable to get pregnant. They have been attempting to conceive for more than 1 year. Your history reveals that the woman has had an irregular menstrual cycle for many years and has had no previous pregnancy. Her husband denies having previously sired any children. After a thorough physical and pelvic exam, what would be the next step in evaluating this couple's infertility?

    (A) The woman should be given a 10-day course of progesterone to see if there is withdrawal bleeding.
    (B) The woman should undergo a hysterosalpingogram.
    (C) The man should have a semen analysis performed.
    (D) The woman should have a sonogram performed to rule out uterine myomata.
    (E) The woman should undergo diagnostic laparoscopy.

130. Symptoms in classic stroke from unilateral carotid artery disease may include

    (A) ipsilateral hemiparesis
    (B) contralateral hemiparesis
    (C) contralateral blindness
    (D) bilateral blindness
    (E) unilateral hearing loss

131. Which of the following characteristics of gastric ulcers indicate the need for surgery?

    (A) spontaneous appearance
    (B) associated with a duodenal ulcer
    (C) small size

(D) less than 30% healing after 3 weeks of medical therapy

(E) symptoms that appear 3 hours after meals

132. The primary pathological effect of acetaminophen poisoning is

(A) bronchospasm

(B) bone marrow suppression

(C) reversible mental status changes

(D) hepatic dysfunction

(E) cardiac dysfunction

133. *Clostridium difficile* colitis may be treated by discontinuing any implicated antibiotics and, if necessary, initiation of therapy with which one of the following?

(A) ampicillin

(B) vancomycin

(C) trimethoprim-sulfamethoxazole

(D) ciprofloxacin

(E) tetracycline

134. Prazosin has the following mechanism of action

(A) calcium-channel blocker

(B) beta-adrenergic blocker

(C) angiotensin-converting enzyme inhibitor

(D) vasodilator

(E) alpha-adrenergic receptor blocker

135. Parathyroid physiology is NOT responsible for the metabolic regulation of

(A) calcium

(B) magnesium

(C) phosphate

(D) chloride

(E) active vitamin D

136. A 5-year-old female presents with a single swollen, firm, non-tender anterior cervical node. The mother states that the child has been healthy the past few months but, upon careful questioning, said she did have some cold symptoms a few weeks ago that resolved without difficulty. There have been no

known exposures to illness, insect bites, or pets. Your differential diagnosis includes

(A) group A beta-streptococcus adenitis

(B) malignancies/Hodgkin's lymphoma

(C) cat scratch fever

(D) atypical mycobacterium

(E) all of the above

DIRECTIONS (Questions 137 through 140): Refer to Figure 9–1 on page 340. Select the ONE lettered answer that is BEST in each case.

Questions 137 through 140

137. The PR interval for the ECG in Figure 9–1 is

(A) indeterminate

(B) 100 ms

(C) 140 ms

(D) 160 ms

(E) 190 ms

138. The axis for the ECG in Figure 9–1 is

(A) +60°

(B) +90°

(C) +110°

(D) –60°

(E) –110°

139. The rhythm for the ECG in Figure 9–1 is

(A) normal sinus rhythm

(B) first-degree atrioventricular (AV) block

(C) Wenkebach phenomenon

(D) Mobitz type II

(E) atrial fibrillation

140. The ECG in the figure can be interpreted as

(A) normal

(B) an acute inferior wall myocardial infarction

(C) lateral wall ischemia

(D) an old anterior wall myocardial infarction

(E) an old inferior wall myocardial infarction

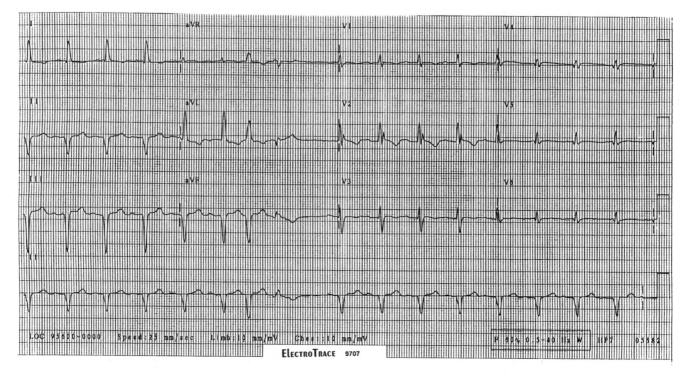

Figure 9–1. ECG.

DIRECTIONS (Questions 141 through 153): Each of the numbered items or incomplete statements in this section is followed by answers or by completions of the statement. Select the ONE lettered answer or completion that is BEST in each case.

Questions 141 through 153

141. Hemorrhage in the acute setting is best controlled by

    (A) manual compression of vessels proximal to the bleeding site
    (B) direct pressure to the bleeding site
    (C) use of vascular clamps
    (D) use of tourniquets

142. Malignant neoplasms of the musculoskeletal system

    (A) generally have a good prognosis
    (B) include osteoblastomas and giant cell tumors
    (C) rarely require surgical excision
    (D) are usually painful
    (E) rarely metastasize

143. Name the correct sequence of events in thyroid hormone secretion.

    (A) TSH-TRH-T_4-T_3
    (B) TRH-TSH-T_3-T_4
    (C) TRH-TSH-T_4-T_3
    (D) TSH-TRH-T_3-T_4
    (E) TRH-T_4-TSH-T_3

144. A patient is determined to be incompetent if he or she

    (A) is psychotic
    (B) is disoriented
    (C) is dangerous to himself/herself and others
    (D) is unable to make decisions in his/her own best interest
    (E) is unable to determine right from wrong

145. Diffuse abdominal pain that is "wave-like" and associated with vomiting is most likely

    (A) cholelithiasis
    (B) bowel obstruction
    (C) appendicitis

(D) peptic ulcer disease

(E) pancreatitis

146. A patient presents with symptoms consistent with infectious mononucleosis. During your workup of this patient you would expect to find all of the following EXCEPT

(A) elevated liver function tests (LFTs)

(B) hepatomegaly

(C) lymphadenopathy

(D) atypical lymphocytes on the differential

(E) pharyngitis

147. A 43-year-old secretary presents to you with a complaint of numbness and tingling of her first three fingers on the right hand. This is particularly noticeable at night, and sometimes the pain extends up the forearm. You can reproduce this pain by having the patient hold her wrist in forcible flexion. Her most likely diagnosis is

(A) bicipital tendinitis

(B) lateral epicondylitis

(C) carpal tunnel syndrome

(D) Raynaud's phenomenon

(E) polymyositis

148. A 58-year-old alcoholic with hepatic encephalopathy has been in the intensive care unit for 10 days. The patient has a sudden onset of fever and cough. The cough is productive of dark brown sputum. On physical exam, the patient appears acutely ill and has the following signs: blood pressure 150/88, pulse 104, respirations 32, and temperature 102.8°F. Chest exam is significant for dullness to percussion and rales over the upper third of the right lung field. Which of the following organisms would you expect to find on a sputum Gram stain?

(A) *Mycoplasma pneumoniae*

(B) a gram-negative bacilli (eg, *Klebsiella pneumoniae)*

(C) respiratory syncytial virus (RSV)

(D) psittacosis

(E) *Clostridium perfringens*

149. Which of the following treatment regimens would you institute for the patient in Question 148?

(A) penicillin IM

(B) ampicillin PO

(C) first-generation cephalosporin IV

(D) aminoglycoside + cephalosporin IV

(E) cough suppressant—no antibiotic at this time

150. Which of the following cerebrospinal fluid (CSF) analyses is an indicator of bacterial meningitis?

(A) white blood cell count between 5 and 100

(B) elevated protein

(C) high glucose

(D) predominant mononuclear cells

(E) numerous red blood cells

151. The most common cause of cirrhosis in the United States is

(A) alcohol

(B) hepatitis C

(C) hepatitis B

(D) hepatitis A

(E) hepatitis D

152. When counseling a sexually active adolescent female about the need for yearly Pap smears, which of the following is NOT a risk factor for developing cervical cancer?

(A) smoking

(B) a family history of cervical cancer

(C) use of oral contraceptives and no other barrier form of contraception

(D) a history of being treated for another sexually transmitted disease

(E) sexual intercourse prior to the age of 18

153. Which of the following is the MOST sensitive indicator of bleeding tendency in a preoperative patient?

   (A) prothrombin time (PT)
   (B) partial thromboplastin time (PTT)
   (C) platelet count
   (D) fibrinogen
   (E) history and physical

DIRECTIONS (Questions 154 through 156): Each group of items in this section consists of lettered headings followed by a set of numbered words or phrases. For each numbered word or phrase, select

   (A) if the item is associated with (A) only
   (B) if the item is associated with (B) only
   (C) if the item is associated with both (A) and (B)
   (D) if the item is associated with neither (A) nor (B)

Questions 154 through 156

   (A) Kawasaki's disease
   (B) Toxic shock syndrome

154. Bilateral, nonpurulent, conjunctival injection

155. Bacterial etiology believed to be the cause

156. Coronary artery involvement in some cases

DIRECTIONS (Questions 157 through 174): Each of the numbered items or incomplete statements in this section is followed by answers or by completions of the statement. Select the ONE lettered answer or completion that is BEST in each case.

Questions 157 through 174

157. All of the following statements regarding chronic lymphocytic leukemia (CLL) are true EXCEPT

   (A) CLL and diffuse, well-differentiated, lymphocytic lymphoma are both neoplasms of B-cell origin and are so similar that they follow essentially the same clinical course.

   (B) CLL, which presents with massive splenomegaly, lymphadenopathy, and lymphocytosis has a median survival of 5 years.

   (C) Combination chemotherapy for CLL is routinely initiated at the time of diagnosis in an attempt to achieve decreased tumor load and possible remission as early in the disease process as possible.

   (D) A Coombs' positive hemolytic anemia occurs in up to 20% of patients with CLL.

   (E) Patients who demonstrate anemia and/or thrombocytopenia at the time of diagnosis of CLL have a 2-year median survival.

158. The syndrome of inappropriate antidiuretic hormone (SIADH) secretion is characterized by all of the following EXCEPT

   (A) serum osmolality greater than urine osmolality
   (B) high urine sodium level
   (C) improvement with fluid restriction
   (D) can be seen in patients with tumors
   (E) responds to demeclocycline

159. A characteristic finding in the presence of an atrial septal defect is

   (A) a diastolic murmur
   (B) a palpable precordial thrill
   (C) a systolic murmur
   (D) cyanosis
   (E) clubbing of the fingers and toes

160. Which of the following statements regarding bladder cancer is true?

   (A) Its most common histology is adenocarcinoma.
   (B) Its most common presenting symptom is painless hematuria.
   (C) Early pulmonary metastases are characteristic.
   (D) Its most common presenting symptom is urinary retention.
   (E) Surgery is the only effective treatment.

161. A 21-year-old Gravida 3, Para 1 female reveals at the time of her first prenatal visit that the father of her baby is an IV-drug user. You advise her to be tested for HIV, and the test results are positive. She is presently 10 weeks' pregnant; what additional counseling/treatment should you now suggest?

    (A) The patient should be advised to undergo immediate abortion because of the detrimental effects of pregnancy on HIV.

    (B) She should be counseled about the greater than 60% chance that she will transmit the HIV virus to her baby.

    (C) She should be given antibiotic prophylaxis for *Pneumocystis carinii* pneumonia (PCP).

    (D) The patient should be reassured that breastfeeding is okay in HIV-positive women.

    (E) The patient should be counseled about the benefits of zidovudine therapy to prevent perinatal transmission of HIV.

162. A careful history, physical examination, and evaluation of the urine can help identify the source of hematuria. Which of the following statements is MOST suggestive of a nonglomerular (extrarenal) source of hematuria?

    (A) red blood cell (RBC) casts

    (B) hematuria with pyuria

    (C) hematuria with proteinuria

    (D) hematuria in a patient with new-onset hypertension and edema

    (E) pattern of persistent microhematuria and intermittent gross hematuria

163. Acetaminophen is commonly ingested by the pediatric population. In a child older than 1 year of age, all of the following statements are true EXCEPT

    (A) The local or national poison control number should be called after determining the age of the patient, amount ingested, and current status of the patient.

    (B) Activated charcoal may be given if less than 6 hours have elapsed since the ingestion.

    (C) During the first 24 hours following ingestion, patients often experience nausea, vomiting, diaphoresis, and general malaise.

    (D) If the initial serum acetaminophen level is in the toxic range, a loading dose of N-acetylcysteine (Mucomyst) should be administered, followed by 17 additional doses.

    (E) Within 72 hours after ingestion, all evidence of toxicity is resolved in most patients.

164. Severe congestive heart failure (CHF) is characterized by

    (A) S4 gallop and jugular venous distension

    (B) low pulmonary capillary wedge pressure

    (C) S3 gallop and jugular venous distension

    (D) generalized vasodilatation

    (E) splenomegaly

165. A 65-year-old patient with generalized atherosclerosis who is 2 days postcardiac catheterization and angioplasty develops an increased blood urea nitrogen (BUN) of 38 mg/dL and creatinine of 2.5 mg/dL. His baseline labs were BUN 20 mg/dL and creatinine 1.3 mg/dL. The patient complains of vague abdominal pain, but no other symptoms. On physical examination, his lower extremities are mottled with several darkened areas on the toes. The MOST likely diagnosis is

    (A) renal vein thrombosis

    (B) renal atheroemboli

    (C) contrast-induced acute tubular necrosis

    (D) interstitial nephritis

    (E) aortic dissection

166. All of the following can be considered as abnormal sexual development EXCEPT

    (A) no sign of puberty in a 13-year-old girl
    (B) onset of puberty in a girl age 9 years
    (C) bilateral or unilateral breast development in a girl prior to age 8 years
    (D) no sign of puberty in a boy age 14 $^1/_2$ years
    (E) absence of menarche in a girl age 16 years

167. *Haemophilus influenzae* type B (HIB) is a common cause of the following types of infections in children EXCEPT

    (A) meningitis
    (B) otitis media
    (C) cellulitis
    (D) epiglottitis
    (E) septic arthritis

168. All of the following statements about patterns of HIV infection in the United States are true EXCEPT

    (A) The cumulative incidence of AIDS cases is disproportionately higher in African Americans and Hispanics than in whites.
    (B) Recent rates of reported AIDS cases are highest in the Northeast and lowest in the Midwest.
    (C) The percentage of reported AIDS cases in women has gradually decreased over time.
    (D) The highest risk of HIV infection in pediatric patients occurs in children born to women who themselves are at risk of HIV infection.
    (E) In the South, more cases of AIDS resulting from heterosexual transmission among adolescents and young adults (ages 13–29 years) occur in towns and rural areas than in towns and rural areas in other parts of the country.

169. The laboratory test that is characteristically elevated in gout is

    (A) serum calcium
    (B) blood urea nitrogen (BUN)
    (C) uric acid
    (D) creatinine
    (E) serum phosphate

170. Antihistamines are a relative contraindication in all of the following medical conditions EXCEPT

    (A) glaucoma
    (B) hypertension
    (C) asthma
    (D) prostatic hypertrophy
    (E) pregnancy

171. Polycystic kidney disease

    (A) is an autosomal dominant disorder
    (B) is associated with an increased risk of cerebral aneurysm
    (C) can progress to end-stage renal failure
    (D) can affect other organs
    (E) all of the above are correct

172. Which of the following is considered the treatment of choice for acute bacterial prostatitis on an outpatient basis?

    (A) penicillin VK
    (B) trimethoprim-sulfamethaxazole
    (C) macrodantin
    (D) doxycycline
    (E) penicillin G

173. Surgical or nonsurgical ablative therapy for arrhythmias is done for all of the following conditions EXCEPT

    (A) chronic atrial fibrillation
    (B) sustained ventricular tachycardia
    (C) paroxysmal supraventricular tachycardia (PSVT)
    (D) acute atrial fibrillation
    (E) Wolff–Parkinson–White (WPW) syndrome

174. Which of the following antidepressant medications would be the safest in a patient with compromised cardiac status?

    (A) Prozac (fluoxetine)
    (B) Elavil (amitriptyline)
    (C) Tofranil (imipramine)
    (D) doxepin
    (E) trazodone

DIRECTIONS (Questions 175 through 178): Each group of items in this section consists of a list of lettered headings followed by a set of numbered words or phrases. For each numbered word or phrase, select the ONE lettered heading that is most closely associated with it. Each lettered heading may be selected once, more than once, or not at all.

Questions 175 through 178
For the number of weeks' gestation, match the events of pregnancy that occur at the time.

    (A) 5.5 to 6 weeks
    (B) 28 weeks
    (C) 20 weeks
    (D) 16 to 20 weeks
    (E) 14 weeks

175. Fundal height at umbilicus

176. Fetal movements first perceived by mother

177. Fetal heart motion first seen on transvaginal sonogram

178. Optimal time to draw maternal serum alpha-fetoprotein

DIRECTIONS (Questions 179 through 193): Each of the numbered items or incomplete statements in this section is followed by answers or by completions of the statement. Select the ONE lettered answer or completion that is BEST in each case.

Questions 179 through 193

179. Frequent causes of cardiac arrest or fibrillation include all of the following EXCEPT

    (A) acute myocardial infarction
    (B) a serum potassium of 5.0 mEq/L
    (C) anoxia
    (D) a serum potassium of 7.0 mEq/L
    (E) drugs

180. Which one of the following tests is used initially to evaluate the presence of HIV infection in a patient?

    (A) HIV antibody status by ELISA
    (B) HIV serum p24 antigen status
    (C) HIV antibody status by Western blot
    (D) T-lymphocyte subset studies
    (E) in vitro culture of HIV from patient's blood

181. At 32 weeks, a 16-year-old Gravida 1, Para 0 presents to the obstetric clinic complaining of headache; her blood pressure is 140/85. According to her prenatal chart, her first-trimester blood pressures were 100/70. At this time she has 2+ protein in her urine and she is hyperreflexic. What is the MOST likely diagnosis?

    (A) chronic hypertension
    (B) migraine headache
    (C) eclampsia
    (D) chronic renal disease
    (E) preeclampsia

182. The patient in Question 181 is admitted to the hospital and placed on bedrest. Instead of improving, her blood pressure increases to 160/100, the proteinuria remains at 2+ to 3+, and she remains hyperreflexic. A decision to deliver her baby is made; what medication must be started at this time?

    (A) hydrochlorothiazide
    (B) hydralazine
    (C) magnesium sulfate
    (D) diazepam
    (E) furosemide

183. Which of the following symptoms would NOT be seen in the patient with Bell's palsy?

    (A) ipsilateral lacrimation
    (B) postauricular pain
    (C) facial weakness involving the upper facial musculature
    (D) paroxysms of stabbing pain on one side of the face
    (E) facial weakness of the lower facial musculature

184. Blindness is a potential complication of

    (A) Takayasu's arteritis
    (B) Behçet's disease
    (C) polyarteritis nodosa
    (D) temporal arteritis
    (E) Sjögren's syndrome

185. Hypercalcemia has numerous etiologies. Which of the following would NOT be considered an etiology for hypercalcemia?

    (A) thyrotoxicosis
    (B) thiazide diuretics
    (C) humoral hypercalcemia of malignancy (HHM)
    (D) loop diuretics
    (E) none of the above

186. Renal failure can be seen in all of the following diseases EXCEPT

    (A) systemic lupus erythematosus (SLE)
    (B) scleroderma
    (C) multiple myeloma
    (D) hemochromatosis
    (E) amyloidosis

187. Innocent murmurs are characterized by which of the following features?

    (A) grade 2/6
    (B) physiologic split S2
    (C) should always be evaluated to exclude the possibility of an underlying cardiac disease
    (D) all of the above
    (E) none of the above

188. The dexamethasone suppression test is used to aid in the diagnosis of

    (A) Graves' disease
    (B) Addison's disease
    (C) Cushing's syndrome
    (D) Reidel's disease
    (E) rheumatoid arthritis

189. In a newborn child, the sudden development of hypotension, shock, and salt wasting is consistent with

    (A) a 15-hydroxylase block
    (B) a 21-hydroxylase block
    (C) a 28-hydroxylase block
    (D) a 32-hydroxylase block
    (E) a 36-hydroxylase block

190. The MOST common cerebral aneurysm

    (A) is usually secondary to trauma
    (B) occurs in the carotid or "anterior" circulation
    (C) is caused by infection
    (D) involves the vertebrobasilar or "posterior" circulation
    (E) involves only the basilar artery

191. Which of the following signs and symptoms are MOST commonly found in a pregnant woman with pyelonephritis?

    (A) lower abdominal pain, fever, and chills
    (B) premature onset of contractions
    (C) fever and chills, nausea and vomiting, and flank pain
    (D) urinary frequency, urgency, and dysuria
    (E) a brownish discoloration of urine

192. Calculate the anion gap in a patient with the following labs: blood urea nitrogen (BUN) 10 mg/dL, creatinine 1.0 mg/dL, sodium 145 mEq/L, potassium 3.0 mEq/L, chloride 105 mEq/L, bicarbonate 15 mEq/L

    (A) 35
    (B) 25

(C) 32

(D) 43

(E) 27

193. A 50-year-old white male presents with complaints of increasing backache, fatigue, and weight loss of at least several weeks' duration, and acute onset 36 hours earlier of fever, loose cough, and dyspnea. Physical exam strongly suggests pneumonia (confirmed on x-ray) and also reveals pallor, petechiae on the face and legs, several recent bruises, mild hepatosplenomegaly, and several small palpable lymph nodes. The LEAST likely diagnosis is

(A) adult T-lymphocyte leukemia (ATL)

(B) aplastic anemia

(C) multiple myeloma

(D) acute myelogenous leukemia (AML)

(E) well-differentiated, lymphocytic lymphoma

DIRECTIONS (Questions 194 through 197): Each group of items in this section consists of a list of lettered headings followed by a set of numbered words or phrases. For each numbered word or phrase, select the ONE lettered heading that is most closely associated with it. Each lettered heading may be selected once, more than once, or not at all.

Questions 194 through 197

(A) esophageal webbing

(B) traumatic esophageal rupture

(C) linear tearing of the gastroesophageal junction

(D) esophageal spasm

(E) associated with long-standing gastro-esophageal reflux

194. Barrett's esophagus

195. Boerhaave syndrome

196. Mallory–Weiss syndrome

197. Plummer–Vinson syndrome

DIRECTIONS (Questions 198 through 200): Each of the numbered items or incomplete statements in this section is followed by answers or by completions of the statement. Select the ONE lettered answer or completion that is BEST in each case.

Questions 198 through 200

198. Syndrome of inappropriate antidiuretic hormone (SIADH) can be seen with

(A) oat cell carcinoma

(B) hyperthyroidism

(C) squamous cell carcinoma

(D) use of thiazide diuretics

(E) excess water intake

199. When lithium is used to treat bipolar affective illness, which lab tests are used in routine monitoring of the patient for side effects?

(A) white blood cell (WBC) count

(B) liver enzymes

(C) glucose

(D) creatinine

(E) electrolytes

200. The incubation of this illness is 2 to 6 weeks. Viral shedding is in the stool, continuously, until the peak of symptoms that generally lasts 1 to 2 weeks. The infection often is clinically silent in children. Adults are often more symptomatic, but rarely develop hepatic failure. The clinical course BEST describes which of the following hepatatrophic viruses?

(A) cytomegalovirus (CMV) infection

(B) hepatitis B

(C) hepatitis E

(D) hepatitis A (HAV)

(E) HIV infection

Practice Test Answers
and Key Phrases

1. **(B)** Pediatrics—characteristics, cardiac anomalies

2. **(B)** Endocrinology—diabetic monitoring

3. **(C)** Pharmacology—side effects of clozapine

4. **(B)** Surgery—complications

5. **(B)** Surgery—physical findings, appendicitis

6. **(C)** Obstetrics & Gynecology—treatment, dysmenorrhea

7. **(B)** Endocrinology—features, Cushing's syndrome

8. **(B)** Infectious Diseases—indications, hepatitis vaccine

9. **(E)** Obstetrics & Gynecology—actions of oral contraceptives

10. **(A)** Pharmacology—action of calcium channel blockers

11. **(E)** Psychiatry—associated conditions

12. **(E)** Pediatrics—nutrition

13. **(D)** Cardiology—physical diagnosis

14. **(D)** Gastroenterology—diagnostic findings

15. **(E)** Obstetrics & Gynecology—indications, RhoGAM

16. **(E)** Dermatology—incidence, basal cell carcinoma

17. **(A)** AIDS—associated conditions

18. **(E)** Surgery—physiology

19. **(B)** Obstetrics & Gynecology—diagnostic studies

20. **(B)** Surgery—physical findings

21. **(A)** Cardiology—arrhythmias

22. **(A)** Neurology—diagnosis of hydrocephalus

23. **(D)** Pharmacology—peak activity, insulin

24. **(A)** Pediatrics—physical diagnosis

25. **(C)** Psychiatry—treatment, ADHD

26. **(B)** Cardiology—causes, aneurysm

27. **(A)** Cardiology—incidence, aneurysm

28. **(E)** Dermatology—treatment of warts

29. **(D)** AIDS—associated diseases

30. **(A)** Pharmacology—contraindications, OCPs

31. **(C)** Endocrinology—diagnosis, hypocalcemia

32. **(D)** Endocrinology—diagnosis, hypercalcemia

33. **(D)** Surgery—associated manifestations, pancreatitis

34. **(E)** Surgery—diagnosis, venous thrombosis

35. **(C)** Pharmacology—drug reaction

36. **(D)** Cardiology—treatment, ventricular tachycardia

37. **(C)** Pediatrics—incidence, otitis media

38. **(B)** Emergency Medicine—treatment, avulsed tooth

39. **(D)** Cardiology—endocarditis prophylaxis

40. **(C)** Surgery—bilirubin metabolism

41. **(E)** Obstetrics & Gynecology—indications for cervical biopsy

42. **(A)** Infectious Diseases—features, genital warts

43. **(C)** Dermatology—morphology, lichen planus

44. **(A)** Surgery—causes, obstruction

45. **(A)** Pulmonary—diagnosis, epiglottitis

46. **(B)** Pulmonary—management, epiglottitis

47. **(B)** Dermatology—clinical features, erythema multiforme

48. **(A)** AIDS—treatment, PCP

49. **(D)** Surgery—clinical features, arterial disease

50. **(B)** Renal—diagnosis, pheochromocytoma

51. **(E)** Neurology—features, brain tumor

52. **(C)** Pediatrics—CPR

53. **(B)** Obstetrics & Gynecology—treatment, UTI

54. **(A)** Infectious Diseases—features, varicella

55. **(B)** Renal—physiology

56. **(C)** Gastroenterology—hormone production

57. **(D)** Pediatrics—pathophysiology, respiratory distress syndrome

58. **(D)** Endocrinology—physical findings, hypercalcemia

59. **(C)** Psychiatry—diagnosis, sleep apnea

60. **(B)** Cardiology—cause, Prinzmetal's angina

61. **(D)** Hematology/Oncology—clinical features, anemia

62. **(C)** Rheumatology—diagnosis, neurologic deficit

63. **(D)** Dermatology—treatment, erysipelas

64. **(E)** Pharmacology—side effects, phenothiazines

65. **(D)** Psychiatry—diagnosis, dementia

66. **(B)** Psychiatry—diagnosis, bipolar affective disorder

67. **(C)** Psychiatry—diagnosis, schizophrenia

68. **(A)** Psychiatry—diagnosis, depression

69. **(B)** Surgery—characteristics, claudication

70. **(C)** Pediatrics—definition, epiphyseal fracture

71. **(B)** Emergency Medicine—characteristics, burns

72. **(D)** Gastroenterology—risk factors, diverticulitis

73. **(D)** Pediatrics—adverse reactions, immunization

74. **(D)** Hematology/Oncology—associated conditions, sickle cell

75. **(E)** Psychiatry—characteristics, narcolepsy

76. **(B)** Surgery—characteristics, bleeding ulcer

77. **(E)** Gastroenterology—characteristics, ulcerative colitis

78. **(A)** Pharmacology—characteristics, steroids

79. **(B)** Rheumatology—classification, arthropathies

80. **(B)** Psychiatry—manifestations, cocaine withdrawal

81. **(A)** Emergency Medicine—techniques, suture

82. **(A)** Emergency Medicine—management, shock

83. **(A)** Surgery—duodenal ulcer repair

84. **(D)** Pediatrics—features, child abuse

85. **(C)** Rheumatology—diagnosis, gout

86–89. **(D), (B), (A), (E)** Obstetrics & Gynecology—clinical features, vaginitis

90. **(E)** Pediatrics—incidence, child neglect

91. **(D)** Obstetrics & Gynecology—prenatal care

92–95. **(C), (B), (E), (D)** Dermatology—diagnosis, skin lesions

96. **(D)** Pediatrics—characteristics, asthma

97. **(D)** Surgery—assesment, vascular injury

98. **(C)** Pediatrics—characteristics, murmurs

99. **(C)** Renal—treatment, nephrotic syndrome

100. **(D)** Pediatrics—developmental screening

101. **(D)** Pulmonary—diagnosis, hyperventilation syndrome

102. **(D)** Pediatrics—Apgar score

103. **(B)** Emergency Medicine—clinical features, mandible fracture

104. **(C)** Cardiology—diagnosis, pericarditis

105. **(C)** Emergency Medicine—diagnosis, peritonsillar abscess

106. **(C)** Neurology—evaluation, seizures

107. **(C)** Surgery—location, vascular disease

108. **(C)** Emergency Medicine—characteristics, frostbite

109. **(E)** Infectious Diseases—characteristics, hepatitis

110. **(D)** Infectious Diseases—clinical manifestations, syphilis

111. **(C)** Pulmonary—diagnosis, pneumothorax

112. **(D)** Pulmonary—treatment, pneumothorax

113. **(B)** Obstetrics & Gynecology—diagnosis, amenorrhea

114. **(C)** Rheumatology—features, ankylosing spondylitis

115. **(C)** Surgery—physical findings, anterior cruciate injury

116. **(C)** Rheumatology—laboratory findings, arthritis

117. **(C)** Obstetrics & Gynecology—patient education, sterilization

118. **(C)** Renal—features, prerenal state

119. **(E)** Surgery—physical findings, bowel obstruction

120. **(C)** Pediatrics—etiology, otitis media

121. **(E)** Cardiology—laboratory findings, infarction

122. **(B)** Dermatology—morphology, skin lesions

123. **(B)** Cardiology—physical findings, mitral stenosis

124. **(E)** Hematology/Oncology—diagnosis, hemolytic anemia

125. **(B)** Pulmonary—diagnosis, asthma

126. **(C)** Gastroenterology—etiology, chronic infection

127. **(D)** Rheumatology—diagnosis, rheumatic fever

128. **(A)** Emergency Medicine—causes, burns in children

129. **(C)** Obstetrics & Gynecology—evaluation, infertility

130. **(B)** Neurology—clinical features, stroke

131. **(B)** Surgery—indications, ulcer repair

132. **(D)** Pharmacology—features, acetaminophen poisoning

133. **(B)** Infectious Diseases—treatment, colitis

134. **(E)** Pharmacology—mechanism of action—prazosin

135. **(D)** Endocrine—physiology, parathyroid gland

136. **(E)** Pediatrics—differential diagnosis, adenopathy

137–140. **(E), (D), (A), (E)** Cardiology—interpretation, ECG

141. **(B)** Emergency Medicine—treatment, hemorrhage

142. **(D)** Hematology/Oncology—features, musculoskeletal neoplasms

143. **(C)** Endocrinology—physiology, thyroid hormone

144. **(D)** Psychiatry—definition, incompetency

145. **(B)** Surgery—clinical manifestations, obstruction

146. **(B)** Infectious Diseases—features, infectious mononucleosis

147. **(C)** Rheumatology—diagnosis, carpal tunnel

148. **(B)** Pulmonary—etiology, pneumonia

149. **(D)** Pulmonary—treatment, pneumonia

150. **(B)** Infectious Diseases—diagnosis, bacterial meningitis

151. **(B)** Gastroenterology—etiology, cirrhosis

152. **(B)** Obstetrics & Gynecology—risk factors, cervical cancer

153. **(E)** Surgery—preoperative evaluation

154–156. **(C), (B), (A)** Infectious Diseases—clinical features, Kawasaki's, and toxic shock

157. **(C)** Hematology/Oncology—features, leukemia

158. **(A)** Renal—features, SIADH

159. **(C)** Cardiology—physical findings, ASD

160. **(B)** Hematology/Oncology—features, bladder cancer

161. **(E)** Obstetrics & Gynecology—prenatal counseling, HIV

162. **(B)** Renal—evaluation, hematuria

163. **(E)** Pediatrics—treatment, acetaminophen poisoning

164. **(C)** Cardiology—characteristics, heart failure

165. **(B)** Renal—diagnosis, renal atheroemboli

166. **(B)** Pediatrics—sexual development

167. **(B)** Pediatrics—etiology, infections

168. **(C)** AIDS—epidemiology, HIV infection

169. **(C)** Rheumatology—evaluation, gout

170. **(B)** Pharmacology—contraindications, antihistamines

171. **(E)** Renal—features, polycystic kidney disease

172. **(B)** Infectious Diseases—treatment, prostatitis

173. **(D)** Surgery—treatment, arrhythmias

174. **(A)** Pharmacology—contraindications, antidepressants

175–178. **(C), (D), (A), (D)** Obstetrics & Gynecology—prenatal care

179. **(B)** Cardiology—etiology, cardiac arrest

180. **(A)** AIDS—laboratory evaluation, HIV

181. **(E)** Obstetrics & Gynecology—diagnosis, preeclampsia

182. **(C)** Obstetrics & Gynecology—treatment, preeclampsia

183. **(D)** Neurology—features, Bell's palsy

184. **(D)** Rheumatology—complications, temporal arteritis

185. **(D)** Endocrinology—etiology, hypercalcemia

186. **(D)** Renal—associated diseases, renal failure

187. **(D)** Cardiology—characteristics, innocent murmurs

188. **(C)** Endocrinology—diagnosis, Cushing's syndrome

189. **(B)** Endocrinology—features, hydroxylase block

190. **(B)** Surgery—features, cerebral aneurysm

191. **(C)** Renal—clinical manifestations, pyelonephritis

192. **(B)** Renal—calculation, anion gap

193. **(B)** Hematology/Oncology—diagnosis, myeloplastic diseases

194–197. **(E), (B), (C), (A)** Surgery—clinical features, esophageal disorders

198. **(A)** Endocrinology—associated disease, SIADH

199. **(D)** Pharmacology—monitoring, lithium therapy

200. **(D)** Infectious Diseases—features, hepatitis

NAME _____
　　　　　　Last　　　　　　　First　　　　　　　　　　　Middle

ADDRESS _____
　　　　　　　　Street

_____
　City　　　　　　　　　　　State　　　　　　　Zip

SOCIAL SECURITY NUMBER

| 0 1 2 3 4 5 6 7 8 9 |
| 0 1 2 3 4 5 6 7 8 9 |
| 0 1 2 3 4 5 6 7 8 9 |
| 0 1 2 3 4 5 6 7 8 9 |
| 0 1 2 3 4 5 6 7 8 9 |
| 0 1 2 3 4 5 6 7 8 9 |
| 0 1 2 3 4 5 6 7 8 9 |
| 0 1 2 3 4 5 6 7 8 9 |
| 0 1 2 3 4 5 6 7 8 9 |

1. (A) (B) (C) (D) (E)　25. (A) (B) (C) (D) (E)　49. (A) (B) (C) (D) (E)　73. (A) (B) (C) (D) (E)
2. (A) (B) (C) (D) (E)　26. (A) (B) (C) (D) (E)　50. (A) (B) (C) (D) (E)　74. (A) (B) (C) (D) (E)
3. (A) (B) (C) (D) (E)　27. (A) (B) (C) (D) (E)　51. (A) (B) (C) (D) (E)　75. (A) (B) (C) (D) (E)
4. (A) (B) (C) (D) (E)　28. (A) (B) (C) (D) (E)　52. (A) (B) (C) (D) (E)　76. (A) (B) (C) (D) (E)
5. (A) (B) (C) (D) (E)　29. (A) (B) (C) (D) (E)　53. (A) (B) (C) (D) (E)　77. (A) (B) (C) (D) (E)
6. (A) (B) (C) (D) (E)　30. (A) (B) (C) (D) (E)　54. (A) (B) (C) (D) (E)　78. (A) (B) (C) (D) (E)
7. (A) (B) (C) (D) (E)　31. (A) (B) (C) (D) (E)　55. (A) (B) (C) (D) (E)　79. (A) (B) (C) (D) (E)
8. (A) (B) (C) (D) (E)　32. (A) (B) (C) (D) (E)　56. (A) (B) (C) (D) (E)　80. (A) (B) (C) (D) (E)
9. (A) (B) (C) (D) (E)　33. (A) (B) (C) (D) (E)　57. (A) (B) (C) (D) (E)　81. (A) (B) (C) (D) (E)
10. (A) (B) (C) (D) (E)　34. (A) (B) (C) (D) (E)　58. (A) (B) (C) (D) (E)　82. (A) (B) (C) (D) (E)
11. (A) (B) (C) (D) (E)　35. (A) (B) (C) (D) (E)　59. (A) (B) (C) (D) (E)　83. (A) (B) (C) (D) (E)
12. (A) (B) (C) (D) (E)　36. (A) (B) (C) (D) (E)　60. (A) (B) (C) (D) (E)　84. (A) (B) (C) (D) (E)
13. (A) (B) (C) (D) (E)　37. (A) (B) (C) (D) (E)　61. (A) (B) (C) (D) (E)　85. (A) (B) (C) (D) (E)
14. (A) (B) (C) (D) (E)　38. (A) (B) (C) (D) (E)　62. (A) (B) (C) (D) (E)　86. (A) (B) (C) (D) (E)
15. (A) (B) (C) (D) (E)　39. (A) (B) (C) (D) (E)　63. (A) (B) (C) (D) (E)　87. (A) (B) (C) (D) (E)
16. (A) (B) (C) (D) (E)　40. (A) (B) (C) (D) (E)　64. (A) (B) (C) (D) (E)　88. (A) (B) (C) (D) (E)
17. (A) (B) (C) (D) (E)　41. (A) (B) (C) (D) (E)　65. (A) (B) (C) (D) (E)　89. (A) (B) (C) (D) (E)
18. (A) (B) (C) (D) (E)　42. (A) (B) (C) (D) (E)　66. (A) (B) (C) (D) (E)　90. (A) (B) (C) (D) (E)
19. (A) (B) (C) (D) (E)　43. (A) (B) (C) (D) (E)　67. (A) (B) (C) (D) (E)　91. (A) (B) (C) (D) (E)
20. (A) (B) (C) (D) (E)　44. (A) (B) (C) (D) (E)　68. (A) (B) (C) (D) (E)　92. (A) (B) (C) (D) (E)
21. (A) (B) (C) (D) (E)　45. (A) (B) (C) (D) (E)　69. (A) (B) (C) (D) (E)　93. (A) (B) (C) (D) (E)
22. (A) (B) (C) (D) (E)　46. (A) (B) (C) (D) (E)　70. (A) (B) (C) (D) (E)　94. (A) (B) (C) (D) (E)
23. (A) (B) (C) (D) (E)　47. (A) (B) (C) (D) (E)　71. (A) (B) (C) (D) (E)　95. (A) (B) (C) (D) (E)
24. (A) (B) (C) (D) (E)　48. (A) (B) (C) (D) (E)　72. (A) (B) (C) (D) (E)　96. (A) (B) (C) (D) (E)

97. (A) (B) (C) (D) (E)	**123.** (A) (B) (C) (D) (E)	**149.** (A) (B) (C) (D) (E)	**175.** (A) (B) (C) (D) (E)
98. (A) (B) (C) (D) (E)	**124.** (A) (B) (C) (D) (E)	**150.** (A) (B) (C) (D) (E)	**176.** (A) (B) (C) (D) (E)
99. (A) (B) (C) (D) (E)	**125.** (A) (B) (C) (D) (E)	**151.** (A) (B) (C) (D) (E)	**177.** (A) (B) (C) (D) (E)
100. (A) (B) (C) (D) (E)	**126.** (A) (B) (C) (D) (E)	**152.** (A) (B) (C) (D) (E)	**178.** (A) (B) (C) (D) (E)
101. (A) (B) (C) (D) (E)	**127.** (A) (B) (C) (D) (E)	**153.** (A) (B) (C) (D) (E)	**179.** (A) (B) (C) (D) (E)
102. (A) (B) (C) (D) (E)	**128.** (A) (B) (C) (D) (E)	**154.** (A) (B) (C) (D) (E)	**180.** (A) (B) (C) (D) (E)
103. (A) (B) (C) (D) (E)	**129.** (A) (B) (C) (D) (E)	**155.** (A) (B) (C) (D) (E)	**181.** (A) (B) (C) (D) (E)
104. (A) (B) (C) (D)	**130.** (A) (B) (C) (D) (E)	**156.** (A) (B) (C) (D) (E)	**182.** (A) (B) (C) (D) (E)
105. (A) (B) (C) (D) (E)	**131.** (A) (B) (C) (D) (E)	**157.** (A) (B) (C) (D) (E)	**183.** (A) (B) (C) (D) (E)
106. (A) (B) (C) (D) (E)	**132.** (A) (B) (C) (D) (E)	**158.** (A) (B) (C) (D) (E)	**184.** (A) (B) (C) (D) (E)
107. (A) (B) (C) (D) (E)	**133.** (A) (B) (C) (D) (E)	**159.** (A) (B) (C) (D) (E)	**185.** (A) (B) (C) (D)
108. (A) (B) (C) (D) (E)	**134.** (A) (B) (C) (D) (E)	**160.** (A) (B) (C) (D) (E)	**186.** (A) (B) (C) (D) (E)
109. (A) (B) (C) (D) (E)	**135.** (A) (B) (C) (D) (E)	**161.** (A) (B) (C) (D) (E)	**187.** (A) (B) (C) (D) (E)
110. (A) (B) (C) (D) (E)	**136.** (A) (B) (C) (D)	**162.** (A) (B) (C) (D) (E)	**188.** (A) (B) (C) (D) (E)
111. (A) (B) (C) (D) (E)	**137.** (A) (B) (C) (D) (E)	**163.** (A) (B) (C) (D) (E)	**189.** (A) (B) (C) (D) (E)
112. (A) (B) (C) (D) (E)	**138.** (A) (B) (C) (D) (E)	**164.** (A) (B) (C) (D) (E)	**190.** (A) (B) (C) (D) (E)
113. (A) (B) (C) (D) (E)	**139.** (A) (B) (C) (D) (E)	**165.** (A) (B) (C) (D) (E)	**191.** (A) (B) (C) (D) (E)
114. (A) (B) (C) (D) (E)	**140.** (A) (B) (C) (D) (E)	**166.** (A) (B) (C) (D) (E)	**192.** (A) (B) (C) (D) (E)
115. (A) (B) (C) (D) (E)	**141.** (A) (B) (C) (D) (E)	**167.** (A) (B) (C) (D) (E)	**193.** (A) (B) (C) (D) (E)
116. (A) (B) (C) (D) (E)	**142.** (A) (B) (C) (D)	**168.** (A) (B) (C) (D) (E)	**194.** (A) (B) (C) (D) (E)
117. (A) (B) (C) (D) (E)	**143.** (A) (B) (C) (D) (E)	**169.** (A) (B) (C) (D) (E)	**195.** (A) (B) (C) (D) (E)
118. (A) (B) (C) (D) (E)	**144.** (A) (B) (C) (D) (E)	**170.** (A) (B) (C) (D) (E)	**196.** (A) (B) (C) (D) (E)
119. (A) (B) (C) (D) (E)	**145.** (A) (B) (C) (D) (E)	**171.** (A) (B) (C) (D) (E)	**197.** (A) (B) (C) (D) (E)
120. (A) (B) (C) (D) (E)	**146.** (A) (B) (C) (D) (E)	**172.** (A) (B) (C) (D) (E)	**198.** (A) (B) (C) (D) (E)
121. (A) (B) (C) (D) (E)	**147.** (A) (B) (C) (D) (E)	**173.** (A) (B) (C) (D) (E)	**199.** (A) (B) (C) (D) (E)
122. (A) (B) (C) (D) (E)	**148.** (A) (B) (C) (D) (E)	**174.** (A) (B) (C) (D) (E)	**200.** (A) (B) (C) (D) (E)

Appleton & Lange Review Titles for Health Professions

A&L/PREP REVIEW SERIES

Appleton & Lange's Review of Cardiovascular-Interventional Technology
Vitanza
1995, ISBN 0-8385-0248-2, A0248-3

Appleton & Lange's Review for the Chiropractic National Boards, Part I
Shanks
1992, ISBN 0-8385-0224-5, A0224-4

Appleton & Lange's Review for the Dental Assistant, 3/e
Andujo
1992, ISBN 0-8385-0135-4, A0135-2

Appleton & Lange's Review for the Dental Hygiene National Board Review, 4/e
Barnes and Waring
1995, ISBN 0-8385-0230-X, A0230-1

Appleton & Lange's Review for the Medical Assistant, 5/e
Palko and Palko
1997, ISBN 0-8385-0285-7, A0285-5

Appleton & Lange's Review of Pharmacy, 6/e
Hall and Reiss
1997, ISBN 0-8385-0281-4, A0281-4

Appleton & Lange's Review for the Physician Assistant, 3/e
Cafferty
1997, ISBN 0-8385-0279-2, A0279-8

Appleton & Lange's Review for the Radiography Examination, 3/e
Saia
1997, ISBN 0-8385-0280-6, A0280-6

Appleton & Lange's Review for the Surgical Technology Examination, 4/e
Allmers and Verderame
1996, ISBN 0-8385-0270-9, A0270-7

Appleton & Lange's Review for the Ultrasonography Examination, 2/e
Odwin
1993, ISBN 0-8385-9073-X, A9073-6

Essentials of Advanced Cardiac Life Support: Program Review & Exam Preparation (PREP)
Brainard
1997, ISBN 0-8385-0259-8, A0259-0

Radiography: Program Review & Exam Preparation (PREP)
Saia
1996, ISBN 0-8385-8244-3, A8244-4

More on reverse ———→

Appleton & Lange Review Titles for Health Professions

MEPC/A&L QUICK REVIEW SERIES

Appleton & Lange's Quick Review: Dental Assistant
Andujo
1997, ISBN 0-8385-1526-6, A1526-1

Appleton & Lange's Quick Review: Massage Therapy
Garofano
1997, ISBN 0-8385-0307-1, A0307-7

Appleton & Lange's Quick Review: Pharmacy, 11/e
Generali
1997, ISBN 0-8385-6342-2, A6342-8

Appleton & Lange's Quick Review: Physician Assistant, 3/e
Rahr and Niebuhr
1996, ISBN 0-8385-8094-7, A8094-3

Dental Assistant: Program Review & Exam Preparation (PREP)
Andujo
1997, ISBN 0-8385-1513-4, A1513-9

Medical Assistant: Program Review & Exam Preparation (PREP)
Hurlbut
1997, ISBN 0-8385-6266-3, A6266-9

MEPC: Medical Assistant *Examination Review*, **4/e**
Dreizen and Audet
1989, ISBN 0-8385-5772-4, A5772-7

MEPC: Medical Record, *Examination Review*, **6/e**
Bailey
1994, ISBN 0-8385-6192-0, A6192-7

MEPC: Obstetrics & Gynecology
Ross
1997, ISBN 0-8385-6328-7, A6328-7

MEPC: Occupational Therapy *Examination Review*, **5/e**
Dundon
1988, ISBN 0-8385-7204-9, A7204-9

MEPC: Optometry *Examination Review*, **4/e**
Casser et al.
1994, ISBN 0-8385-7449-1, A7449-0

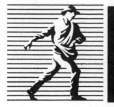